Rare Kidney Diseases

Rare Kidney Diseases

New Translational Research Approach to Improve Diagnosis and Therapy

Editors

Gianluigi Zaza
Giovanni Gambaro

MDPI • Basel • Beijing • Wuhan • Barcelona • Belgrade • Manchester • Tokyo • Cluj • Tianjin

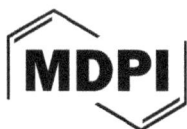

Editors
Gianluigi Zaza
University of Verona
Italy

Giovanni Gambaro
University of Verona
Italy

Editorial Office
MDPI
St. Alban-Anlage 66
4052 Basel, Switzerland

This is a reprint of articles from the Special Issue published online in the open access journal *International Journal of Molecular Sciences* (ISSN 1422-0067) (available at: https://www.mdpi.com/journal/ijms/special_issues/rare_kidney_diseases).

For citation purposes, cite each article independently as indicated on the article page online and as indicated below:

LastName, A.A.; LastName, B.B.; LastName, C.C. Article Title. *Journal Name* **Year**, *Article Number*, Page Range.

ISBN 978-3-03936-782-5 (Hbk)
ISBN 978-3-03936-783-2 (PDF)

© 2020 by the authors. Articles in this book are Open Access and distributed under the Creative Commons Attribution (CC BY) license, which allows users to download, copy and build upon published articles, as long as the author and publisher are properly credited, which ensures maximum dissemination and a wider impact of our publications.

The book as a whole is distributed by MDPI under the terms and conditions of the Creative Commons license CC BY-NC-ND.

Contents

About the Editors vii

Gianluigi Zaza and Giovanni Gambaro
Editorial of Special Issue "Rare Kidney Diseases: New Translational Research Approach to Improve Diagnosis and Therapy"
Reprinted from: *Int. J. Mol. Sci.* **2020**, *21*, 4244, doi:10.3390/ijms21124244 1

Maurizio Bruschi, Simona Granata, Giovanni Candiano, Antonia Fabris, Andrea Petretto, Gian Marco Ghiggeri, Giovanni Gambaro and Gianluigi Zaza
Proteomic Analysis of Urinary Extracellular Vesicles Reveals a Role for the Complement System in Medullary Sponge Kidney Disease
Reprinted from: *Int. J. Mol. Sci.* **2019**, *20*, 5517, doi:10.3390/ijms20215517 5

Lisa Gianesello, Monica Ceol, Loris Bertoldi, Liliana Terrin, Giovanna Priante, Luisa Murer, Licia Peruzzi, Mario Giordano, Fabio Paglialonga, Vincenzo Cantaluppi, Claudio Musetti, Giorgio Valle, Dorella Del Prete, Franca Anglani and Dent Disease Italian Network
Genetic Analyses in Dent Disease and Characterization of *CLCN5* Mutations in Kidney Biopsies
Reprinted from: *Int. J. Mol. Sci.* **2020**, *21*, 516, doi:10.3390/ijms21020516 21

Claudia Muhle-Goll, Philipp Eisenmann, Burkhard Luy, Stefan Kölker, Burkhard Tönshoff, Alexander Fichtner and Jens H. Westhoff
Urinary NMR Profiling in Pediatric Acute Kidney Injury—A Pilot Study
Reprinted from: *Int. J. Mol. Sci.* **2020**, *21*, 1187, doi:10.3390/ijms21041187 41

Domenico De Rasmo, Anna Signorile, Ester De Leo, Elena V. Polishchuk, Anna Ferretta, Roberto Raso, Silvia Russo, Roman Polishchuk, Francesco Emma and Francesco Bellomo
Mitochondrial Dynamics of Proximal Tubular Epithelial Cells in Nephropathic Cystinosis
Reprinted from: *Int. J. Mol. Sci.* **2020**, *21*, 192, doi:10.3390/ijms21010192 57

Ronak Jagdeep Shah, Lisa E. Vaughan, Felicity T. Enders, Dawn S. Milliner and John C. Lieske
Plasma Oxalate as a Predictor of Kidney Function Decline in a Primary Hyperoxaluria Cohort
Reprinted from: *Int. J. Mol. Sci.* **2020**, *21*, 3608, doi:10.3390/ijms21103608 69

Sofia Andrighetto, Jeremy Leventhal, Gianluigi Zaza and Paolo Cravedi
Complement and Complement Targeting Therapies in Glomerular Diseases
Reprinted from: *Int. J. Mol. Sci.* **2019**, *20*, 6336, doi:10.3390/ijms20246336 79

Francesco Paolo Schena, Pasquale Esposito and Michele Rossini
A Narrative Review on C3 Glomerulopathy: A Rare Renal Disease
Reprinted from: *Int. J. Mol. Sci.* **2020**, *21*, 525, doi:10.3390/ijms21020525 95

Fay J. Dickson and John A. Sayer
Nephrocalcinosis: A Review of Monogenic Causes and Insights They Provide into This Heterogeneous Condition
Reprinted from: *Int. J. Mol. Sci.* **2020**, *21*, 369, doi:10.3390/ijms21010369 115

Fabio Sallustio, Claudia Curci, Vincenzo Di Leo, Anna Gallone, Francesco Pesce and Loreto Gesualdo
A New Vision of IgA Nephropathy: The Missing Link
Reprinted from: *Int. J. Mol. Sci.* **2020**, *21*, 189, doi:10.3390/ijms21010189 131

Emmanuel Letavernier, Elise Bouderlique, Jeremy Zaworski, Ludovic Martin and Michel Daudon
Pseudoxanthoma Elasticum, Kidney Stones and Pyrophosphate: From a Rare Disease to Urolithiasis and Vascular Calcifications
Reprinted from: *Int. J. Mol. Sci.* **2019**, *20*, 6353, doi:10.3390/ijms20246353 . . . . **147**

About the Editors

Gianluigi Zaza, Associate Professor in Nephrology. Biography text: Prof. Gianluigi Zaza studied medicine at the University of Bari in 2000. He did his clinical training in Nephrology at the Division of Nephrology, Dialysis and Transplantation, University of Bari (2000–2005). From 2002 to 2005, he was a post-doctoral research fellow in the Department of Pharmacology, St. Jude Children's Research Hospital Memphis, TN, USA. In 2010, he completed his PhD in Clinical Pharmacology and Medicine. In 2011, he began as Assistant Professor at the Renal Unit, Department of Medicine, School of Medicine, University of Verona, Italy, where he was appointed as Associate Professor in 2017. The scientific activity of Prof. Zaza resulted in several publications in international journals (more than 100 articles published in peer-reviewed journals). Moreover, he obtained many national and international awards/honors. Prof. Zaza continues his clinical activities as a medical doctor primarily involved in clinical nephrology and transplant medicine. Additionally, his research interests include translational medicine, proteomics and transcriptomics.

Giovanni Gambaro, Full Professor in Nephrology. Biography text: Prof. Giovanni Gambaro graduated in medicine at the University of Padova in 1979. He did his clinical training in Nephrology and Internal Medicine at the University of Padova. In 1993, he completed his PhD in Nephro-Urological Science. The scientific activity of Prof. Gambaro resulted in more than 400 publications in international journals (h-index: 45). He is a full professor in nephrology and Director of the Renal Unit, Department of Medicine, University of Verona, Italy. His main research interests include nephrolithiasis, the epidemiology of chronic kidney disease, diabetic nephropathy and genetic kidney disorders.

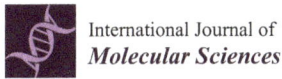

Editorial

Editorial of Special Issue "Rare Kidney Diseases: New Translational Research Approach to Improve Diagnosis and Therapy"

Gianluigi Zaza * and Giovanni Gambaro

Renal Unit, Department of Medicine, University-Hospital of Verona, 37126 Verona, Italy; giovanni.gambaro@univr.it
* Correspondence: gianluigi.zaza@univr.it

Received: 8 June 2020; Accepted: 11 June 2020; Published: 14 June 2020

In this Special Issue entitled "Rare Kidney Diseases: New Translational Research Approach to Improve Diagnosis and Therapy", of the International Journal of Molecular Sciences, that includes original articles and reviews, authors have underlined the role of biomedical research in providing new insights into the pathologies of complex kidney diseases.

Rare kidney diseases comprise a group of more than one hundred different life-threatening or chronically debilitating disorders affecting a small number of patients worldwide (approximately <1 in 2000 individuals in Europe and <200,000 in USA) [1] with different local and/or systemic clinical manifestations/complications. Most of them have a genetic basis, often affecting patients early in childhood, and are frequently progressive, disabling and life-threatening [2]. These features can have an overwhelming psychological impact on the families of children affected by these diseases.

However, although often perceived by the public opinion and media as a prime target of national health care systems, the research in this area has been, for many years, neglected in favor of more common diseases. Main reasons for the lack of interest in this field could be due to the small number of patients available and the consequent limited epidemiological data regarding many of these disorders.

Additionally, rare diseases can affect people in different ways. Even patients with the same disorder can exhibit very different signs and symptoms, or there may be many subtypes of the same condition. This diversity comprises a significant challenge to healthcare practitioners and scientists alike in terms of being able to gain sufficient experience for the most proper and timely definition, diagnosis and management.

A step forward in this field has been obtained by the advances in biotechnologies and "omics" methodologies [3–6] that have led to the discovery of previously unrecognized disease-associated biological processes and identified new potential diagnostic biomarkers and drug targets.

In this issue Bruschi et al. [7], by using a comprehensive comparative proteomic analysis (by mass spectrometry) of urinary microvesicles and exosomes, reported, for the first time, that several urinary proteins (some of them implicated in complement pathway regulation) may be able to clearly identify patients with medullary sponge kidney (MSK) disease, a rare kidney condition often associated with nephrocalcinosis/nephrolithiasis and cystic anomalies in the precalyceal ducts, from idiopathic calcium nephrolithiasis (ICN) as a control group.

The analysis of urinary extracellular vesicles is ideal because they can be easily obtained without invasive procedures, and they contain elevated levels of cell-specific proteins from every segment of the nephron, representing diverse cellular processes including metabolic, immunity-related and coagulation responses [8,9]. These intrinsic characteristics of extracellular vesicles could, therefore, provide a panel of informative marker proteins that not only allow the diagnosis and monitoring of MSK but could also provide insight into the underlying pathophysiological and biochemical processes.

Gianesello et al. [10] investigated allelic and locus heterogeneity in Dent disease (DD), an X-linked renal tubulopathy mainly caused by loss-of-function mutations in CLCN5 (DD1) and OCRL genes, and analyzed ClC-5, megalin, and cubilin expression in DD1 kidney biopsies. They further expanded the spectrum of CLCN5 mutations in DD by describing 23 novel mutations. In DD1 kidney biopsies, they showed that the loss of ClC-5 tubular expression caused defective megalin and cubilin trafficking. In DD3 patients (who have neither CLCN5 nor OCRL gene mutations) whole exome sequencing (WES) did not detect a new disease-causing gene. Instead, it revealed the concomitant presence of likely pathogenic variants in genes encoding proximal tubular endocytic apparatus components, suggesting that they may have had a role in determining the DD3 phenotype.

Furthermore, Muhle-Goll C et al. [11] investigated the accuracy of nuclear magnetic resonance (NMR)-based urine metabolomics for the diagnosis of acute kidney injury (AKI) in a pilot cohort study of neonates and children with established Kidney Disease: Improving Global Outcomes (KDIGO) AKI of heterogeneous etiology. They further explored if metabolomic fingerprints and biomarkers allow for a differentiation of specific AKI subtypes.

Multivariate analysis identified a panel of four metabolites that allowed diagnosis of AKI with an area under the receiver operating characteristics curve (AUC-ROC) of 0.95 (95% confidence interval 0.86–1.00). Especially urinary citrate levels were significantly reduced whereas leucine and valine levels were elevated. Metabolomic differentiation of AKI causes appeared promising but these results need to be validated in larger studies.

De Rasmo D et al. [12] analyzed molecular aspects of nephropathic cystinosis, a rare inherited metabolic disease characterized by an impaired transport of the amino acid cystine out of lysosomes due to the reduced or absent function of the specific carrier cystinosin, which is encoded by the CTNS gene.

In particular, authors investigated mitochondrial dynamics in $CTNS^{-/-}$ conditionally immortalized proximal tubular epithelial cells (ciPTEC) carrying the classical homozygous 57-kb deletion with the intent of identifying new therapeutic targets and biomarkers for treatment follow-up.

Interestingly, their results clearly demonstrated that $CTNS^{-/-}$ cells showed an overexpression of parkin associated with the deregulation of ubiquitination of mitofusin 2 and fission 1 proteins, an altered proteolytic processing of optic atrophy 1 (OPA1) and a decreased OPA1 oligomerization. According to molecular findings, the analysis of electron microscopy images showed a decrease in the mitochondrial cristae number and an increase in the cristae lumen and cristae junction width. Cysteamine treatment restored mitochondrial size, cristae number and lumen, but had no effect on cristae junction width, making tubular cells more susceptible to apoptotic stimuli.

Based on their results, authors concluded that several cellular mediators of mitochondrial dynamics could be useful to develop new therapeutic interventions in this disease. This could be assessed by a future multicenter translational study.

The retrospective analysis of John C. Lieske group [13] investigated plasma oxalate (POx) as a potential predictor of end-stage kidney disease (ESKD) among primary hyperoxaluria (PH) patients. PH is a rare inherited autosomal recessive genetic disease caused by defects in genes that encode proteins important for glyoxylate metabolism [14].

Notably, results of this study demonstrated that in patients with PH, higher POx concentration was a risk factor for ESKD, particularly in advanced chronic kidney disease stages.

Together with the aforementioned original articles, this issue also includes five literature reviews.

Andrighetto et al. [15] reviewed the role of the complement cascade in a wide spectrum of rare renal diseases (including antibody-related glomerulopathies and non-antibody-mediated kidney diseases, such as C3 glomerular disease, atypical hemolytic uremic syndrome and focal segmental glomerulosclerosis) and the potential therapeutic effects of new selective complement-targeting drugs.

Schena FP group [16], describing recent research findings on C3 glomerulopathy, emphasized the importance of a multidisciplinary approach (that involves nephrologists, renal pathologists, molecular biologists and geneticists) to optimize the diagnosis and the treatment of this rare and neglected disease.

Fay J. Dickson and John A. Sayer [17] elegantly reviewed recent literature evidences regarding the employment of a novel precision-medicine approach to ensure patients affected by nephrocalcinosis and their families receive prompt diagnosis (that may slow down the progression to CKD), tailored treatment and accurate prognostic information (it is also useful to screen other family members).

Next, Sallustio et al. [18], based on recent literature evidences, have suggested a new vision of IgA Nephropathy, a primary glomerulonephritis that affects people mainly in the 2nd and 3rd decade of life. Whole-genome genomic studies revealed that this disorder is influenced by several environmental and behavioral factors that, if promptly corrected, may change the course of the disease.

Finally, Letavernier E et al., in an interesting narrative review [19], summarized recent discoveries concerning the pathophysiology of Pseudoxanthoma elasticum, a rare mendelian disease responsible for both cardiovascular and renal papillary calcifications, and discussed the potential implications of pyrophosphate deficiency as a promoter of vascular calcifications in kidney stone formers and in patients affected by CKD.

Overall, the 10 contributions have clearly shown that, in the future, molecular biology will certainly impact clinical decision making in nephrology and will become part of the day-to-day clinical practice.

Funding: This research received no external funding.

Conflicts of Interest: The authors declare no conflict of interest.

References

1. Devuyst, O.; Knoers, N.V.; Remuzzi, G.; Schaefer, F.; Board of the working group for inherited kidney diseases of the European renal association and European dialysis and transplant association. Rare inherited kidney diseases: Challenges, opportunities, and perspectives. *Lancet* **2014**, *383*, 1844–1859. [CrossRef]
2. Bakurov, I.; Castelli, M.; Vanneschi, L.; Freitas, M.J. Supporting medical decisions for treating rare diseases through genetic programming. In *Applications of Evolutionary Computation. EvoApplications 2019*; Kaufmann, P., Castillo, P., Eds.; Springer: Berlin/Heidelberg, Germany, 2019.
3. Xie, J.; Liu, L.; Mladkova, N.; Li, Y.; Ren, H.; Wang, W.; Cui, Z.; Lin, L.; Hu, X.; Yu, X.; et al. The genetic architecture of membranous nephropathy and its potential to improve non-invasive diagnosis. *Nat. Commun.* **2020**, *11*, 1–18. [CrossRef] [PubMed]
4. Sanna-Cherchi, S.; Khan, K.; Westland, R.; Krithivasan, P.; Fievet, L.; Rasouly, H.M.; Ionita-Laza, I.; Capone, V.P.; Fasel, D.A.; Kiryluk, K.; et al. Exome-wide Association Study Identifies GREB1L Mutations in Congenital Kidney Malformations. *Am. J. Hum. Genet.* **2017**, *101*, 789–802. [CrossRef] [PubMed]
5. Fabris, A.; Bruschi, M.; Santucci, L.; Candiano, G.; Granata, S.; Gassa, A.D.; Antonucci, N.; Petretto, A.; Ghiggeri, G.M.; Gambaro, G.; et al. Proteomic-based research strategy identified laminin subunit alpha 2 as a potential urinary-specific biomarker for the medullary sponge kidney disease. *Kidney Int.* **2017**, *91*, 459–468. [CrossRef] [PubMed]
6. Bruschi, M.; Granata, S.; Santucci, L.; Candiano, G.; Fabris, A.; Antonucci, N.; Petretto, A.; Bartolucci, M.; Del Zotto, G.; Antonini, F.; et al. Proteomic Analysis of Urinary Microvesicles and Exosomes in Medullary Sponge Kidney Disease and Autosomal Dominant Polycystic Kidney Disease. *Clin. J. Am. Soc. Nephrol.* **2019**, *14*, 834–843. [CrossRef] [PubMed]
7. Bruschi, M.; Granata, S.; Candiano, G.; Fabris, A.; Petretto, A.; Ghiggeri, G.M.; Gambaro, G.; Zaza, G. Proteomic analysis of urinary extracellular vesicles reveals a role for the complement system in medullary sponge kidney disease. *Int. J. Mol. Sci.* **2019**, *20*, 5517. [CrossRef] [PubMed]
8. Pisitkun, T.; Shen, R.-F.; Knepper, M.A. Identification and proteomic profiling of exosomes in human urine. *Proc. Natl. Acad. Sci. USA* **2004**, *101*, 13368–13373. [CrossRef] [PubMed]
9. Moon, P.-G.; You, S.; Lee, J.; Hwang, D.; Baek, M.-C. Urinary exosomes and proteomics. *Mass Spectrom. Rev.* **2011**, *30*, 1185–1202. [CrossRef] [PubMed]
10. Gianesello, L.; Ceol, M.; Bertoldi, L.; Terrin, L.; Priante, G.; Murer, L.; Peruzzi, L.; Giordano, M.; Paglialonga, F.; Cantaluppi, V.; et al. Genetic analyses in dent disease and characterization of CLCN5 mutations in kidney biopsies. *Int. J. Mol. Sci.* **2020**, *21*, 516. [CrossRef] [PubMed]
11. Muhle-Goll, C.; Eisenmann, P.; Luy, B.; Kölker, S.; Tönshoff, B.; Fichtner, A.; Westhoff, J. Urinary NMR profiling in pediatric acute kidney injury—A pilot study. *Int. J. Mol. Sci.* **2020**, *21*, 1187. [CrossRef] [PubMed]

12. De Rasmo, D.; Signorile, A.; De Leo, E.; Polishchuk, E.; Ferretta, A.; Raso, R.; Russo, S.; Polishchuk, R.; Emma, F.; Bellomo, F. Mitochondrial Dynamics of Proximal Tubular Epithelial Cells in Nephropathic Cystinosis. *Int. J. Mol. Sci.* **2020**, *21*, 192. [CrossRef] [PubMed]
13. Shah, R.J.; Vaughan, L.; Enders, F.; Milliner, D.; Lieske, J.C. Plasma oxalate as a predictor of kidney function decline in a primary hyperoxaluria cohort. *Int. J. Mol. Sci.* **2020**, *21*, 3608. [CrossRef] [PubMed]
14. Cochat, P.; Rumsby, G. Primary hyperoxaluria. *New Engl. J. Med.* **2013**, *369*, 649–658. [CrossRef] [PubMed]
15. Andrighetto, S.; Leventhal, J.; Zaza, G.; Cravedi, P. Complement and complement targeting therapies in glomerular diseases. *Int. J. Mol. Sci.* **2019**, *20*, 6336. [CrossRef] [PubMed]
16. Schena, F.P.; Esposito, P.; Rossini, M. A Narrative review on C3 glomerulopathy: A rare renal disease. *Int. J. Mol. Sci.* **2020**, *21*, 525. [CrossRef] [PubMed]
17. Dickson, F.; Sayer, J.A. Nephrocalcinosis: A review of monogenic causes and insights they provide into this heterogeneous condition. *Int. J. Mol. Sci.* **2020**, *21*, 369. [CrossRef] [PubMed]
18. Sallustio, F.; Curci, C.; Di Leo, V.; Gallone, A.; Pesce, F.; Gesualdo, L. A new vision of IgA nephropathy: The missing link. *Int. J. Mol. Sci.* **2010**, *21*, 189. [CrossRef] [PubMed]
19. Letavernier, E.; Bouderlique, E.; Zaworski, J.; Martin, L.; Daudon, M. Pseudoxanthoma elasticum, kidney stones and pyrophosphate: From a rare disease to urolithiasis and vascular calcifications. *Int. J. Mol. Sci.* **2019**, *20*, 6353. [CrossRef] [PubMed]

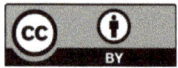

© 2020 by the authors. Licensee MDPI, Basel, Switzerland. This article is an open access article distributed under the terms and conditions of the Creative Commons Attribution (CC BY) license (http://creativecommons.org/licenses/by/4.0/).

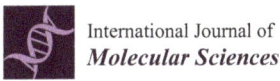

Article

Proteomic Analysis of Urinary Extracellular Vesicles Reveals a Role for the Complement System in Medullary Sponge Kidney Disease

Maurizio Bruschi [1,†], Simona Granata [2,†], Giovanni Candiano [1], Antonia Fabris [2], Andrea Petretto [3], Gian Marco Ghiggeri [4], Giovanni Gambaro [2] and Gianluigi Zaza [2,*]

1. Laboratory of Molecular Nephrology, IRCCS Istituto Giannina Gaslini, 16147 Genova, Italy; maurizibruschi@gaslini.org (M.B.); giovannicandiano@gaslini.org (G.C.)
2. Renal Unit, Department of Medicine, University/Hospital of Verona, Piazzale A. Stefani 1, 37126 Verona, Italy; simona.granata@univr.it (S.G.); antoniafabris21@gmail.com (A.F.); giovanni.gambaro@univr.it (G.G.)
3. Laboratory of Mass Spectrometry—Core Facilities, IRCCS Istituto Giannina Gaslini, 16147 Genova, Italy; a.petretto@gmail.com
4. Division of Nephrology, Dialysis and Transplantation, IRCCS Istituto Giannina Gaslini, 16147 Genova, Italy; GMarcoGhiggeri@gaslini.org
* Correspondence: gianluigi.zaza@univr.it; Tel.: +39-045-8122528; Fax: +39-045-8027311
† These authors contributed equally to the study.

Received: 12 September 2019; Accepted: 4 November 2019; Published: 5 November 2019

Abstract: Medullary sponge kidney (MSK) disease is a rare and neglected kidney condition often associated with nephrocalcinosis/nephrolithiasis and cystic anomalies in the precalyceal ducts. Little is known about the pathogenesis of this disease, so we addressed the knowledge gap using a proteomics approach. The protein content of microvesicles/exosomes isolated from urine of 15 MSK and 15 idiopathic calcium nephrolithiasis (ICN) patients was investigated by mass spectrometry, followed by weighted gene co-expression network analysis, support vector machine (SVM) learning, and partial least squares discriminant analysis (PLS-DA) to select the most discriminative proteins. Proteomic data were verified by ELISA. We identified 2998 proteins in total, 1764 (58.9%) of which were present in both vesicle types in both diseases. Among the MSK samples, only 65 (2.2%) and 137 (4.6%) proteins were exclusively found in the microvesicles and exosomes, respectively. Similarly, among the ICN samples, only 75 (2.5%) and 94 (3.1%) proteins were exclusively found in the microvesicles and exosomes, respectively. SVM learning and PLS-DA revealed a core panel of 20 proteins that distinguished extracellular vesicles representing each clinical condition with an accuracy of 100%. Among them, three exosome proteins involved in the lectin complement pathway maximized the discrimination between MSK and ICN: Ficolin 1, Mannan-binding lectin serine protease 2, and Complement component 4-binding protein β. ELISA confirmed the proteomic results. Our data show that the complement pathway is involved in the MSK, revealing a new range of potential therapeutic targets and early diagnostic biomarkers.

Keywords: medullary sponge kidney; idiopathic calcium nephrolithiasis; complement system; proteomics

1. Introduction

In the last decade, great efforts have been undertaken to characterize the biological networking associated with medullary sponge kidney (MSK) disease, a rare clinical condition (prevalence of approximately 5 cases per 100,000 in the general population) often associated with nephrocalcinosis and nephrolithiasis, urinary acidification and concentration defects, and cystic anomalies in the precalyceal ducts [1]. Most of these studies, based on clinical observations, as well as molecular analysis, have provided evidence that supports the genetic transmission of MSK and an association with metabolic disorders (such as hyperparathyroidism) and bone diseases [2–11].

More recently, we used proteomic analysis to catalog the MSK-specific protein profile, as well as the protein content of urinary extracellular vesicles [12]. This revealed the presence of several key regulators of epithelial cell differentiation, kidney development, cell migration/adhesion, and extracellular matrix organization, providing a new insight into the pathophysiology of MSK [12]. The most abundant protein found in MSK urinary extracellular vesicles was laminin subunit α2 (LAMA2, Merosin), a well-characterized member of the laminin family of at least 15 αβγ heterotrimeric proteins, which contributes to the extracellular matrix and is a major component of the basement membrane [12,13]. This protein is thought to promote cyst formation [14–16]. It also regulates extracellular laminin assembly, and the laminin then determines the orientation of the apical pole [17].

In our most recent publication [18], we compared the protein content of extracellular vesicles (exosomes and microvesicles) from MSK and autosomal dominant polycystic kidney disease (ADPKD) patients by mass spectrometry (MS) and identified a profile including 34 proteins that discriminate between the two clinical conditions. The most abundant protein in MSK vesicles was SPP1, also known as osteopontin, which is implicated in physiological/pathological bone mineralization and kidney stone formation [19]. This protein is synthesized in the kidney and secreted into the urine by epithelial cells, including those lining the loop of Henle, distal convoluted tubule, and papillary duct [20]. SPP1 inhibits the nucleation, growth, and aggregation of calcium oxalate crystals [21] and the binding of these crystals to kidney epithelial cells [22]. Although it has been recently found that osteopontin was up-regulated in the kidney from established rat models for polycystic kidney disease compared with wild-type mice [23,24], no data are available for MSK (no animal model is available for this disease). Therefore, based on our in vivo data, we can assume that in MSK patients, osteopontin could be also more up-regulated than ADPKD. A reason could be that in MSK, this biological element may be implicated not only in cystic development, but also in nephrolithiasis, a major clinical condition associated with medullary sponge kidney.

The diagnostic accuracy for MSK is currently low because it depends on personal experience (MSK is often confused with other causes of nephrocalcinosis or with papillary ductal plugging) and diagnosis requires invasive radiation and/or nephrotoxic contrast agents for medical imaging. Although the studies described above have shed light on the biological mechanisms associated with MSK, the pathogenesis of this disorder is only partially defined and further studies are necessary to identify suitable diagnostic biomarkers. To address this knowledge gap, we carried out a comprehensive comparative proteomic analysis of urinary microvesicles and exosomes to identify biological differences between MSK and idiopathic calcium nephrolithiasis (ICN) as a control group. The analysis of urinary extracellular vesicles is ideal because they can be obtained without invasive procedures and they contain elevated levels of cell-specific proteins from every segment of the nephron, representing diverse cellular processes including metabolic, immunity-related, and coagulation responses [25,26]. These intrinsic characteristics of extracellular vesicles could, therefore, provide a panel of informative marker proteins that not only allow the diagnosis and monitoring of MSK but could also provide insight into the underlying pathophysiological and biochemical processes.

2. Results

2.1. Characterization of Exosomes and Microvesicles

The size and purity of the microvesicles and exosomes isolated by ultracentrifugation were confirmed by dynamic light scattering (DLS), revealing a Gaussian distribution profile with peak means at 1000 ± 65 and 90 ± 5 nm, the typical size for microvesicles and exosomes, respectively (Figure S1A). There was no difference in size between the MSK and ICN patients for either type of vesicle. Western blot analysis revealed that the exosomes were positive for CD63 and CD81 but not CD45, whereas the microvesicles showed the opposite antigen profile (Figure S1B).

2.2. Protein Composition of Exosomes and Microvesicles

The protein composition of microvesicles and exosomes from the urine of ICN and MSK patients was determined by MS analysis. We identified 2998 proteins in total, 1764 (58.9%) of which were present in all four sample types. Among the ICN samples, only 75 (2.5%) and 94 (3.1%) proteins were exclusively found in the microvesicles and exosomes, respectively. Similarly, among the MSK samples, only 65 (2.2%) and 137 (4.6%) proteins were exclusively found in the microvesicles and exosomes, respectively (Figure 1).

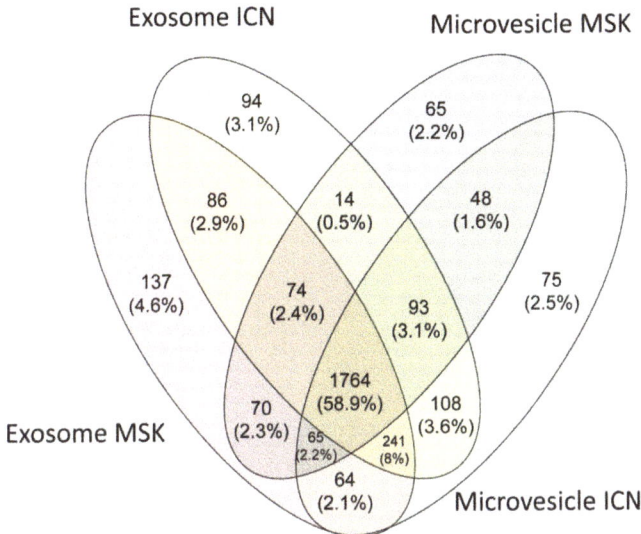

Figure 1. Venn diagram showing all the proteins identified in exosomes and microvesicles isolated from the urine of idiopathic calcium nephrolithiasis (ICN) and medullary sponge kidney (MSK) patients. Venn diagram shows common and exclusive proteins in the ICN and MSK groups. The numbers (and percentages) of proteins in the overlapping and non-overlapping areas are indicated.

About 2% of the total proteins found in extracellular vesicles were associated with one or both kidney diseases according to the DisGeNET database [27]. Among these associated proteins, 40% were found in the ICN and 100% in the MSK samples (Figure S2). The cellular origins of the proteins in the microvesicles were very similar in the ICN and MSK disease samples, with 35% of proteins originating from membranes, 25% from the cytoplasm, 7% from the nucleus, and 33% from other organelles. Similar results were observed for the exosome proteins, with 19% originating from membranes, 31% from the cytoplasm, 11% from the nucleus, and 38% from other organelles.

The overlapping protein content of each sample was confirmed by constructing a two-dimensional scatter plot of the multidimensional scaling (MDS) analysis (Figure S3). No samples were excluded during the quality check, performed by non-hierarchical clustering. We used weighted-gene co-expression network analysis (WGCNA) to identify proteins associated with each type of extracellular vesicle and disease, revealing a total of 14 modules comprising proteins with similar expression profiles. To distinguish between modules, we chose an arbitrary color for each module. The number of proteins included in each module ranged from 31 (salmon) to 950 (turquoise). The lime, pink, violet, and tan modules showed closer relationships with the microvesicles or exosomes from the ICN samples, whereas the gray, yellow, and green modules showed closer relationships with the microvesicles from the MSK samples (Figure 2).

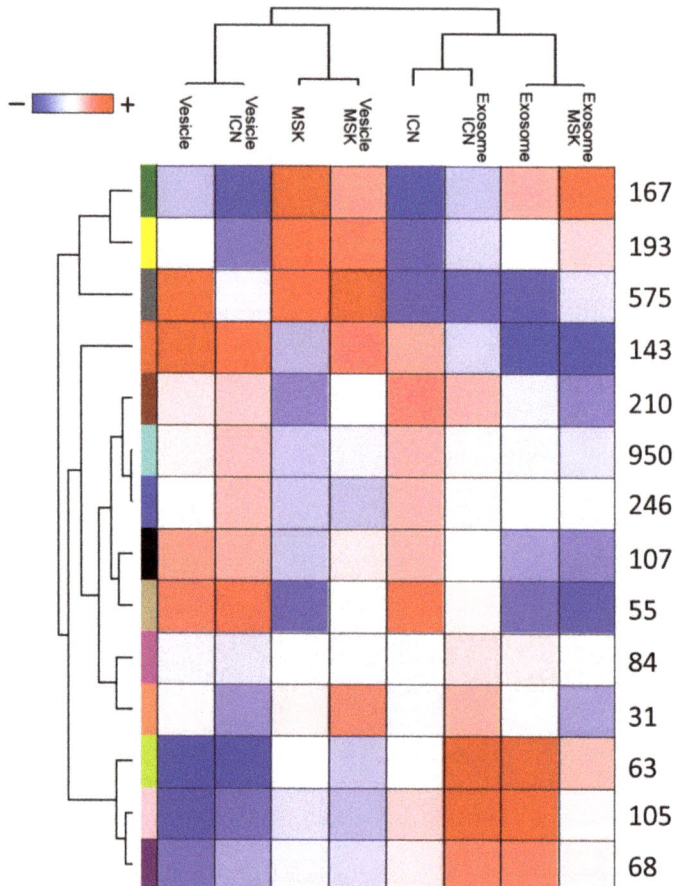

Figure 2. Module identification and relationships with clinical traits. Heat map of the relationships between module eigengenes and the trait indicator of each sample. The grade of the relationship ranges from −1 (blue) to 1 (red), where blue represents a perfect negative correlation and red a perfect positive correlation.

Next, we applied the Mann–Whitney *U*-test to identify the proteins that best distinguish the type of disease in the microvesicles or exosomes (Figure 3A,B).

This revealed a total of 142 discriminatory proteins (Tables S1 and S2): 105 distinguished between ICN and MSK microvesicles and 43 distinguished between ICN and MSK exosomes, with six featuring in both vesicle types (Figure S4A). Their expression profiles after Z-score analysis are shown in Figure S4B. support vector machine (SVM) learning and partial least squares discriminant analysis (PLS-DA) were then used to highlight the proteins that maximize the discrimination between different sample types, revealing a core panel of 20 proteins that identified the four sample types with an accuracy of 100% (Figure 4A). Following the Z-score analysis, we built a heat map of the corresponding expression profiles (Figure 4B).

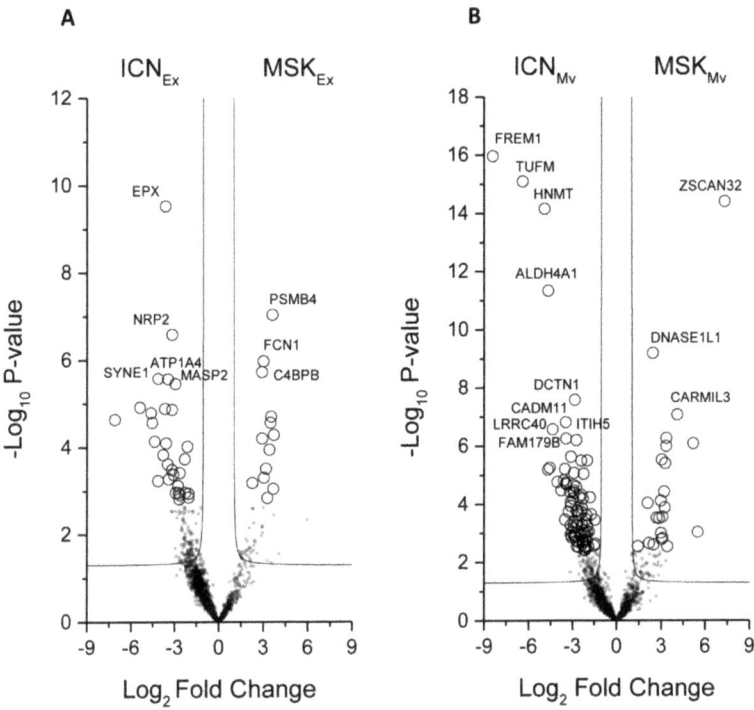

Figure 3. Volcano plot showing the univariate statistical analysis of urinary exosome (**A**) and microvesicle (**B**) fractions from ICN and MSK patients. The plot is based on the fold change (log$_2$) and p-value (–log$_{10}$) of all proteins identified in all samples. White circles indicate proteins with statistically significant differences in abundance between the two groups of patients.

The diversity of expression profiles among the proteins that showed significant and high levels of sample discrimination indicated an equally diverse range of functions, so we assigned Gene Ontology (GO) functional annotations to build a network of biochemical pathways among the different groups (Figure S5). In this network, circles and lines represent the biochemical pathways and their interconnections, respectively. In addition, the different pathways were clustered into 12 functional groups based on their GO annotations (ellipses): immune system, production of reactive oxygen species, IL-8 regulation, transport, regulation of ERBB signaling, tyrosine phosphorylation, receptor activity, peptidyl serine modification, hydrolase activity, DNA regulation, nucleoside metabolism, and cell and organ development. These 12 clusters were grouped into four macro-areas: regulation of metabolism, signal transduction, inflammation, and regulation of cell development. To generate a more concise picture of the biochemical process associated with the three proteins that maximize the discrimination between the exosomes of ICN and MSK samples [Mannan-binding lectin serine protease 2 (MASP2), Ficolin 1 (FCN1), and Complement component 4-binding protein β (C4BPB)], we explored the enrichment of GO annotations in greater detail. This highlighted the lectin-based complement activation pathway as the perturbed biochemical process most likely associated with all three potential biomarkers (Figure 5). The diagram shows the pathway mapped as a network of proteins (nodes) and their interactions (edges). Node color represents the fold change in protein abundance in the urinary exosome fraction of MSK (red) versus ICN (blue) patients, and the node size represents the corresponding p-values.

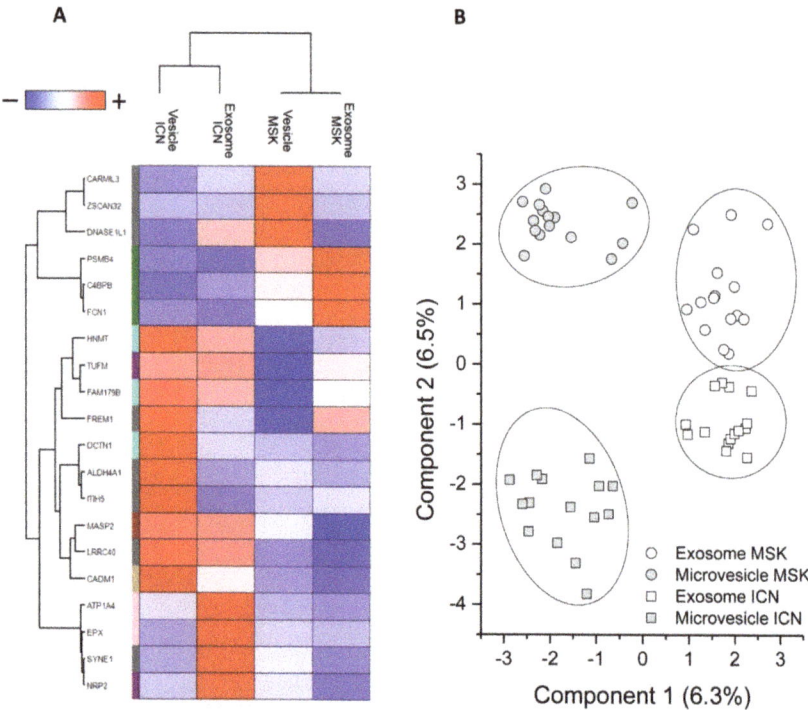

Figure 4. Proteins that achieve maximum discrimination between the exosome and microvesicle fractions of ICN and MSK patients. (**A**) Heat map of 20 core proteins identified through the combined use of univariate statistical analysis, machine learning, and partial least squares discriminant analysis. In the heat map, each row represents a protein, and each column corresponds to a sample type (exosome and microvesicle fractions from ICN and MSK patients). Normalized Z-scores of protein abundance are depicted by a pseudocolor scale with red indicating positive expression, white equal expression, and blue negative expression compared to each protein value, whereas the dendrogram displays the outcome of unsupervised hierarchical clustering, placing similar proteome profile values near each other. (**B**) Two-dimensional scatter plot representing the partial least squares discriminant analysis of exosomes (white symbols) and microvesicles (gray symbols) from MSK (circle) and ICN (square) patients, using the 20 core proteins. The ellipsis indicates 95% confidence interval. Visual inspection of the dendrogram, heat map, and scatter plot confirm the ability of these proteins to clearly distinguish among the four different sample types.

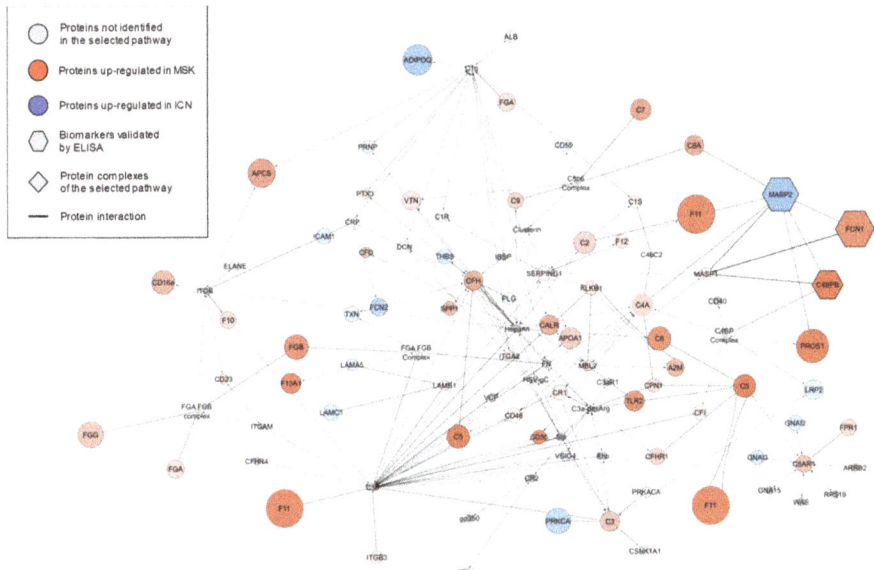

Figure 5. Complement lectin pathway activation. The diagram shows the zoom-in of the immune system enrichment results mapped as a network. Nodes and edges represent, respectively, the proteins and their interaction in the pathway of complement lectin activation. The color intensity of each protein (node) indicates the fold change increment in the urinary exosome fraction of MSK (red) versus ICN (blue) patients and the node size is representative of their p-value. The gray nodes represent unidentified proteins (circle) and protein complexes (diamonds) in the lectin pathway. The hexagons indicate the three proteins that maximize the discrimination between ICN and MSK samples as highlighted by the combined use of univariate/multivariate statistical analysis and machine learning algorithms.

2.3. ELISA Analysis of MASP2, FCN1, and C4BPB to Confirm the MS Data

The mass spectrometry (MS) results were verified by ELISA for all patients enrolled in the study using an in-house assay setup (Figure 6). We found that MASP2 was expressed more strongly in ICN patients compared to MSK patients (Figure 6A, black circle). The median (and interquartile range) values for ICN and MSK were 1.05 (0.41–1.4) and 0.2 (0.1–0.4), respectively ($p < 0.0001$). Received operating characteristic (ROC) analysis revealed that the expression of MASP2 in the urinary exosome can distinguish between ICN and MSK patients (Figure 6B, black line). The area under the curve (AUC), 95% confidence interval (CI), and p-value for the ROC analysis were 0.89, 0.81–0.97, and $p < 0.0001$, respectively. The cutoff, sensitivity, specificity, and likelihood ratio were 0.62, 67%, 97%, and 20, respectively.

In contrast to MASP2, FCN1 (Figure 6A, red circle) and C4BPB (Figure 6A, green circle) were more strongly expressed in MSK patients compared to ICN patients. For FCN1, the median (and interquartile range) values for ICN and MSK were 0.34 (0.28–0.47) and 1.06 (0.59–1.5), respectively ($p < 0.0001$). ROC analysis revealed that the expression of FCN1 in the urinary exosome can distinguish between ICN and MSK patients (Figure 6B, red line). The AUC, 95% CI and p-values for the ROC analysis were 0.9, 0.82–0.98, and $p < 0.0001$, respectively. The cutoff, sensitivity, specificity, and likelihood ratio were 0.55, 77%, 87%, and 5.7, respectively. For C4BPB, the median (and interquartile range) values for ICN and MSK were 0.45 (0.3–0.59) and 1.2 (0.67–1.67), respectively ($p < 0.0001$). ROC analysis revealed that the expression of C4BPB in the urinary exosome can distinguish between ICN and MSK patients (Figure 6B, green line). The AUC, 95% CI, and p-values for the ROC analysis were 0.9, 0.82–0.98, and $p < 0.0001$, respectively. The cutoff, sensitivity, specificity, and likelihood ratio were 0.62, 77%, 87%, and 5.7, respectively.

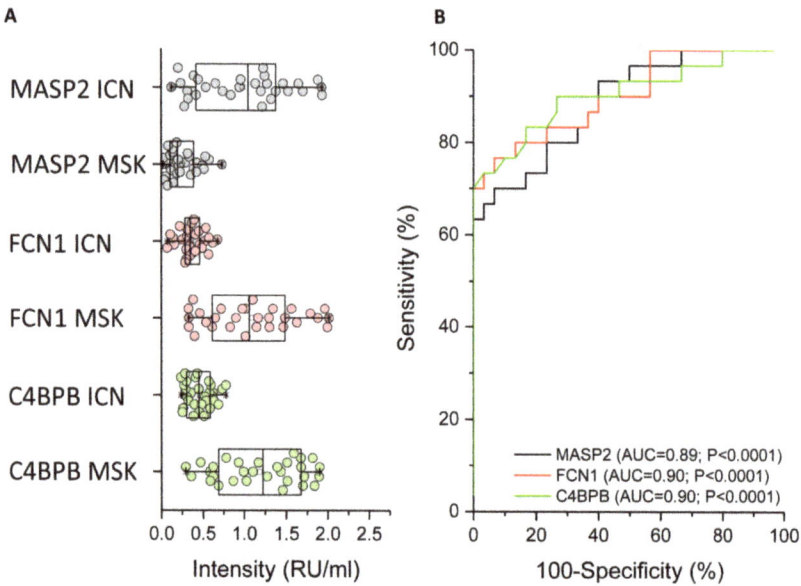

Figure 6. ELISA experiments to verify the proteomic data. (**A**) Box plot showing the median and interquartile range values of MASP (black), FCN1 (red), and C4BPB (green) in the urinary exosome of all patients. In particular, MASP2 was strongly expressed in the urinary exosome of ICN compared to MSK patients, whereas FCN1 and C4BPB showed the opposite profile. (**B**) Received operating characteristic (ROC) curve analysis confirming that the expression of all three proteins discriminates between ICN and MSK patients.

3. Discussion

MSK is a rare kidney disease that is currently difficult to diagnose because the molecular basis of pathogenesis is unclear and robust diagnostic biomarkers are not available in the clinic. We, therefore, carried out a comprehensive comparative proteomic analysis of urinary microvesicles and exosomes from MSK patients and a control group with the distinct kidney disorder ICN. We defined the protein profiles of both vesicles in both diseases and applied innovative statistical methods (including SVM learning and PLS-DA) to identify specific proteins (and the corresponding biological networks) that can accurately discriminate between patients with each disease. These proteins and networks not only represent a source of novel biomarker candidates and potential therapeutic targets but should also shed light on the molecular basis of MSK.

Statistical analysis identified a core panel of 20 highly discriminative proteins, the most promising were FCN1, MASP2, and C4BPB, all of which are major functional or regulatory components of the lectin complement pathway. These three proteins were not associated with either MSK or ICN according to the DisGeNET, a database containing one of the largest publicly available collections of genes and variants associated with human diseases [27]. FCN1 and C4BPB were more abundant in the exosomes of MSK patients compared to ICN controls, whereas MASP2 showed the opposite profile. It is possible that all three proteins, because of their molecular weight and the absence of proteinuria and/or renal impairment in our enrolled patients, did not pass through an intact glomerular membrane but were instead derived from renal epithelial cells [28].

FCN1 (also known as M-ficolin) is an oligomeric pattern-recognition protein consisting of an N-terminal collagen-like domain and a C-terminal globular fibrinogen-like domain [29,30]. It can form complexes with MASP2 to activate the lectin complement pathway [31]. FCN1 may also interact with C-reactive protein (CRP) via a conformational change induced by mild acidosis at the local site of infection [32,33], and with pentraxin 3 (PTX3) in a Ca^{2+}-dependent manner [34]. The high level of FCN1 in urinary exosomes isolated from our MSK patients suggests that the lectin complement pathway may be involved in the complex biological process leading to the growth of cysts. This agrees with previous studies based on mouse models deficient in complement factors, which develop fewer kidney cysts and suffer less severe pericystic tissue inflammation, helping to preserve normal renal functions [35]. Further evidence that the complement pathway is involved in cystic disorders has been gathered from patients affected by ADPKD, whose urine and cyst fluids were found to be enriched for complement proteins [36–38].

The downregulation of MASP2 in our MSK patients was accompanied by the upregulation of C4BPB, a multimeric protein that inhibits the activation of the complement cascade by preventing the formation of the classical C3 and C5 convertases [39]. This may reflect the physiological attempt of the kidneys to mitigate the activation of the lectin complement pathway. This could also explain the contra-regulation of FCN1 and MASP2. However, additional studies are necessary to confirm this effect. Indeed, the hyperactivation of complement may induce glomerular and tubulointerstitial injury [40].

Taken together, our data suggest for the first time that the lectin complement pathway may be involved in the complex biological machinery associated with MSK, but it is clearly not associated with nephrolithiasis. Extracellular vesicles may, therefore, be part of the pathological machinery leading to the growth of cysts. Although we cannot exclude that the complement system could be a secondary response to the disease, this might offer a therapeutic option for progression blockade. Additionally, urinary vesicles may provide a source of valuable clinical biomarkers allowing MSK to be distinguished from other cystic disorders (including ADPKD) and types of nephrolithiasis.

However, our results must be validated using a larger cohort of patients, and additional functional studies are required to better define the biological role of the lectin complement cascade in the pathogenesis of MSK.

4. Materials and Methods

4.1. Patients

Having obtained informed written consent, we enrolled 15 adult MSK patients and 15 adult ICN patients matched for age, gender, and geographical origin, followed up at our renal unit. The inclusion criteria for the MSK group were the same as described in our previous study [12]. Particularly, patients had both kidneys involved, nephrocalcinosis and/or cysts in at least 2 papillae in each kidney. For MSK, patients had papillary precalyceal ectasias on films obtained at least 10 min after contrast medium injection in the absence of compression maneuvers and signs of obstruction. The X-ray films were reviewed by an independent radiologist to confirm the diagnosis. For ICN patients the inclusion criteria were calcium stone disease, normal serum creatinine and electrolyte concentrations, and urinary pH ≤ 5.5 measured in spot morning urine (after overnight fasting) to exclude tubular acidosis. Exclusion criteria for ICN patients were: the presence of endocrine diseases and cystic kidney disorders, nephrocalcinosis, and obstructive nephropathy. In all ICN patients, the MSK disease was ruled out by careful clinical examination.

Clinical data were registered in an electronic database. Informed consent was obtained from all patients in accordance with the Declaration of Helsinki and the ethical board of the University Hospital of Verona approved the study (1312CESC, 24 May 2017).

4.2. Isolation of Microvesicles and Exosomes

Second morning urine samples were obtained from all patients. Microvesicles and exosomes were isolated by centrifugation as previously reported [18]. Briefly, 16 ml aliquots of urine were centrifuged at 16,000× g for 30 min at 16 °C in order to remove alive and dead cells and organelles. The obtained supernatant was centrifuged for 120 min at 22,000× g at 16 °C to obtain the microvesicle fraction. The microvesicle-containing pellet was washed in phosphate-buffered saline (PBS) and repelleted as above for a total of five wash cycles to obtain a clean microvesicle fraction. To obtain the exosome, the supernatant was centrifuged for 120 min at 100,000× g at 16 °C. Then one-step sucrose cushion ultracentrifugation for 120 min at 100,000× g at 16 °C was performed to further purify exosomes according to their density. The exosome-containing pellet was washed in PBS and repelleted as above for a total of five wash cycles to obtain a clean exosome fraction. This procedure was carried out for each sample and the microvesicle and exosome fractions were stored at −80 °C until use.

4.3. Dynamic Light Scattering

The size of the exosomes and microvesicles was determined by dynamic light scattering (DLS) using a Zetasizer nano ZS90 particle sizer (Malvern Instruments, Worcestershire, UK) at a 90° fixed angle. The particle diameter was calculated using the Stokes–Einstein equation. For particle sizing in solution, exosome and microvesicle aliquots were diluted in 10% PBS and analyzed at a constant 25 °C.

4.4. Western Blot

Microvesicle and exosome fractions from 16 ml urine samples were separated by SDS-PAGE (8–16% acrylamide gradient) and then transferred to a nitrocellulose membrane. The membrane was blocked with 1% bovine serum albumin (BSA) in PBS plus 0.1% Tween-20 (PBST), rinsed in PBST, and labeled with one of the following primary human antibodies diluted in 1% BSA in PBST: anti-CD63 (Novus Biological, Littleton, CA, USA), anti-CD81 (Novus Biological, Littleton, CA, USA), or anti-CD45 (LifeSpan BioSciences, Seattle, WA, USA) [41]. After rinsing again in PBST, the membrane was incubated with horseradish peroxidase (HRP)-conjugated anti-mouse secondary antibodies (Novus Biological, Littleton, CA, USA). Chemiluminescence was detected and quantified using the ChemiDoc Touch Imaging System and Image Lab software (Bio-Rad, Hercules, CA, USA).

4.5. Mass Spectrometry

Samples were processed with in-StageTip (iST) method with two poly (styrene divinylbenzene) reversed-phase sulfonate (SDB-RPS) disks. The microvesicle- and exosome-containing pellets were solubilized with a solution containing 10 mM Tris(2-carboxyethyl)phosphine, 40 mM chloro-acetamide, 100 mM Tris (pH 8.5), and 2% sodium deoxycholate. Lysis, reduction, and alkylation of the samples were performed in a single step and then loaded into the StageTip. The samples were then diluted with a buffer containing 25 mM Tris (pH 8.5) and 1 µg of trypsin. After the acidification step with 1% trifluoroacetic acid (TFA), the samples were washed with 0.2% TFA three times. The proteins were eluted in 60 µl 5% v/v ammonium hydroxide containing 80% v/v acetonitrile. The desalted peptides were dried in a speed vacuum and resuspended in 2% acetonitrile containing 0.2% formic acid (FA). They were then separated on a 50-cm reversed-phase Easy Spray column (75-µm internal diameter × 50 cm; 2 µm/100 Å C18) on an Ultimate 3000 RSLCnano device (Thermo Fisher Scientific, Waltham, MA, USA) with a binary buffer system comprising buffer A (0.1% FA) and buffer B (80% acetonitrile, 5% dimethylsulfoxide, 0.1% FA). The program consisted of a 70-min gradient (2–45% buffer B) at a flow rate of 250 µl/min, with the column temperature maintained at 60 °C. The chromatography system was coupled to an Orbitrap Fusion Tribrid mass spectrometer (Thermo Fisher Scientific, Waltham, MA, USA), acquiring data in Charge Ordered Parallel Ion aNalysis (CHOPIN) mode. The precursors were ionized using an EASY-spray source held at +2.2 kV and the iICNet capillary temperature was held at 300 °C. Single MS survey scans were performed over the mass window 375–1500 m/z with an AGC target of 250,000, a maximum injection time of 50 ms, and a resolution of 120,000 at 200 *m/z*. Monoisotopic precursor selection was enabled for peptide isotopic distributions, precursors of z = 2–5 were selected for 2 s of cycle time, and dynamic exclusion was set to 25 s with a ± 10 ppm window set around the precursor. The following CHOPIN conditions were applied: a) if the precursor charge state is 2, then follow with collision-induced dissociation (CID) and scan in the ion trap with an isolation window of 1.8, CID energy of 35%, and a rapid ion trap scan rate; b) if the precursor charge state is 3–5 and precursor intensity >500,000, then follow with higher-energy C-trap dissociation (HCD) and scan in the Orbitrap with an isolation window of 1.8, HCD energy of 28%, and a resolution of 15,000; c) if the precursor charge state is 3–5 and precursor intensity < 500,000, then follow with CID as described for option (a). For all MS^2 events, the following options were set: "Injection Ions for All Available Parallelizable Time" with an AGC target value of 4000 and a maximum injection time of 250 ms for CID, or an AGC target value of 10,000 and a maximum injection time of 40 ms for HCD.

4.6. MS Data Analysis

Raw MS files were processed in the MaxQuant v1.6.0.16 environment using the MaxLFQ algorithm for label-free quantification and Andromeda search engine. Peptide and protein false discovery rate (FDRs) were both set at < 0.01. The search contained variable modifications for the oxidation of methionine (M), N-terminal protein acetylation (protein N-terminus), and fixed carbamidomethyl modifications (C). For protease digestion, up to two missed cleavages were allowed. Peptides of length greater than six amino acids have been considered for the identification. The "match between runs" algorithm with a setting of 1 min time window was used for the quantification of MS missed data in each individual measurement. UniProt FASTA Homo sapiens database (access August 2017) was used for the identification of peptides and proteins.

4.7. ELISA

MASP2, FNC1, and C4BPB levels were determined using an in-house ELISA setup. Briefly, polyclonal antibody anti-MASP2, anti-FCN1, or anti-C4BPB (LifeSpan Biosciences) was used to coat overnight at 4 °C 96-well MaxiSorp Nunc plates (Thermo Fisher Scientific, Waltham, MA, USA). The plates were then blocked with 3% BSA in PBS. Exosome fractions were solubilized in 10 µl of mild detergent solution (1% Nonidet P-40, 0.5% Tween-20 in PBS), supplemented with 90 µl 3% BSA in PBST and incubated at 4 °C overnight. After three washes in PBST, the plates were incubated for 4h with the corresponding monoclonal antibody (anti-MASP2, anti-FCN1, or anti-C4BPB, all from LifeSpan Biosciences, Seattle, WA, USA) diluted 1:1000 with 1% BSA in PBST. After three washes with PBST, the plates were incubated with HRP-conjugated anti-mouse IgG diluted 1:5000 in 1% BSA in PBST for 1h. After washing, the peroxidase substrate (TMB, Bio-Rad, Hercules, CA, USA) was added. The reaction was stopped with an H_2SO_4 solution. The absorbance at 450 nm was measured using an iMark microplate reader (Bio-Rad, Hercules, CA, USA). To standardize the response of the antibodies, we used a pool of strongly positive controls. The optical density results were expressed as relative units per milliliter (RU/ml).

4.8. Statistical Analysis

After normalization, unsupervised hierarchical clustering and multidimensional scaling (MDS) with Spearman's rank correlation and *k*-means were used to recognize outliers and sample dissimilarity. Weighted-gene co-expression network analysis (WGCNA) package in *R* was used for building the co-expression network with the normalized expression profiles of the identified proteins. A weighted adjacency matrix was constructed using the power function. After choosing the appropriate beta parameter of power (with the value of independence scale set to 0.8), the adjacency matrix was transformed into a topological overlap matrix (TOM), which measures the network connectivity of all the proteins. To classify proteins with co-expression profiles into protein modules, hierarchical clustering analysis was conducted according to the TOM dissimilarity with a minimum size of

30 proteins per module. To identify the relationship between each module and clinical trait, we used module eigengenes (MEs) and calculated the correlation between MEs and each clinical trait and their statistical significance corrected for multiple interactions. A heat map was then used to visualize the degree and significance of each relationship.

A non-parametric Mann–Whitney U-test, machine learning methods, such as non-linear support vector machine (SVM) learning, and partial least squares discriminant analysis (PLS-DA) were used to identify the hub proteins of modules that maximize the discrimination between the selected clinical traits. For the Mann–Whitney U-test, proteins were considered to be significantly differentially expressed between the two conditions with power of 80% and an adjusted p-value ≤ 0.05 after correction for multiple interactions (Benjamini–Hochberg) and a fold change of ≥ 2. In addition, the proteins needed to show at least 70% identity in the samples in one of two conditions. Volcano plots were used to visualize this analysis. In SVM learning, a fourfold cross-validation approach was applied to estimate the prediction and classification accuracy. The whole matrix was also randomly divided into two parts, one for learning (65%) and the other to verify the accuracy of the prediction (35%). Finally, the resulting core panel of hub proteins was uploaded to Cytoscape using the EnrichmentMap, ClusterMaker2, and AutoAnnotate apps to construct a protein–protein interaction network and identify the principal biological processes and pathways involved in each condition. Gene Ontology (GO) annotations were extracted from the Gene Ontology Consortium (http://www.geneontology.org/).

For ELISA data analysis, the Mann–Whitney U-test was used to assess differences in MASP2, FCN1, or C4BPB protein levels between the two study groups, and the results were expressed as medians and interquartile ranges. A value of $p < 0.05$ was considered to be statistically significant. Received operating characteristic (ROC) curves were generated to assess the diagnostic efficiency of each assay. Youden's index and likelihood ratio were used, to identify the cutoff and the diagnostic performance of the tests, respectively. All statistical tests were performed using the latest version of the software package R available at the time of the experiments.

Supplementary Materials: Supplementary materials can be found at http://www.mdpi.com/1422-0067/20/21/5517/s1. Figure S1. Characterization of exosome and microvesicle fractions purified from the urine samples of ICN and MSK patients. Figure S2. Venn diagram of all proteins identified in exosomes and microvesicles isolated from the urine of ICN and MSK patients, and proteins associated with ICN and MSK. Figure S3. Multidimensional scaling analysis of extracellular vesicles from the urine of ICN and MSK patients. Figure S4. Exosome and microvesicle proteins that show significant differences in abundance between ICN and MSK patients. Figure S5. Enrichment network map of the significant proteins found in urinary microvesicles and exosomes from MSK and ICN patients. Table S1. List of identification values for all significant proteins between MSK and ICN in exosome and microvesicle fraction. Table S2. List of all significant proteins between MSK and ICN in exosome and microvesicle fraction.

Author Contributions: Conceptualization: S.G. and G.Z.; data curation: M.B., S.G., and G.Z.; formal analysis: M.B., G.M.G., G.G., and G.Z.; methodology: M.B., S.G., G.C., A.F., and A.P.; supervision: G.Z.; validation: M.B. and G.C.; writing—original draft preparation: M.B., S.G., and G.Z.; writing—review and editing: G.M.G. and G.G.

Acknowledgments: This study was performed (in part) in the LURM (Laboratorio Universitario di Ricerca Medica) Research Center, University of Verona.

Conflicts of Interest: The authors have no conflict of interest to declare.

Abbreviations

MSK	medullary sponge kidney
ICN	idiopathic calcium nephrolithiasis
LAMA2	laminin subunit α2
SVM	support vector machine
PLS-DA	partial least squares discriminant analysis
ADPKD	autosomal dominant polycystic kidney disease
MS	mass spectrometry

SPP1	osteopontin
PBS	phosphate-buffered saline
DLS	dynamic light scattering
iST	in-StageTip
SDB-RPS	poly (styrene divinylbenzene) reversed-phase sulfonate
TFA	trifluoroacetic acid
BSA	bovine serum albumin
PBST	PBS plus 0.1% Tween-20
HRP	horseradish peroxidase
ROC	Received operating characteristic
AUC	area under the curve
CI	confidence interval
FCN1	Ficolin 1
MASP2	Mannan-binding lectin serine protease 2
C4BPB	Complement component 4-binding protein β
PTX3	pentraxin 3
CRP	C-reactive protein

References

1. Fabris, A.; Anglani, F.; Lupo, A.; Gambaro, G. Medullary sponge kidney: State of the art. *Nephrol. Dial. Transplant.* **2013**, *28*, 1111–1119. [CrossRef] [PubMed]
2. Indridason, O.S.; Thomas, L.; Berkoben, M. Medullary sponge kidney associated with congenital hemihypertrophy. *J. Am. Soc. Nephrol.* **1996**, *7*, 1123–1130. [PubMed]
3. El-Sawi, M.; Shahein, A.R. Medullary sponge kidney presenting in a neonate with distal renal tubular acidosis and failure to thrive: A case report. *J. Med. Case Rep.* **2009**, *3*, 6656. [CrossRef] [PubMed]
4. Patriquin, H.B.; O'Regan, S. Medullary sponge kidney in childhood. *AJR Am. J. Roentgenol.* **1985**, *145*, 315–319. [CrossRef] [PubMed]
5. Lambrianides, A.L.; John, D.R. Medullary sponge disease in horseshoe kidney. *Urology* **1987**, *29*, 426–427. [CrossRef]
6. Gambaro, G.; Fabris, A.; Citron, L.; Tosetto, E.; Anglani, F.; Bellan, F.; Conte, M.; Bonfante, L.; Lupo, A.; D'Angelo, A. An unusual association of contralateral congenital small kidney reduced renal function and hyperparathyroidism in sponge kidney patients: On the track of the molecular basis. *Nephrol. Dial. Transplant.* **2005**, *20*, 1042–1047. [CrossRef] [PubMed]
7. Janjua, M.U.; Long, X.D.; Mo, Z.H.; Dong, C.S.; Jin, P. Association of medullary sponge kidney and hyperparathyroidism with RET G691S/S904S polymorphism: A case report. *J. Med. Case Rep.* **2018**, *12*, 197. [CrossRef]
8. Ria, P.; Fabris, A.; Dalla Gassa, A.; Zaza, G.; Lupo, A.; Gambaro, G. New non-renal congenital disorders associated with medullary sponge kidney (MSK) support the pathogenic role of GDNF and point to the diagnosis of MSK in recurrent stone formers. *Urolithiasis* **2017**, *45*, 359–362. [CrossRef]
9. Osther, P.J.; Hansen, A.B.; Røhl, H.F. Renal acidification defects in medullary sponge kidney. *Br. J. Urol.* **1988**, *61*, 392–394. [CrossRef]
10. Fabris, A.; Bernich, P.; Abaterusso, C.; Marchionna, N.; Canciani, C.; Nouvenne, A.; Zamboni, M.; Lupo, A.; Gambaro, G. Bone disease in medullary sponge kidney and effect of potassium citrate treatment. *Clin. J. Am. Soc. Nephrol.* **2009**, *4*, 1974–1979. [CrossRef]
11. McPhail, E.F.; Gettman, M.T.; Patterson, D.E.; Rangel, L.J.; Krambeck, A.E. Nephrolithiasis in medullary sponge kidney: Evaluation of clinical and metabolic features. *Urology* **2012**, *79*, 277–281. [CrossRef] [PubMed]
12. Fabris, A.; Bruschi, M.; Santucci, L.; Candiano, G.; Granata, S.; Dalla Gassa, A.; Antonucci, N.; Petretto, A.; Ghiggeri, G.M.; Gambaro, G.; et al. Proteomic-based research strategy identified laminin subunit alpha 2 as a potential urinary-specific biomarker for the medullary sponge kidney disease. *Kidney Int.* **2017**, *91*, 459–468. [CrossRef] [PubMed]
13. Colognato, H.; Yurchenco, P.D. Form and function: The laminin family of heterotrimers. *Dev. Dyn.* **2000**, *218*, 213–234. [CrossRef]

14. Vijayakumar, S.; Dang, S.; Marinkovich, M.P.; Lazarova, Z.; Yoder, B.; Torres, V.E.; Wallace, D.P. Aberrant expression of laminin-332 promotes cell proliferation and cyst growth in ARPKD. *Am. J. Physiol. Renal. Physiol.* **2014**, *306*, F640–F654. [CrossRef] [PubMed]
15. Joly, D.; Berissi, S.; Bertrand, A.; Strehl, L.; Patey, N.; Knebelmann, B. Laminin 5 regulates polycystic kidney cell proliferation and cyst formation. *J. Biol. Chem.* **2006**, *281*, 29181–29189. [CrossRef]
16. Shannon, M.B.; Patton, B.L.; Harvey, S.J.; Miner, J.H. A hypomorphic mutation in the mouse laminin alpha5 gene causes polycystic kidney disease. *J. Am. Soc. Nephrol.* **2006**, *17*, 1913–1922. [CrossRef]
17. Weir, M.L.; Oppizzi, M.L.; Henry, M.D.; Onishi, A.; Campbell, K.P.; Bissell, M.J.; Muschler, J.L. Dystroglycan loss disrupts polarity and beta-casein induction in mammary epithelial cells by perturbing laminin anchoring. *J. Cell Sci.* **2006**, *119 (Pt 19)*, 4047–4058. [CrossRef]
18. Bruschi, M.; Granata, S.; Santucci, L.; Candiano, G.; Fabris, A.; Antonucci, N.; Petretto, A.; Bartolucci, M.; Del Zotto, G.; Antonini, F.; et al. Proteomic Analysis of Urinary Microvesicles and Exosomes in Medullary Sponge Kidney Disease and Autosomal Dominant Polycystic Kidney Disease. *Clin. J. Am. Soc. Nephrol.* **2019**, *14*, 834–843. [CrossRef]
19. Kleinman, J.G.; Wesson, J.A.; Hughes, J. Osteopontin and calcium stone formation. *Nephron Physiol.* **2004**, *98*, 43–47. [CrossRef]
20. Verhulst, A.; Persy, V.P.; Van Rompay, A.R.; Verstrepen, W.A.; Helbert, M.F.; De Broe, M.E. Osteopontin synthesis and localization along the human Nephron. *J. Am. Soc. Nephrol.* **2002**, *13*, 1210–1218.
21. Worcester, E.M.; Beshensky, A.M. Osteopontin inhibits nucleation of calcium oxalate crystals. *Ann. N. Y. Acad. Sci.* **1995**, *760*, 375–387. [CrossRef] [PubMed]
22. Wesson, J.A.; Worcester, E. Formation of hydrated calcium oxalates in the presence of poly-L-aspartic acid. *Scan. Microsc.* **1996**, *10*, 415–424.
23. Cowley, B.D., Jr.; Ricardo, S.D.; Nagao, S.; Diamond, J.R. Increased renal expression of monocyte chemoattractant protein-1 and osteopontin in ADPKD in rats. *Kidney Int.* **2001**, *60*, 2087–2096. [CrossRef] [PubMed]
24. Gauer, S.; Urbschat, A.; Gretz, N.; Hoffmann, S.C.; Kränzlin, B.; Geiger, H.; Obermüller, N. Kidney Injury Molecule-1 Is Specifically Expressed in Cystically-Transformed Proximal Tubules of the PKD/Mhm (cy/+) Rat Model of Polycystic Kidney Disease. *Int. J. Mol. Sci.* **2016**, *17*, 802. [CrossRef] [PubMed]
25. Pisitkun, T.; Shen, R.F.; Knepper, M.A. Identification and proteomic profiling of exosomes in human urine. *Proc. Natl. Acad. Sci. USA* **2004**, *101*, 13368–13373. [CrossRef]
26. Moon, P.G.; You, S.; Lee, J.E.; Hwang, D.; Baek, M.C. Urinary exosomes and proteomics. *Mass Spectrom. Rev.* **2011**, *30*, 1185–1202. [CrossRef]
27. Piñero, J.; Bravo, À.; Queralt-Rosinach, N.; Gutiérrez-Sacristán, A.; Deu-Pons, J.; Centeno, E.; García-García, J.; Sanz, F.; Furlong, L.I. DisGeNET: A comprehensive platform integrating information on human disease-associated genes and variants. *Nucleic Acids Res.* **2017**, *45*, D833–D839. [CrossRef]
28. Salih, M.; Demmers, J.A.; Bezstarosti, K.; Leonhard, W.N.; Losekoot, M.; van Kooten, C.; Gansevoort, R.T.; Peters, D.J.; Zietse, R.; Hoorn, E.J.; et al. Proteomics of Urinary Vesicles Links Plakins and Complement to Polycystic Kidney Disease. *J. Am. Soc. Nephrol.* **2016**, *27*, 3079–3092. [CrossRef]
29. Runza, V.L.; Schwaeble, W.; Männel, D.N. Ficolins: Novel pattern recognition molecules of the innate immune response. *Immunobiology* **2008**, *213*, 297–306. [CrossRef]
30. Kjaer, T.R.; Hansen, A.G.; Sørensen, U.B.; Nielsen, O.; Thiel, S.; Jensenius, J.C. Investigations on the pattern recognition molecule M-ficolin: Quantitative aspects of bacterial binding and leukocyte association. *J. Leukoc. Biol.* **2011**, *90*, 425–437. [CrossRef]
31. Thiel, S. Complement activating soluble pattern recognition molecules with collagen-like regions, mannan-binding lectin, ficolins and associated proteins. *Mol. Immunol.* **2007**, *44*, 3875–3888. [CrossRef] [PubMed]
32. Zhang, J.; Yang, L.; Ang, Z.; Yoong, S.L.; Tran, T.T.; Anand, G.S.; Tan, N.S.; Ho, B.; Ding, J.L. Secreted M-ficolin anchors onto monocyte transmembrane G protein-coupled receptor 43 and cross talks with plasma C-reactive protein to mediate immune signaling and regulate host defense. *J. Immunol.* **2010**, *185*, 6899–6910. [CrossRef] [PubMed]
33. Tanio, M.; Wakamatsu, K.; Kohno, T. Binding site of C-reactive protein on M-ficolin. *Mol. Immunol.* **2009**, *47*, 215–221. [CrossRef] [PubMed]

34. Gout, E.; Moriscot, C.; Doni, A.; Dumestre-Pérard, C.; Lacroix, M.; Pérard, J.; Schoehn, G.; Mantovani, A.; Arlaud, G.J.; Thielens, N.M. M-ficolin interacts with the long pentraxin PTX3: A novel case of cross-talk between soluble pattern-recognition molecules. *J. Immunol.* **2011**, *186*, 5815–5822. [CrossRef]
35. Zhou, J.; Ouyang, X.; Schoeb, T.R.; Bolisetty, S.; Cui, X.; Mrug, S.; Yoder, B.K.; Johnson, M.R.; Szalai, A.J.; Mrug, M. Kidney injury accelerates cystogenesis via pathways modulated by heme oxygenase and complement. *J. Am. Soc. Nephrol.* **2012**, *23*, 1161–1171. [CrossRef] [PubMed]
36. Su, Z.; Wang, X.; Gao, X.; Liu, Y.; Pan, C.; Hu, H.; Beyer, R.P.; Shi, M.; Zhou, J.; Zhang, J.; et al. Excessive activation of the alternative complement pathway in autosomal dominant polycystic kidney disease. *J. Intern. Med.* **2014**, *276*, 470–485. [CrossRef]
37. Lai, X.; Bacallao, R.L.; Blazer-Yost, B.L.; Hong, D.; Mason, S.B.; Witzmann, F.A. Characterization of the renal cyst fluid proteome in autosomal dominant polycystic kidney disease (ADPKD) patients. *Proteom. Clin. Appl.* **2008**, *2*, 1140–1152. [CrossRef]
38. Bakun, M.; Niemczyk, M.; Domanski, D.; Jazwiec, R.; Perzanowska, A.; Niemczyk, S.; Kistowski, M.; Fabijanska, A.; Borowiec, A.; Paczek, L.; et al. Urine proteome of autosomal dominant polycystic kidney disease patients. *Clin. Proteom.* **2012**, *9*, 13. [CrossRef]
39. Rawal, N.; Rajagopalan, R.; Salvi, V.P. Stringent regulation of complement lectin pathway C3/C5 convertase by C4b-binding protein (C4BP). *Mol. Immunol.* **2009**, *46*, 2902–2910. [CrossRef]
40. Salvadori, M.; Rosso, G.; Bertoni, E. Complement involvement in kidney diseases: From physiopathology to therapeutical targeting. *World J. Nephrol.* **2015**, *4*, 169–184. [CrossRef]
41. Nolan, J.P.; Duggan, E. Analysis of Individual Extracellular Vesicles by Flow Cytometry. *Methods Mol. Biol.* **2018**, *1678*, 79–92. [PubMed]

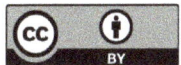

© 2019 by the authors. Licensee MDPI, Basel, Switzerland. This article is an open access article distributed under the terms and conditions of the Creative Commons Attribution (CC BY) license (http://creativecommons.org/licenses/by/4.0/).

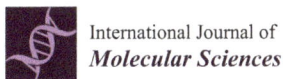

Article

Genetic Analyses in Dent Disease and Characterization of *CLCN5* Mutations in Kidney Biopsies

Lisa Gianesello [1,†], Monica Ceol [1,†], Loris Bertoldi [2,†], Liliana Terrin [1], Giovanna Priante [1], Luisa Murer [3], Licia Peruzzi [4], Mario Giordano [5], Fabio Paglialonga [6], Vincenzo Cantaluppi [7], Claudio Musetti [7], Giorgio Valle [2], Dorella Del Prete [1], Franca Anglani [1,2,*] and Dent Disease Italian Network [‡]

[1] Laboratory of Histomorphology and Molecular Biology of the Kidney, Clinical Nephrology, Department of Medicine—DIMED, University of Padua, 35128 Padua, Italy; lisa.gianesello@unipd.it (L.G.); monica.ceol@unipd.it (M.C.); liliana.terrin@gmail.com (L.T.); giovanna.priante@unipd.it (G.P.); dorella.delprete@unipd.it (D.D.P.)
[2] CRIBI Biotechnology Centre, University of Padua, 35131 Padua, Italy; loris.bertoldi@phd.unipd.it (L.B.); giorgio.valle@unipd.it (G.V.)
[3] Pediatric Nephrology, Dialysis and Transplant Unit, Department of Women's and Children's Health, Padua University Hospital, 35128 Padua, Italy; luisa.murer@aopd.veneto.it
[4] Pediatric Nephrology Unit, Regina Margherita Children's Hospital, 10126 CDSS Turin, Italy; licia.peruzzi@unito.it
[5] Pediatric Nephrology Unit, University Hospital, P.O. Giovanni XXIII, 70126 Bari, Italy; mario.giordano@policlinico.ba.it
[6] Pediatric Nephrology, Dialysis and Transplant Unit, Fondazione IRCCS, Ca' Granda Ospedale Maggiore Policlinico, 20122 Milan, Italy; fabio.paglialonga@policlinico.mi.it
[7] Nephrology and Kidney Transplantation Unit, Department of Translational Medicine, University of Piemonte Orientale (UPO), 28100 Novara, Italy; vincenzo.cantaluppi@med.uniupo.it (V.C.); claudio.musetti@med.uniupo.it (C.M.)
* Correspondence: franca.anglani@unipd.it; Tel.: +39-049-8212-155
† These authors contributed equally to this work.
‡ Membership of the Dent Disease Italian Network is provided in the Acknowledgments.

Received: 4 December 2019; Accepted: 10 January 2020; Published: 14 January 2020

Abstract: Dent disease (DD), an X-linked renal tubulopathy, is mainly caused by loss-of-function mutations in *CLCN5* (DD1) and *OCRL* genes. *CLCN5* encodes the ClC-5 antiporter that in proximal tubules (PT) participates in the receptor-mediated endocytosis of low molecular weight proteins. Few studies have analyzed the PT expression of ClC-5 and of megalin and cubilin receptors in DD1 kidney biopsies. About 25% of DD cases lack mutations in either *CLCN5* or *OCRL* genes (DD3), and no other disease genes have been discovered so far. Sanger sequencing was used for *CLCN5* gene analysis in 158 unrelated males clinically suspected of having DD. The tubular expression of ClC-5, megalin, and cubilin was assessed by immunolabeling in 10 DD1 kidney biopsies. Whole exome sequencing (WES) was performed in eight DD3 patients. Twenty-three novel *CLCN5* mutations were identified. ClC-5, megalin, and cubilin were significantly lower in DD1 than in control biopsies. The tubular expression of ClC-5 when detected was irrespective of the type of mutation. In four DD3 patients, WES revealed 12 potentially pathogenic variants in three novel genes (*SLC17A1*, *SLC9A3*, and *PDZK1*), and in three genes known to be associated with monogenic forms of renal proximal tubulopathies (*SLC3A*, *LRP2*, and *CUBN*). The supposed third Dent disease-causing gene was not discovered.

Keywords: dent disease; *CLCN5* gene mutations; proximal tubular ClC-5 expression; megalin; cubilin; kidney biopsies; immunohistochemistry; whole exome sequencing

1. Introduction

The term Dent disease (DD) identifies a group of X-linked renal disorders characterized by features of incomplete Fanconi syndrome including low-molecular-weight proteinuria (LMWP), and more or less severe hypercalciuria, nephrocalcinosis and/or nephrolithiasis. This triad of symptoms has been variously named in the past as X-linked recessive nephrolithiasis with renal failure (OMIM 310468), X-linked recessive hypophosphatemic rickets (OMIM 300554), or the idiopathic LMWP of Japanese children (OMIM 308990), testifying to the disease's phenotypic variability [1,2]. DD usually presents in children or young adults, progressing to chronic kidney disease (CKD) between the third and fifth decades of life in 30–80% of cases [3,4].

The most common genetic cause of DD is a mutated *CLCN5* gene encoding the ClC-5 chloride channel Cl-/H+ antiporter (DD1; MIM#300009) [5–9]. In the kidney, ClC-5 is expressed primarily in the proximal tubular cells (PTCs) located mainly in the subapical endosomes. Together with megalin and cubilin synergistic receptors, it is involved in the endocytic reabsorption of albumin and LMW proteins [10,11]. ClC-5 expression levels are lower in the α intercalated cells of the cortical collecting duct and in the cortical and medullary thick ascending limb of Henle's loop [12].

DD1 features a marked allelic heterogeneity, with more than 200 *CLCN5* mutations described so far [9]. Functional investigations in Xenopus Levis oocytes and mammalian cells enabled these *CLCN5* mutations to be classified. The most common mutations lead to a defective protein folding and processing, resulting in endoplasmic reticulum (ER) retention of the mutant protein for further degradation by the proteasome [13–17]. Few studies have investigated ClC-5 expression in DD1 kidney biopsies.

OCRL gene mutations, which are usually associated with Lowe syndrome (OMIM #309000), have been identified in about 10–15% of DD patients (DD2; MIM#300555). Approximately 25% of DD patients (DD3) have neither *CLCN5* nor *OCRL* gene mutations [18–21].

This study aimed to investigate allelic and locus heterogeneity in DD and to analyze ClC-5, megalin, and cubilin expression in DD1 kidney biopsies. We further expanded the spectrum of *CLCN5* mutations in DD by describing 23 novel mutations. In DD1 kidney biopsies, we showed that the loss of ClC-5 tubular expression caused defective megalin and cubilin trafficking. In DD3, whole exome sequencing (WES) did not detect a new disease-causing gene. Instead, it revealed the concomitant presence of likely pathogenic variants in genes encoding proximal tubular (PT) endocytic apparatus components, suggesting that they may have had a role in determining the DD3 phenotype.

2. Results

2.1. CLCN5 Gene Mutation Analysis

The 85% of the 158 patients analyzed for the presence of *CLCN5* mutations were of Italian origin, 6% were non-Italian European (Balcanic and English), and the remaining 9% were extra-European (Figure 1).

DNA sequence analysis of the *CLCN5* gene revealed 50 different mutations in 56 unrelated patients. Six different mutations were found twice. Among the detected mutations, the most common types were missense mutations (21 cases), followed by frameshift mutations (14 cases), nonsense mutations (13 cases), and splicing mutations (eight cases) (Figure 2).

Twenty-three mutations were not previously described, which were judged potentially pathogenic by in silico tools and classified as pathogenic or likely pathogenic according to American College of Medical Genetics and American College of Pathologists (ACMG/AMP) guidelines [22] (Table 1). The novel frameshift, nonsense, and missense mutations were mapped onto ClC-5 protein domains (Table 1). Table S1 summarizes the clinical details of 20 patients with novel *CLCN5* mutations (clinical data were unavailable for three). LMWP and hypercalciuria were the most common signs at the time of their molecular diagnosis, and their clinical phenotypic variability reflected that of patients with known *CLCN5* mutations [9].

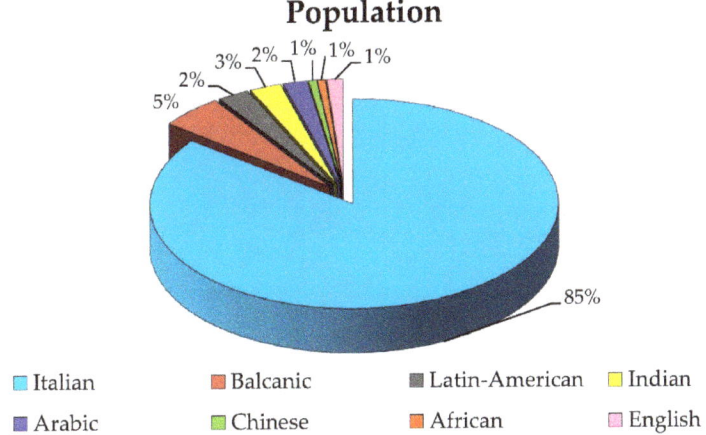

Figure 1. Ethnical distribution of the 158 analyzed patients.

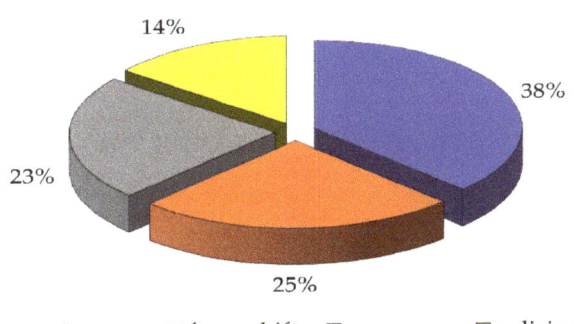

Figure 2. Percentages of mutations of *CLCN5* gene by type.

Table 1. Novel mutations in the *CLCN5* gene.

Type of Mutation	Nucleotide	Exon-Intron	Protein	Pathogenicity Assessment	Protein Domain
Frameshift	c.100_101insG	Exon 2	p.(Glu35fs)	Pathogenic (Ib)	A helix, stop in Loop A-B
Frameshift	c.125delA	Exon 3	p.(Glu42fs)	Pathogenic (Ib)	Loop A-B
Frameshift	c.266_267insT	Exon 4	p.(Ile89fs)	Pathogenic (Ib)	B helix, stop in Loop B-C
Frameshift	c.518delT	Exon 6	p.(Ile173fs)	Pathogenic (Ib)	D helix, stop in Loop D-E
Frameshift [§]	c.691delA	Exon 6	p.(Lys231fs)	Pathogenic (Ia)	Loop F-G, stop at the end of helix G
Frameshift	c.1164_1165insAG	Exon 8	p.(Lys388fs)	Pathogenic (Ib)	L helix, stop in helix M
Frameshift	c.1635_1638delCAAG	Exon 10	p.(Ser545fs)	Pathogenic (Ib)	Q helix, stop in cytoplasmic
Frameshift	c.1657delG	Exon 10	p.(Arg554fs)	Pathogenic (Ib)	Cytoplasmic, stop at the beginning of CBS1 cytoplasmic domain
Frameshift	c.1920delC	Exon 10	p.(Ile641fs)	Pathogenic (Ib)	CBS1 cytoplasmic domain, stop in cytoplasmic
Nonsense	c.1287G>A	Exon 8	p.(Trp429*)	Pathogenic (Ib)	M helix

Table 1. Cont.

Type of Mutation	Nucleotide	Exon-Intron	Protein	Pathogenicity Assessment	Protein Domain
Nonsense	c.2016C>G	Exon 11	p.(Tyr672*)	Pathogenic (Ib)	Cytoplasmic
Nonsense	c.2128C>T	Exon 11	p.(Gln710*)	Pathogenic (Ib)	Cytoplasmic-beta strand in CBS2 domain
Missense	c.262G>A	Exon 4	p.(Gly88Ser)	Likely pathogenic (IV)	B helix
Missense	c.305G>T	Exon 4	p.(Cys102Phe)	Likely pathogenic (V)	Loop B-C
Missense	c.518T>A	Exon 6	p.(Ile173Lys)	Likely pathogenic (V)	D helix
Missense §	c.608C>G	Exon 6	p.(Ser203Trp)	Pathogenic (II)	E helix
Missense	c.809G>A	Exon 8	p.(Ser270Asn)	Likely pathogenic (IV)	Loop H-I
Missense §	c.922G>A	Exon 8	p.(Val308Met)	Pathogenic (IIIb)	Loop I-J
Missense	c.1565T>A	Exon 10	p.(Val522Asp)	Likely pathogenic (V)	P helix
Missense	c.1619C>T	Exon 10	p.(Ala540Val)	Likely pathogenic (IV)	Q helix
Missense	c.2192A>C	Exon 12	p.(His731Pro)	Likely pathogenic (V)	Cytoplasmic-CBS2 domain
Splicing	c.105+5G>C	Intron 2-splice site	p.?	Likely pathogenic (II)	
Splicing	c.1348-1G>A	Intron 8-splice site	p.?	Pathogenic (Ic)	

§ CLCN5 mutations also analyzed in patients' kidney biopsies.

2.2. ClC-5, Megalin, and Cubilin Immunolabeling in DD1 Kidney Biopsies

Renal tubular ClC-5 expression was analyzed by immunohistochemistry (IHC) in 10 patients carrying *CLCN5* stop codon (frameshift and nonsense mutations) or missense mutations (Table 2). In control biopsies, ClC-5 immunostaining was mainly apical and subapical (Figure 3). Our antibody has around 66% overall epitope sequence similarity to ClC-3 and ClC-4, which are both expressed in the membranes of intracellular organelles [23], so cross-reactivity can be expected. Immunolabeling for ClC-3, ClC-4, and ClC-5 in serial sections of a control sample showed that tubular apical staining was almost exclusively attributable to ClC-5 expression, while cytoplasmic staining was due largely to ClC-3 and ClC-5, and much less to ClC-4 (Figure S1).

In DD1 biopsies, ClC-5 apical immunolabeling was negligible in most tubules, whatever the type of mutation (Figure 3). As expected, ClC-5 expression was very significantly downregulated (Figure 4) in DD1 biopsies compared with control biopsies (median CTRL 8.69% [Interquartile range (IQR) 1.94–15.97%], DD1 0.01% [IQR 0.00–0.12%]; $p < 0.01$).

Table 2 shows the morphometric findings on ClC-5 immunostaining for each mutation. Notably, two patients (Pt3 and Pt4) carried the same very premature nonsense mutation p.(Arg34*), but with a completely different pattern of expression: ClC-5 immunolabeling was completely absent in one, while in the other, it stained 0.12% of the whole biopsy area, which was more than in any of the other biopsies analyzed (Figure 3).

Analyzing megalin and cubilin immunofluorescence (IF) in the same patients (Figure 5) revealed that both receptors were significantly downregulated by comparison with control biopsies (median megalin: CTRL 4.52% [IQR 3.64–8.39%], DD1 1.67% [IQR 0.09–3.91%], $p = 0.019$; median cubilin: CTRL 10.87% [IQR 1.54–19.85%], DD1 1.01% [IQR 0.83–2.67%], $p = 0.003$) (Figure 4).

Table 2. Morphometric evaluation of tubular ClC-5 immunolabeling in 10 DD1 patients' kidney biopsies.

Patient	CLCN5 Mutation	Age at Biopsy (Years)	Indication for Biopsy	Histopathological Findings	ClC-5 Immunolabeling Morphometric Evaluation (% Positive Area)
1	p.(Thr44fs)	2	Proteinuria	Minimal changes	0.01
2	p.(Lys231fs) (novel)	14	Proteinuria	Normal	0.00
3	p.(Arg34*)	11	Nephrotic syndrome	Chronic interstitial nephritis with global glomerulosclerosis	0.12
4	p.(Arg34*)	6	Proteinuria	Global glomerulosclerosis and IgM nephropathy	0.00
5	p.(Gln600*)	6	Proteinuria	Tubulointerstitial injury with focal glomerulosclerosis	0.05
6	p.(Ser203Trp) (novel)	3	Proteinuria	Normal	0.01
7	p.(Ser261Arg)	4	Heavy proteinuria	Proliferative mesangial glomerulonephritis	0.07
8	p.(Tyr272Cys)	NA	Proteinuria	Normal	0.01
9	p.(Val308Met) (novel)	9	Proteinuria and hematuria	Normal	0.08
10	p.(Trp547Arg)	1	Proteinuria	Normal	0.00

NA: not available.

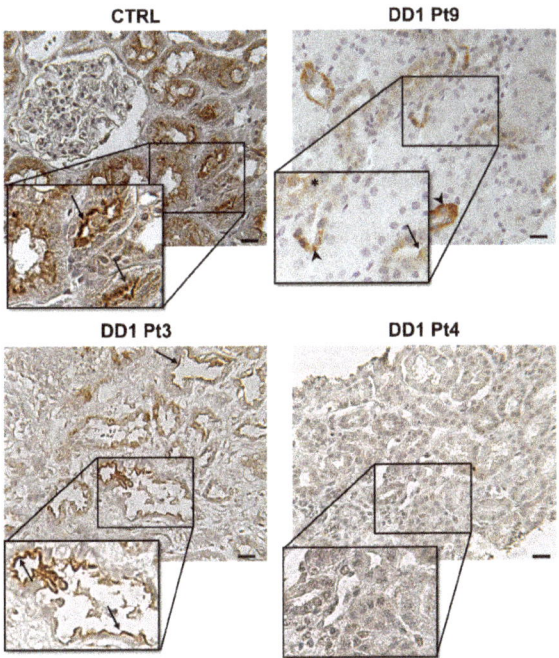

Figure 3. ClC-5 immunolabeling in control and DD1 kidneys. Representative images disclosing ClC-5 positivity in control and DD1 kidneys. In CTRL, ClC-5 staining was located mainly in tubular apical and subapical positions. In DD1 patients, some tubules presented basolateral or cytoplasmic ClC-5 positivity (Pt9), and very few showed apical staining (Pt9, Pt3). ClC-5 immunostaining was negligible in most DD1 tubules (Pt4), whatever the type of mutation. The asterisk indicates a cytoplasmic signal, arrows indicate apical and subapical signals, the arrowhead indicates a basolateral signal. Scale bar = 50 µm. CTRL= control, Pt = patient.

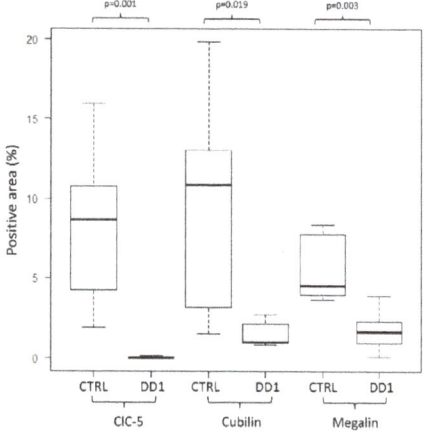

Figure 4. ClC-5, cubilin, and megalin quantitative analysis. Morphometric analysis showed a significant decrease in the percentage of positive area in kidneys of DD1 patients than in control kidneys for all molecules examined. Data were analyzed using the Mann–Whitney U-test. CTRL = control.

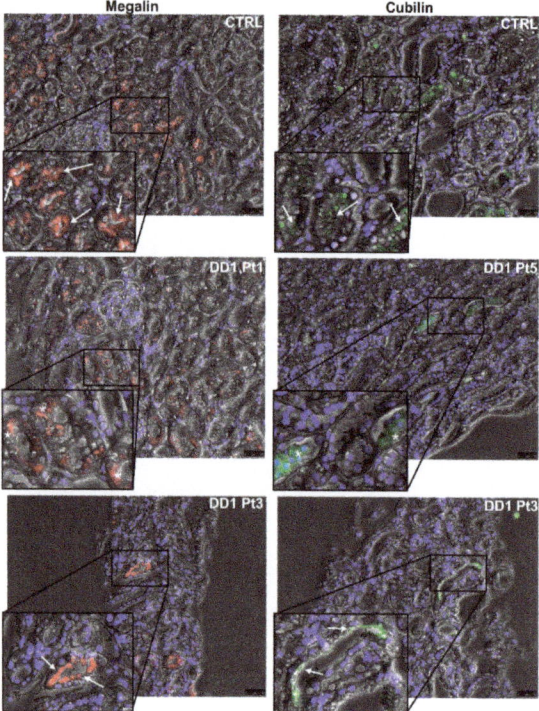

Figure 5. Megalin and cubilin immunolabeling in control and DD1 kidneys. Representative images disclosing megalin and cubilin positivity in control and DD1 kidneys. In CTRL, megalin (red) and cubilin (green) staining was located mainly in tubular apical and subapical positions. Immunolabeling for both receptors was rarely apical in DD1 patients (Pt3), while it was more frequently found in the cytoplasm (Pt1 and Pt5). The asterisk indicates a cytoplasmic signal, arrows indicate apical and subapical signals. Blue indicates counter-staining of nuclei with 4′,6-diamidino-2-phenylindole (DAPI). Scale bar = 50 µm. CTRL = control, Pt = patient.

2.3. Whole Exome Sequencing (WES) Study

Among *CLCN5* negative patients, 34 underwent mutational screening of the *OCRL* gene, and 19 patients were found to not carry mutations. In eight out of 19 *CLCN5* and *OCRL*-negative patients (four children and four adults), we performed WES.

We first searched for mutations in phenocopy genes. Known monogenic forms of nephrolithiasis and nephrocalcinosis as well as of proximal and distal tubulopathy, for a total of 62 genes including known genes of the PT endocytic pathway (Table S2), were firstly evaluated in these patients. Furthermore, the first 100 genes prioritized for their association with *CLCN5* or *OCRL* genes using the Scalable kernel-based gene prioritization (SCUBA) were investigated [24] (Table S3).

Unexpectedly, in two children, we detected *CLCN5* or *OCRL* known disease-causing mutations, p.(Lys231fs) and p.(Arg318Cys), respectively. If on one hand this finding was disturbing because it meant that by previous Sanger sequencing we had missed two causative mutations in the two known genes, on the other hand, it confirmed that our pool of DD3 cases was well representative of DD patients based on disease phenotype.

In four patients (three adults and one child), we detected 12 variants in three genes known to be associated either with monogenic forms of proximal renal tubulopathy (*SLC3A1*) or with monogenic syndromes involving proximal tubule dysfunction (*LRP2*, *CUBN*), as well as in novel genes not related to monogenic nephropathies (*SLC17A1*, *SLC9A3*, and *PDZK1*). These last genes could be candidates for DD-like phenotypes for their function in PT, and detected variants were predicted to be pathogenic or likely pathogenic by in silico tools (although with a different degree of concordance), except for one in the *SLC17A1* gene (Table 3). Table S4 summarizes the four patients' clinical phenotypes.

In two adults patients (AMS and BDA), we detected biallelic likely pathogenic variants in *SLC3A1* and *LRP2* genes whose mutations are responsible for the recessive diseases Cystinuria (MIM#220100) and Donnai–Barrow/Facio-oculo-acoustico-renal syndrome (DB/FOAR, MIM#222448), respectively.

In AMS, we also identified a very rare missense variant classified as a variant of uncertain significance (VUS) in the *SLC17A1* gene encoding sodium/phosphate cotransporter 1 (NPT1), which occurs at the apical pole of PTCs [25] and participates in renal urate export [26,27]. The same patient was found to be homozygous for the very rare nonsense variant p.(Arg8*) in the *PDKZ1* gene. This gene encodes the Na(+)/H(+) exchange regulatory cofactor NHE-RF3, which is a PDZ domain-containing scaffolding protein and one of the key molecules of the urate transportsome [28,29].

The already known pathogenic *LRP2* mutation p.(Asp2054Asn) [30] was detected in AMV. In this patient, we also found an in-frame indel variant of the *CUBN* gene encoding for cubilin. *CUBN* gene mutations are known to cause Imerslund–Gräsbeck syndrome (IGS, MIM#261100), which is an autosomal recessive disorder involving selective intestinal vitamin B12 malabsorption and LMWP. The p.(Val2347del) variant in *CUBN* is very rare (TOPmed 0.0000001); Mutation Taster (MT) and PROVEAN predicted its pathogenicity, and it was classified as VUS according to ACMG/AMP guidelines [22].

Among eight different *LRP2* uncommon coding variants with a minor allele frequency (MAF) < 0.05 detected in our DD3 patients, four were identified in one patient (AMT) of which two were predicted to be pathogenic by in silico tools (Table 3). Similar to AMV, this patient carried an uncommon *CUBN* missense variant that was considered pathogenic by MT, PROVEAN, and DANN, but classified as benign according to ACMG/AMP guidelines. He also harbored a very rare variant in the *SLC9A3* gene, which was predicted as pathogenic by in silico tools, and classified as VUS. The *SLC9A3* gene encodes sodium/hydrogen exchanger 3 (NHE3), which is the main apical Na+/H+ exchanger in adult kidneys [31], and part of the macromolecular endocytic complex at the brush border of PTCs [32,33].

Table 3. Candidate variants for DD3 phenotypes detected by whole-exome sequencing (WES).

Pt ID	Transcript Level Variation	Codon Substitution	Frequency ExAC (European)	Mutation Taster	PROVEAN	DANN	ClinVar	ACMG/AMP Variant Interpretation
SLC17A1 (NM_005074.3)								
AMS	c.1309G>A	p.(Ala437Thr)	rs1189357572 0.000003 (GnomAD) (0.000008)	Polymorphism (1.000)	Neutral (−1.97)	0.967	NA	VUS
PDZK1 (NM_002614.4)								
AMS	c.22C>T	p.(Arg8*) homozygous	rs191362962 0.0001157 (0.0001799)	Disease causing automatic	NA	0.998	NA	VUS
LRP2 (NM_004525.2)								
BDA	c.6727C>T	p.(Arg2243*)	novel	Disease causing automatic (1.000)	NA	0.996	NA	Pathogenic (Ib)
BDA	c.242T>A	p.(Ile81Asn)	novel	Disease causing (1.000)	Damaging (−4.62)	0.993	NA	Likely pathogenic (V)
AMV	c.6160G>A	p.(Asp2054Asn)	rs138269726 0.0011 (0.0017)	Disease causing (1.000)	Neutral (−1.85)	0.999	Pathogenic allele	Likely pathogenic (II)
AMT	c.2006G>A	p.(Gly669Asp)	rs34291900 0.0285 (0.0434)	Disease causing (1.000)	Damaging (−5.44)	0.998	Likely benign allele	Likely benign
AMT	c.7894A>G	p.(Asn2632Asp)	rs17848169 0.02951 (0.0426)	Disease causing (1.000)	Neutral (−1.73)	0.452	Likely benign allele	Likely benign
SLC3A1 (NM_000341.4)								
AMS	c.680G>A	p.(Arg227Gln)	rs142469446 0.0002 (0.0002)	Disease causing (1.000)	Neutral (−1.63)	1	NA	Likely pathogenic (IV)
AMS	c.797T>C	p.(Phe266Ser)	rs141587158 0.003 (0.004)	Disease causing (1.000)	Damaging (−4.7)	0.998	NA	Likely pathogenic (IIIb)
CUBN (NM_001081.3)								
AMT	c.10265C>T	p.(Thr3422Ile)	rs1801230 0.01832 (0.02829)	Disease causing (1.000)	Damaging (−2.94)	0.985	Likely benign allele	Benign
AMV	c.7040_7042del	p.(Val2347del)	rs1279549461 (TOPmed) 0.0000001	Disease causing (0.998)	Deleterious (−9.81)	NA	NA	VUS
SLC9A3 (NM_004174.3)								
AMT	c.848G>A	p.(Arg283His)	rs146899318 0.00033 (0.00036)	Disease causing (0.853)	Damaging (−3.85)	0.999	NA	VUS

Pt: patient, ACMG/AMP: American College of Medical Genetics and American College of Pathologists, NA: not available, VUS: Variant of uncertain significance.

3. Discussion

Dent disease 1 is a worldwide disease, and this is further confirmed by our cohort of patients which included persons from all over the word. More than 220 *CLCN5* pathogenic mutations have been reported so far. Mutations were found scattered along all exons of the gene and in different protein domains [9,34–45]. Mansour-Hendili et al. [9] reported that the majority were missense and frameshift mutations (33.33% and 29.05% respectively) followed by nonsense mutations (17.52%), splicing mutations (12.39%), and large deletions (4.70%). In our cohort of patients, missense and frameshift mutations were also the most frequent, but with a lower proportion (38% and 25% respectively), while we observed more nonsense mutations compared to the previously reported data (23%).

In our study, DNA sequence analysis of the *CLCN5* gene revealed 50 different mutations, 23 of which have never been described before. ACMG/AMP guidelines classify the nine missense novel mutations in *CLCN5* as likely pathogenic. They were mapped onto ClC-5 protein domains (Table 1).

The p.(Ile173Lys) missense mutation is in the D helix, which is one of the four helixes (D, F, N, and R) brought together near the channel center to form the Cl-selectivity filter [46] and consequently believed to alter ClC-5 conductance.

The p.(His731Pro) missense mutation affects the ClC-5 carboxy-terminus cytoplasmic domain. All eukaryotic ClCs have a large cytoplasmic C-terminus containing a pair of cystathionine beta-synthase (CBS) domains. Several authors have shown that CBS domains are involved in regulating the activity of ClCs, including ClC-5 [47–49]. Mutations affecting the two CBS domains were reported correctly targeted to the plasma membrane and early endosomes, but with altered ClC-5 electrical activity [14]. The nonsense mutation p.(Arg718*) truncating the ClC-5 protein near the C-terminus reportedly results in ER retention, underscoring the importance of the C-terminus in passing protein quality control in ER [50]. These findings suggest that truncated ClC-5 proteins at the C-terminus could cause function loss through defective protein processing. However, three different truncated mutations at the C-terminus—p.(Tyr617*), p.(Arg648*), and p.(Arg704*)—targeted the cell surface (albeit only one with residual activity) [50], so we cannot say whether our stop codon mutations at the C-terminus of ClC-5 protein (Table 1) could exhibit residual activity targeting the plasma membrane.

The p.(Ser203Trp) missense mutation affects the E helix, whose role in ClC-5 function is still unclear. The nearby p.(Leu200Arg) mutation reportedly produced a loss of Cl- conductance [1], and the p.(Ser203Leu) was found to cause current failures due to ER retention [50]. Taken together, these findings indicate that the p.(Ser203Trp) mutation is probably pathogenic.

Six missense mutations map in the major helixes (B, H, I, O, P, and Q) involved in dimer interface formation [9,46], or in the intervening loops, suggesting an impaired physical contact between the two subunits that might disrupt proper pore configuration [50,51]. In addition, for the p.(Ala540Val), a pathogenic missense in the same position in a Dent family from New Zealand has already been reported [38], confirming the possible damaging role of the alteration of this residue. The p.(Ser270Asn) missense mutation maps in the loop between helixes H and I, near the "proton glutamate" (Glu 268), which is crucial to the Cl-/H+ transport function [9]. Since the p.(Ser270Arg) mutation was reportedly associated with chloride current abolition [52], we hypothesize a similar effect of this new mutation.

Very few studies investigated ClC-5 expression in kidney biopsies [10,53]. We analyzed ClC-5 protein expression in kidney biopsies from 10 patients carrying three novel and seven known *CLCN5* mutations and in eight control biopsies. In controls, ClC-5 immunolabeling was mainly apical and subapical in tubular cells, and it was not co-localized with ClC-3 or ClC-4 staining. The few studies on ClC-5 expression in human kidney reported similar staining findings [10,53], which are justified by the well-accepted ClC-5 localization in early and recycling endosomes and the plasma membrane [54,55].

Our study is the first to demonstrate the loss of ClC-5 protein expression in DD1 kidneys. However, an apical staining was detected in very few tubules in 7/10 DD1 biopsies, including those with the novel p.(Val308Met) and p.(Ser203Trp) mutations. Therefore, we speculate that the expression of these ClC-5 mutants is regulated post-translationally, and mutated proteins can very rarely reach the plasma membrane. This is consistent with previous findings in ClC-5 mutant models. Both missense and nonsense ClC-5 mutants could be either targeted to early endosomes or plasma membrane, but with a limited activity, or confined to the ER [50]. In fact, some DD1 tubules were only labeled at the basolateral pole (probably a sign of ER retention) (Figure 3 Pt 9).

Apical staining was unexpectedly detected for the very premature truncated ClC-5 protein at codon 34. Premature stop codons (PSCs) account for one in two *CLCN5* mutations, and cause three distinct molecular alterations: (1) the production of a truncated, usually non-functional, protein; (2) degradation of the transcripts containing PSCs via the nonsense-mediated decay (NMD) pathway; and (3) exon skipping due to alternative cryptic acceptor or donor sites being used in the exon encompassing the stop codon [56]. The first molecular change can be excluded, because our ClC-5 antibody recognized an epitope at the C-terminus of the protein. The second and third might apply because (1) NMD may occasionally be bypassed when translational read-through allows the decoding of stop codons as sense codons, thus enabling protein translation; (2) PSCs can also prompt exon skipping by altering exonic splicing enhancer (ESE) or exonic splicing silencer (ESS) motifs. PSCs have even been found to be statistically inclined to induce exon skipping more than other exon mutations [57]. If this is true of the p.(Arg34*) mutation, we can expect exon skipping to be in frame, thus enabling complete protein synthesis and allowing the mutated protein to be detected by immunolabeling. However, such explanations for this ClC-5 mutant protein's presence in one biopsy should be considered with caution, as the ClC-5 protein was not found in most tubules, nor in another biopsy carrying the same mutation. This could mean that how PSCs are processed by cell transcriptional and translational apparatus might depend on the context (meaning the cell environment and/or the genomic context).

As in *Clcn5* knock-out (KO) animal models [58], ClC-5 loss in human kidney causes defective cubilin and megalin recycling, leading to LMWP. All the ClC-5 mutants studied here triggered both their defective expression at the brush border of PTCs and their downregulation. The presence of a megalin signal at the apical border of some tubules in the biopsy carrying the p.(Arg34*) mutation (Figure 5, Pt3) suggests a residual ClC-5 activity enabling a normal endocytic process and consequent megalin recycling.

Few studies have examined megalin and cubilin expression in DD1. Urinary megalin excretion was found to be significantly lower in DD1 patients than in normal individuals [59]. IHC on kidney biopsies from two patients carrying different *CLCN5* mutations revealed a defective megalin, cubilin, and Dab2 expression in PTCs [60,61]. Studies on megalin recycling in conditionally immortalized proximal tubular epithelial cell lines from three patients with *CLCN5* mutations showed defects in cell surface expression and internalization [62]. Our data definitively corroborate previous findings and suggest that a reduced intracellular megalin and cubilin synthesis may also contribute to their defective apical exposure.

Approximately one in four DD patients have no *CLCN5* or *OCRL* gene mutations. Whether mutations in a third, as yet unknown gene can cause DD3 remains to be seen, but—judging from our WES study on six DD3 patients—this seems unlikely. Instead, as we previously suggested [63], WES data point to DD3 patients having atypical phenotypes of known hereditary nephropathies or blended phenotypes. In fact, we identified in two patients (AMS and BDA) biallelic likely pathogenic variants in two genes (*SLC3A1*, *LRP2*) whose mutations are known to cause cystinuria and DB/FOAR. Our findings suggest that probably these patients were misdiagnosed as DD because of the presence renal Fanconi syndrome. Indeed, several disorders are caused by mutations of genes coding for components of the endolysosomal system in the PT. Besides *CLCN5* (DD1) and *OCRL* (Lowe syndrome and Dent disease type 2) genes, they include *LRP2* (DB/FOAR), *CUBN*, *AMN* (Imerslund–Gräsbeck syndrome), and *CTNS* (nephropathic cystinosis). Typically, these recessive disorders cause proximal tubular dysfunction and lead to inappropriate urinary loss of LMW proteins and solutes (e.g., phosphate, glucose, amino acids, urate), and they often lead to renal failure. The clinical entity of generalized proximal tubular dysfunction is referred to as renal Fanconi syndrome.

However, apart from BDA who was found to carry biallelic pathogenic variants in the *LRP2* gene and, for this reason, and after a careful clinical revaluation, was assessed to suffer from an atypical form of DB/FOAR syndrome [64], the other patient (AMS) did not suffer from cystinuria, despite carrying biallelic variants in the *SLC3A1* gene that were classified as likely pathogenic according to ACMG/AMP variant interpretation. Indeed, in this patient, the urinary level of cysteine was found to be normal even after repeated measurements. Two hypotheses may explain these findings: (1) the variants may be hypomorphic, thereby allowing a limited gene product activity, and (2) the two variants are in the same allele (complex allele), although their MAF was highly different, suggesting the absence of a linkage disequilibrium.

Instead, what appears relevant from this study is finding in three patients (comprising AMS) possible pathogenic variants in more than one gene connected in functional networks (*PDZK1*, *SLC17A1*, *CUBN*, *SLC3A9*, and *LRP2*), which we considered important for explaining patients' phenotypes, thus suggesting digenic or oligogenic disorders.

The major finding of WES study is the discovery in AMS of a homozygous truncating mutation in the *PDZK1* gene. This is a new gene that has never been related before to human diseases, although it is one of the loci of strongest effect on serum urate level and gut [65–67]. NHE-RF3 encoded by *PDZK1* is a major scaffolder protein in the brush border of kidney PTCs [68], interacting through its PDZ domain with key molecules of urate transport, including NPT1 [29]. Furthermore, NHE-RF3 is one of the several proteins interacting with the type-2a sodium phosphate cotransporter (NaPi-2a), which is the major inorganic phosphate cotransporter of the PTCs [69]. Targeted disruption of the *Pdzk1* gene by homologous recombination in mice induced modulation of the expression of selective ion channels in the kidney, including NaPi-2a. The steady-state levels of NaPi-2a were found to be reduced under a phosphorus (Pi)-rich diet, and this was paralleled by higher urinary total and fractional Pi excretion [69]. In these KO mice, serum urate was not measured, nor were urate transporters investigated. However, urine and serum analysis did not reveal any significant difference between KO and wild-type mice except for a significant increase in the cholesterol levels [69]. Interestingly, in *Pdzk1* KO mice under a high-Pi diet, the PDZ scaffolding protein NHE-RF1 was increased at the bush border of proximal tubules. NHE-RF1 was demonstrated to localize with megalin in the brush border, because it bounds to its internal C-terminal PDZ binding motif [70]. It was also showed that NHE-RF1 silencing in PTCs increased megalin expression [70].

In the same patient, we also detected a very rare missense variant in the *SLC17A1* gene, which is classified as VUS due to its extreme rarity in the human population (data from gnomAD: 1 allele out of 250846). The *SLC17A1* gene is one of the loci associated with serum urate level and gout [71] and encodes NPT1, which is a Cl-dependent urate transport interacting with NHE-RF3 encoded by the *PDZK1* gene [26]. The clinical phenotype of patient AMS involves multiple tubular defects (particularly hyperphosphaturia, hypercalciuria, and severe hypouricemia), which might be consistent with a partial renal Fanconi syndrome and had led to a clinical suspicion of renal hypouricemia (MIM#220150 and 612076) and atypical DD. By WES, we excluded the presence of pathogenic variants in both *SLC22A12* and *SLC2A9* genes encoding URAT1 and GLUT9, respectively. It is tempting to speculate that the *PDZK1* and the *SLC17A1* gene variants might have had a role in determining AMS clinical phenotype for their direct interaction with urate and phosphate transport. Family studies will help clarify these aspects.

Since megalin and cubilin PTC expression is altered in DD1, it is conceivable that *LRP2* and/or *CUBN* mutations can cause or contribute to a DD-like nephropathy. WES results seem to support this hypothesis. In addition to BDA, who has already been described as carrying biallelic mutations in the *LRP2* gene [64], AMV was also found to carry a known pathogenic *LRP2* allele and a very rare inframe deletion in the *CUBN* gene. *CUBN* variants have recently been associated with proteinuria with no signs of IGS. It was shown that a homozygous frameshift mutation in exon 53 of *CUBN* (p.Ser2785fs) only caused proteinuria [72]. Moreover, a missense variant in exon 57 (p.Ile2984Val) was associated with albuminuria [73]. Mutations in the *CUBN* gene cause IGS apparently only when they affect the cubilin–amnionless interaction domain (exons 1–20) or the IF-Cbl binding site (exons 21–29) [74]. In our patient, *CUBN* mutation is localized in exon 46. Follow-up showed that our patient's LMWP was intermittent while his proteinuria started at 1 year old and ranged between 0.4 and 1 g/24 h.

True digenic inheritance (DI) is the simplest form for oligogenic disease [75], but it is also encountered when pathogenic mutations responsible for two different diseases are co-inherited, leading to a blended phenotype [76]. The two heterozygous mutations in the *LRP2* and *CUBN* genes, encoding proteins working close together on the same endocytic pathway, might plausibly be responsible for patient AMV's disease phenotype. Further studies on his kidney biopsy and/or urinary proteoma might confirm this hypothesis. Family studies may help to solve these questions.

We detected two *LRP2* coding variants associated with two likely pathogenic missense variants in the *CUBN* and *SLC9A3* genes in the genome of a single patient (AMT). It is noteworthy that these genes respectively encode megalin, cubilin, and NHE3, which are located—together with ClC-5, amnionless, and Dab2—at the cell surface of PTCs, forming its endocytic apparatus [54,55].

SLC9A3 homozygous or compound heterozygous disease-causing mutations have recently been reported in nine patients from eight families with congenital secretory sodium diarrhea (MIM#616868) [77]. No association has been found as yet between *SLC9A3* variants and renal proximal tubulopathies, but a defective Nhe3 exposure was found in *Clcn5* KO mice [55,78]. Studies by Gekle et al. [33] support a crucial role for NHE3 in proximal tubular receptor-mediated endocytosis by demonstrating in Nhe3 KO mice that Nhe3 deficiency led to a reduced protein reabsorption: the urinary protein patterns resembled those of mice deficient in megalin or ClC-5. Recent evidence also highlights the importance of NHE3 for calcium reabsorption. Nhe3 KO mice revealed significant urinary calcium wasting and a low cortical bone mineral density and trabecular bone mass [79].

The genetic data of the AMT patient are puzzling and raise some questions. With the advent of high-throughput sequencing, we are bound to discover more patients suffering from oligogenic diseases and learn more about how complex interactions between allelic and locus heterogeneity affect disease phenotypes [80]. The presence of multiple coding variants in the same gene, either in cis or in trans, may also conceivably cause defective protein functioning, although this needs to be demonstrated in animal and in vitro models [81]. The genotype–phenotype correlation in the AMT patient is worth investigating, because it seems to reveal such an impact on disease phenotype. This patient was 26 years old when referred to a nephrologist for kidney stones. His height (158 cm) and weight (42 kg) were below the third percentile. His renal phenotype mainly featured proximal tubulopathy manifesting as Fanconi syndrome with LMWP, hypercalciuria, hyperphosphaturia, glycosuria, natriuresis, and hypercitraturia. Therefore, the patient's presenting phenotype was mainly related to an impaired renal calcium and phosphate metabolism. WES detected no relevant variants in genes known to be responsible for monogenic forms of nephrolithiasis and renal tubulopathies. We hypothesized that the AMT patient's phenotype was due to the variants in *LRP2*, *CUBN*, and *SLC9A3*, whose products work on the same cellular pathways as ClC-5, or pathways related thereto, but this hypothesis needs to be evaluated by in vitro studies. From the point of view of the referring clinicians, tubular abnormalities might be a real challenge: indeed, clinical characteristics of different diseases sometimes overlap, and a full-blown classical phenotype (in the case of AMS, a renal Fanconi syndrome) is rare. Therefore, when multiple tubular defects (i.e., alteration in tubular handling of 2–4 different solutes) coexist, the chance of a blended phenotype becomes more plausible, and a next-generation sequencing (NGS) approach might be a good strategy to identify multiple (and possibly interacting) genetic defects that may explain each individual phenotype.

4. Material and Methods

4.1. Patients

4.1.1. DNA Samples

From 2006 to 2018, DNA samples were collected from 158 unrelated pediatric and adult males with clinically suspected DD according to the criteria described in our previous study [82]. Patients should have encountered at least two of the above-mentioned criteria for being referred to our laboratory for a molecular diagnosis. Since proteinuria was recently reported as one of the DD symptoms in concomitance with signs of incomplete Fanconi tubulopathy [83], and because of the cost of urinary assessment of LMW proteins, we decided to include in the diagnostic workflow also patients presenting with proteinuria, although in the absence of documented LMWP. Informed consent to the genetic study was obtained from all probands or their parents.

DNA samples from eight patients (four children and four adults) with no detectable *CLCN5* or *OCRL* gene mutations underwent WES. The selection was based on the presence of a likely DD phenotype (i.e., the presence of LMWP and/or proteinuria, hypercalciuria, and at least one of the following: nephrocalcinosis, kidney stones, hypophosphataemia, renal failure, aminoaciduria, rickets, or a positive family history) with or without extra-renal symptoms. The study was approved by Padua University Hospital's Ethical Committee, protocol 0028285 (11 May 2016)

4.1.2. Biopsies

Ten kidney biopsies were collected from patients carrying nine different *CLCN5* mutations (Table 2). All biopsies were performed for diagnostic purposes and available for immunolabeling studies subject to informed consent.

Eight control cortical tissues were obtained from nephrectomies for renal cancer (sites remote from the tumor-bearing renal tissue), disclosing a normal morphology and no immunofluorescence. The study was approved by Padua University Hospital's Ethical Committee, protocol 0007452 (1 February 2018).

4.2. Sanger Sequencing

CLCN5 gene mutation analysis was performed by Sanger sequencing. Genomic DNA was extracted from peripheral blood using the QIAamp DNA Blood Minikit (Qiagen, Milan, Italy) according to the manufacturer's instructions. The primers and PCR conditions for amplifying the *CLCN5* gene-coding region and intron–exon boundaries are described elsewhere [82]. The PCR products were analyzed using the Bioanalyzer 2100 (Agilent Technologies, Milan, Italy) and purified with the MinElute PCR Purification Kit (Qiagen, Milan, Italy). Sanger sequencing was done with the BigDye Terminator v1.1 Cycle Sequencing Kit (ThermoFisher Scientific, Milan, Italy) and the ABI-PRISM 3100 Genetic Analyzer (ThermoFisher Scientific, Milan, Italy). The nomenclature of mutations is based on the *CLCN5* cDNA sequence NM_0000844. Missense and splicing mutations were interpreted using the Mutation Taster (MT) [84], and classified according to the American College of Medical Genetics and American College of Pathologists (ACMG/AMP) variant classification guidelines [22]. Mutations were confirmed by sequencing a second independent PCR product.

4.3. Whole-Exome Sequencing (WES)

WES was performed at Padua University's Centro di Ricerca Interdipartimentale per le Biotecnologie Innovative (CRIBI) sequencing center using the Ion Proton System (ThermoFisher Scientific, Milan, Italy), obtaining an average reads coverage of 80X for each sample. Data were analyzed as suggested by the manufacturer, with read alignment using TMAP and variant calling with TSVC, which are both included in the Ion Proton Suite (v 5.0). QueryOR (http://queryor.cribi.unipd.it, accessed on 27 November 2019) [85] was used to analyze and prioritize short-nucleotide variants (SNV). This web-based query platform enables quick, easy, in-depth variant prioritization by aggregating several functional annotations of both genes and variants. The prioritization strategy entails a ranking that sorts results by the number and weight of the criteria met (see below).

Two main approaches were initially used to identify the most promising variants: (1) a gene-centered search, considering known details of genes and associated pathways, and information about the disease and related disorders; and (2) a variant-centered search, focusing on the intrinsic characteristics of variants, such as type (indel, snp, mnp), codon effect (frameshift, missense, and nonsense variants), and genomic position.

In a subsequent prioritization step, variants were ranked by sequencing coverage, minor allele frequency (MAF) values ≤ 0.05, and predicted possible–probable deleteriousness. For this purpose, QueryOR provides coding variant predictions based on several tools, including the well-known SIFT, PolyPhen2, and MT, and the more recent PROVEAN, CADD, and DANN scores [84,86–90]. Sanger sequencing was used to validate variants identified by the in silico prioritization strategy during WES. Table S5 shows the gene names, NCBI reference sequences, primers, and PCR amplification conditions.

Identified variants were checked against relevant database such as Clinvar (https://www.ncbi.nlm.nih.gov/clinvar/, accessed on 27 November 2019) and The Human Gene Mutation Database (HGMD) (http://www.hgmd.cf.ac.uk/ac/index.php, accessed on 27 November 2019), and were classified according to ACMG/AMP guidelines [22].

4.4. Immunohistochemistry (IHC)

IHC was conducted on formalin-fixed, paraffin-embedded sections using an indirect immunoperoxidase method. Specimens were treated as previously described [91], and incubated overnight with rabbit anti-human ClC-5 (Sigma-Aldrich, Milan, Italy, cat. HPA000401) diluted 1:200, goat anti-human ClC-3 (Santa Cruz Biotechnologies, Heidelberg, Germany, cat. sc-17572) diluted 1:150, and rabbit anti-human ClC-4 (Sigma-Aldrich, Milan, Italy, cat. HPA063637) diluted 1:50 in PBS at 4 °C in a humidified chamber. A donkey anti-goat IgG-HRP secondary antibody (Santa Cruz Biotechnologies, Heidelberg, Germany, cat. sc-2020) diluted 1:100 was used for ClC-3. Immunolabeling specificity was confirmed by incubating without any primary antibody. Images were acquired with the Diaplan light microscope (Leitz, Como, Italy) and 20X/0.45 objective using a Micropublisher 5.0 RTV camera (Teledyne QImaging, Surrey, BC, Canada).

4.5. Immunofluorescence (IF)

IF analyses were performed on serial sections of kidney biopsies. Samples were treated as previously described [92] and incubated overnight with primary antibody (sheep anti-human cubilin [R&D Systems, Minneapolis, MN, USA, cat. AF3700], rabbit anti-human megalin [LS-Bio, Seattle, WA, USA, cat. LS-B105]) diluted 1:100 in PBS 5% BSA at 4 °C. Sections were incubated with the appropriate fluorescent secondary antibody [92]. Nuclei were counterstained with 4′,6-diamidino-2-phenylindole (DAPI). Negative controls were run by omitting the primary antibody. Images were acquired with a DMI6000CS-TCS SP8 fluorescence microscope (Leica Microsystems, Milan, Italy) with a 20X/0.4 objective using a DFC365FX camera (Leica Microsystems, Milan, Italy) and analyzed with the LAS-AF software (Leica Microsystems, Milan, Italy).

4.6. Morphometric Analysis

ClC-5, megalin, and cubilin signals on kidney biopsies were quantified by morphometric analysis using Image-Pro Plus 7.0 (Media Cybernetics, Abingdon, United Kingdom). Signals were acquired at 200X with the same time exposure, gain, and intensity for all patients, and quantified excluding the glomerular compartment. For ClC-5, only apical or subapical tubular staining was considered as positive. Quantities were expressed as the mean area covered by pixels (%).

4.7. Statistical Analysis

Non-parametric tests (Mann–Whitney U-test) were used due to the small sample size. Results with $p < 0.05$ were considered significant and given as median ± IQR. All analyses were performed with R software version 3.5.1 (R Foundation for Statistical Computing, Vienna, Austria) [93].

5. Conclusions

By describing 23 novel *CLCN5* mutations, this study extends the allelic heterogeneity of DD1. Our results on DD1 kidney biopsies provide evidence that ClC-5 is lost in PTCs, and this, in turn, leads to a defective trafficking of megalin and cubilin in these cells.

Using WES to investigate DD3 patients, we did not identify the supposed third Dent disease-causing gene. Instead, our study suggests that likely pathogenic variants in genes encoding components of the endocytic apparatus of tubular cells (megalin, cubilin, NHE3, and NHE-RF3) may have determined DD3 phenotypes. However, except for one patient in whom we identified a known monogenic disease, in the other patients, the presence of variants in more than one gene related in functional networks suggest that we are probably facing oligogenic disorders. Furthermore, our study suggests that DD3 patients are a pool of patients with DD-like phenotypes, which may present atypical phenotypes of known hereditary nephropathies or blended phenotypes.

Supplementary Materials: Supplementary materials can be found at http://www.mdpi.com/1422-0067/21/2/516/s1. Figure S1: ClC-5, ClC-4 and ClC-3 immunolabeling in serial sections of a control kidney. Tubular staining was almost exclusively apical (arrows) for ClC-5, while cytoplasmic staining (arrowheads) was seen for ClC-3, and ClC-5 and much less for ClC-4. Scale bar = 50 µm. Table S1: Clinical phenotypes of 20 patients carrying novel CLCN5 mutations. Table S2: List of phenocopy genes. Table S3: List of the genes prioritized according to scalable kernel-based gene prioritization (SCUBA) [24]. Table S4: DD-like phenotype of patients carrying likely pathogenic variants as detected by whole exome sequencing. Table S5: PCR primer sequences and amplification conditions.

Author Contributions: Study conception, design of experiments, and critical review of the results: F.A., G.V., M.C., L.B.; WES experiments: L.B.; WES data analyses: F.A., L.B., and L.T.; Sanger experiments: L.G., L.T., and M.C.; IHC experiments: M.C. and G.P.; IF experiments: L.G. and G.P.; Statistical analysis: L.G.; Morphometric analysis: M.C. and D.D.P.; Drafting of the paper: F.A., L.B., L.G., and M.C.; Supervision of clinical cases and clinical data collection: D.D.P., V.C. and C.M.; Histopathological data reporting on kidney biopsies: L.M., M.G., L.P., F.P., and F.A. F.A. conceived the paper's structure, supervised its writing, and thoroughly reviewed all content. All authors have read and agreed to the published version of the manuscript.

Funding: This work was supported by the University of Padua, Strategic Project BIOINFOGEN prot. STPD11F33L, and by the Rare Kidney Stone Consortium (U54DK83908), which is part of the Rare Diseases Clinical Research Network (RDCRN), an initiative of the Office of Rare Diseases Research (ORDR), NCATS, as Grant number PAD-182824 awarded to L.G. This consortium is funded through collaboration between NCATS, and the National Institute of Diabetes and Digestive and Kidney Diseases.

Acknowledgments: This work was performed with the contribution of the Italian Network of Dent Disease researchers: Gian Marco Ghiggeri and Giancarlo Barbano (Division of Nephrology, Dialysis and Kidney Transplantation, G. Gaslini Pediatric Institute, Genova), Francesco Emma and Gianluca Vergine (Division of Nephrology and Dialysis, Bambin Gesù Pediatric Hospital, Rome), Giuseppe Vezzoli (Division of Nephrology, Dialysis and Hypertension, IRCCS San Raffaele Hospital, Milan), Marilena Cara (Nephrology Division, Camposampiero General Hospital, Camposampiero) Gabriele Ripanti (Pediatrics and Neonatology Division, San Salvatore Hospital, Pesaro), Anita Ammenti (Pediatric Institute, University of Parma), Licia Peruzzi (Division of Nephrology, Dialysis and Transplantation, Regina Margherita Hospital, Turin), Giacomo Colussi (Nephrology Unit, Varese Hospital, Varese), Mario Giordano (Nephrology and Pediatric Dialysis, Pediatric Hospital, Bari) Maria Rosa Caruso (Nephrology Unit, Bergamo Hospital, Bergamo), Ilse Maria Ratsch (Pediatric Institute, University of Ancona), Giuseppina Marra and Fabio Paglialonga (Nephrology Unit, IRCCS Foundation, Ca' Granda Ospedale Maggiore Policlinico, University of Milan), Angela La Manna (Department of Pediatrics, 2nd University of Napoli), Caterina Canavese (Nephrology and Kidney Transplantation Unit, Department of Translational Medicine, University of Piemonte Orientale (UPO), Novara), Diego Bellino (Division of Nephrology, Dialysis and Kidney Transplantation, San Martino University Hospital, Genova), Luisa Murer (Pediatric Nephrology, Dialysis and Transplant Unit, Department of Women's and Children's Health, Padua University Hospital), Milena Brugnara (Pediatric Division, Department of Life and Reproduction Sciences, University of Verona), Andrea Pasini and Claudio La Scola (Nephrology and Dialysis Unit, Department of Pediatrics, Azienda Ospedaliero Universitaria Sant'Orsola-Malpighi, Bologna).

Conflicts of Interest: The authors declare no conflict of interest.

References

1. Lloyd, S.E.; Pearce, S.H.; Fisher, S.E.; Steinmeyer, K.; Schwappach, B.; Scheinman, S.J.; Harding, B.; Bolino, A.; Devoto, M.; Goodyer, P.; et al. A common molecular basis for three inherited kidney stone diseases. *Nature* **1996**, *379*, 445–449. [CrossRef] [PubMed]
2. Thakker, R.V. Pathogenesis of Dent's disease and related syndromes of X-linked nephrolithiasis. *Kidney Int.* **2000**, *57*, 787–793. [CrossRef] [PubMed]
3. Wrong, O.M.; Norden, A.G.; Feest, T.G. Dent's disease; a familial proximal renal tubular syndrome with low-molecular-weight proteinuria, hypercalciuria, nephrocalcinosis, metabolic bone disease, progressive renal failure and a marked male predominance. *Q. J. Med.* **1994**, *87*, 473–493.
4. Reinhart, S.C.; Norden, A.G.; Lapsley, M.; Thakker, R.V.; Pang, J.; Moses, A.M.; Frymoyer, P.A.; Favus, M.J.; Hoepner, J.A.; Scheinman, S.J. Characterization of carrier females and affected males with X-linked recessive nephrolithiasis. *J. Am. Soc. Nephrol.* **1995**, *5*, 1451–1461. [CrossRef] [PubMed]
5. Lloyd, S.E.; Gunther, W.; Pearce, S.H.; Thomson, A.; Bianchi, M.L.; Bosio, M.; Craig, I.W.; Fisher, S.E.; Scheinman, S.J.; Wrong, O.; et al. Characterization of renal chloride channel, CLCN5, mutations in hypercalciuric nephrolithiasis (kidney stones) disorders. *Hum. Mol. Genet.* **1997**, *6*, 1233–1239. [CrossRef] [PubMed]
6. Jentsch, T.J.; Günther, W.; Pusch, M.; Schwappach, B. Properties of voltage-gated chloride channels of the ClC gene family. *J. Physiol.* **1995**, *482*, 19S–25S. [CrossRef]
7. Thakker, R.V. Chloride channels cough up. *Nat. Genet.* **1997**, *17*, 125. [CrossRef]
8. Picollo, A.; Pusch, M. Chloride/proton antiporter activity of mammalian CLC proteins ClC-4 and ClC-5. *Nature* **2005**, *436*, 420–423. [CrossRef]
9. Mansour-Hendili, L.; Blanchard, A.; Le Pottier, N.; Roncelin, I.; Lourdel, S.; Treard, C.; González, W.; Vergara-Jaque, A.; Morin, G.; Colin, E.; et al. Mutation update of the CLCN5 gene responsible for Dent disease 1. *Hum. Mutat.* **2015**, *36*, 743–752. [CrossRef]
10. Jouret, F.; Igarashi, T.; Gofflot, F.; Wilson, P.D.; Karet, F.E.; Thakker, R.V.; Devuyst, O. Comparative ontogeny; processing; and segmental distribution of the renal chloride channel; ClC-5. *Kidney Int.* **2004**, *65*, 198–208. [CrossRef]
11. Christensen, E.I.; Devuyst, O.; Dom, G.; Nielsen, R.; Van Der Smissen, P.; Verroust, P.; Leruth, M.; Guggino, W.B.; Courtoy, P.J. Loss of chloride channel ClC-5 impairs endocytosis by defective trafficking of megalin and cubilin in kidney proximal tubules. *Proc. Natl. Acad. Sci. USA* **2003**, *100*, 8472–8477. [CrossRef] [PubMed]
12. Gunther, W.; Luchow, A.; Cluzeaud, F.; Vandewalle, A.; Jentsch, T.J. ClC-5, the chloride channel mutated in Dent's disease; colocalizes with the proton pump in endocytically active kidney cells. *Proc. Natl. Acad. Sci. USA* **1998**, *95*, 8075–8080. [CrossRef] [PubMed]
13. D'Antonio, C.; Molinski, S.; Ahmadi, S.; Huan, L.J.; Wellhauser, L.; Bear, C.E. Conformational defects underlie proteasomal degradation of Dent's disease-causing mutants of ClC-5. *Biochem. J.* **2013**, *452*, 391–400. [CrossRef] [PubMed]
14. Lourdel, S.; Grand, T.; Burgos, J.; González, W.; Sepúlveda, F.V.; Teulon, J. ClC-5 mutations associated with Dent's disease: A major role of the dimer interface. *Pflug. Arch.* **2012**, *463*, 247–256. [CrossRef] [PubMed]
15. Grand, T.; L'Hoste, S.; Mordasini, D.; Defontaine, N.; Keck, M.; Pennaforte, T.; Genete, M.; Laghmani, K.; Teulon, J.; Lourdel, S. Heterogeneity in the processing of CLCN5 mutants related to Dent disease. *Hum. Mutat.* **2011**, *32*, 476–483. [CrossRef] [PubMed]
16. Smith, A.J.; Reed, A.A.; Loh, N.Y.; Thakker, R.V.; Lippiat, J.D. Characterization of Dent's disease mutations of CLC-5 reveals a correlation between functional and cell biological consequences and protein structure. *Am. J. Physiol. Ren. Physiol.* **2009**, *296*, F390–F397. [CrossRef]
17. Ludwig, M.; Doroszewicz, J.; Seyberth, H.W.; Bökenkamp, A.; Balluch, B.; Nuutinen, M.; Utsch, B.; Waldegger, S. Functional evaluation of Dent's disease-causing mutations: Implications for ClC-5 channel trafficking and internalization. *Hum. Genet.* **2005**, *117*, 228–237. [CrossRef]
18. Hoopes, R.R., Jr.; Raja, K.M.; Koich, A.; Hueber, P.; Reid, R.; Knohl, S.J.; Scheinman, S.J. Evidence for genetic heterogeneity in Dent's disease. *Kidney Int.* **2004**, *65*, 1615–1620. [CrossRef]

19. Hoopes, R.R., Jr.; Shrimpton, A.E.; Knohl, S.J.; Hueber, P.; Reed, A.A.; Christie, P.T.; Igarashi, T.; Lee, P.; Lehman, A.; White, C.; et al. Dent disease with mutations in OCRL1. *Am. J. Hum. Genet.* **2005**, *76*, 260–267. [CrossRef]
20. Hichri, H.; Rendu, J.; Monnier, N.; Coutton, C.; Dorseuil, O.; Poussou, R.V.; Baujat, G.; Blanchard, A.; Nobili, F.; Ranchin, B.; et al. From Lowe syndrome to Dent disease: Correlations between mutations of the OCRL1 gene and clinical and biochemical phenotypes. *Hum. Mutat.* **2011**, *32*, 379–388. [CrossRef]
21. Shrimpton, A.E.; Hoopes, R.R., Jr.; Knohl, S.J.; Hueber, P.; Reed, A.A.; Christie, P.T.; Igarashi, T.; Lee, P.; Lehman, A.; White, C.; et al. OCRL1 mutations in Dent 2 patients suggest a mechanism for phenotypic variability. *Nephron Physiol.* **2009**, *112*, 27–36. [CrossRef] [PubMed]
22. Richards, S.; Aziz, N.; Bale, S.; Bick, D.; Das, S.; Gastier-Foster, J.; Grody, W.W.; Hegde, M.; Lyon, E.; Spector, E.; et al. ACMG Laboratory Quality Assurance Committee. Standards and guidelines for the interpretation of sequence variants: A joint consensus recommendation of the American College of Medical Genetics and Genomics and the Association for Molecular Pathology. *Genet. Med.* **2015**, *17*, 405–424. [CrossRef] [PubMed]
23. Jentsch, T.J. Chloride channels are different. *Nature* **2002**, *415*, 276–277. [CrossRef] [PubMed]
24. Zampieri, G.; Tran, D.V.; Donini, M.; Navarin, N.; Aiolli, F.; Sperduti, A.; Valle, G. Scuba: Scalable kernel-based gene prioritization. *BMC Bioinform.* **2018**, *19*, 23. [CrossRef]
25. Merriman, T.R.; Dalbeth, N. The genetic basis of hyperuricaemia and gout. *Jt. Bone Spine* **2011**, *78*, 35–40. [CrossRef]
26. Iharada, M.; Miyaji, T.; Fujimoto, T.; Hiasa, M.; Anzai, N.; Omote, H.; Moriyama, Y. Type 1 sodium-dependent phosphate transporter (SLC17A1 Protein) is a Cl(-)-dependent urate exporter. *J. Biol. Chem.* **2010**, *285*, 26107–26113. [CrossRef] [PubMed]
27. Chiba, T.; Matsuo, H.; Kawamura, Y.; Nagamori, S.; Nishiyama, T.; Wei, L.; Nakayama, A.; Nakamura, T.; Sakiyama, M.; Takada, T.; et al. NPT1/SLC17A1 is a renal urate exporter in humans and its common gain-of-function variant decreases the risk of renal under-excretion gout. *Arthritis Rheumatol.* **2015**, *67*, 281–287. [CrossRef]
28. Higashino, T.; Matsuo, H.; Sakiyama, M.; Nakayama, A.; Nakamura, T.; Takada, T.; Ogata, H.; Kawamura, Y.; Kawaguchi, M.; Naito, M.; et al. Common variant of PDZ domain containing 1 (PDZK1) gene is associated with gout susceptibility: A replication study and meta-analysis in Japanese population. *Drug Metab. Pharm.* **2016**, *31*, 464–466. [CrossRef]
29. Anzai, N.; Kanai, Y.; Endou, H. New insights into renal transport of urate. *Curr. Opin. Rheumatol.* **2007**, *19*, 151–157. [CrossRef]
30. De Ligt, J.; Willemsen, M.H.; van Bon, B.W.; Kleefstra, T.; Yntema, H.G.; Kroes, T.; Vulto-van Silfhout, A.T.; Koolen, D.A.; de Vries, P.; Gilissen, C.; et al. Diagnostic exome sequencing in persons with severe intellectual disability. *N. Engl. J. Med.* **2012**, *367*, 1921–1929. [CrossRef]
31. Alexander, R.T.; Dimke, H.; Cordat, E. Proximal tubular NHEs: Sodium, protons and calcium? *Am. J. Physiol. Ren. Physiol.* **2013**, *305*, F229–F236. [CrossRef] [PubMed]
32. Biemesderfer, D.; Nagy, T.; DeGray, B.; Aronson, P. Specific association of megalin and the Na+/H+ exchanger isoform NHE3 in the proximal tubule. *J. Biol. Chem.* **1999**, *274*, 17518–17524. [CrossRef]
33. Gekle, M.; Völker, K.; Mildenberger, S.; Freudinger, R.; Shull, G.E.; Wiemann, M. NHE3 Na+/H+ exchanger supports proximal tubular protein reabsorption in vivo. *Am. J. Physiol. Ren. Physiol.* **2004**, *287*, F469–F473. [CrossRef] [PubMed]
34. Szczepanska, M.; Zaniew, M.; Recker, F.; Mizerska-Wasiak, M.; Zaluska-Lesniewska, I.; Kilis-Pstrusinska, K.; Adamczyk, P.; Zawadzki, J.; Pawlaczyk, K.; Ludwig, M.; et al. Dent disease in children: Diagnostic and therapeutic considerations. *Clin. Nephrol.* **2015**, *84*, 222–230. [CrossRef] [PubMed]
35. Tang, X.; Brown, M.R.; Cogal, A.G.; Gauvin, D.; Harris, P.C.; Lieske, J.C.; Romero, M.F.; Chang, M.H. Functional and transport analyses of CLCN5 genetic changes identified in Dent disease patients. *Physiol. Rep.* **2016**, *4*, e12776. [CrossRef] [PubMed]
36. Li, F.; Yue, Z.; Xu, T.; Chen, M.; Zhong, L.; Liu, T.; Jing, X.; Deng, J.; Hu, B.; Liu, Y.; et al. Dent Disease in Chinese Children and Findings from Heterozygous Mothers: Phenotypic Heterogeneity, Fetal Growth, and 10 Novel Mutations. *J. Pediatr.* **2016**, *174*, 204–210.e1. [CrossRef]
37. Kubo, K.; Aizawa, T.; Watanabe, S.; Tsugawa, K.; Tsuruga, K.; Ito, E.; Joh, K.; Tanaka, H. Does Dent disease remain an underrecognized cause for young boys with focal glomerulosclerosis? *Pediatr. Int.* **2016**, *58*, 747–749. [CrossRef]

38. Wong, W.; Poke, G.; Stack, M.; Kara, T.; Prestidge, C.; Flintoff, K. Phenotypic variability of Dent disease in a large New Zealand kindred. *Pediatr. Nephrol.* **2017**, *32*, 365–369. [CrossRef]
39. Guven, A.; Al-Rijjal, R.A.; BinEssa, H.A.; Dogan, D.; Kor, Y.; Zou, M.; Kaya, N.; Alenezi, A.F.; Hancili, S.; Tarım, Ö.; et al. Mutational analysis of PHEX, FGF23 and CLCN5 in patients with hypophosphataemic rickets. *Clin. Endocrinol.* **2017**, *87*, 103–112. [CrossRef]
40. Günthner, R.; Wagner, M.; Thurm, T.; Ponsel, S.; Höfele, J.; Lange-Sperandio, B. Identification of co-occurrence in a patient with Dent's disease and ADA2-deficiency by exome sequencing. *Gene* **2018**, *649*, 23–26. [CrossRef]
41. Sancakli, O.; Kulu, B.; Sakallioglu, O. A novel mutation of Dent's disease in an 11-year-old male with nephrolithiasis and nephrocalcinosis. *Arch. Argent. Pediatr.* **2018**, *116*, e442–e444.
42. Bignon, Y.; Alekov, A.; Frachon, N.; Lahuna, O.; Jean-Baptiste Doh-Egueli, C.; Deschênes, G.; Vargas-Poussou, R.; Lourdel, S. A novel CLCN5 pathogenic mutation supports Dent disease with normal endosomal acidification. *Hum. Mutat.* **2018**, *39*, 1139–1149. [CrossRef] [PubMed]
43. Wen, M.; Shen, T.; Wang, Y.; Li, Y.; Shi, X.; Dang, X. Next-Generation Sequencing in Early Diagnosis of Dent Disease 1: Two Case Reports. *Front. Med.* **2018**, *5*, 347. [CrossRef] [PubMed]
44. Matsumoto, A.; Matsui, I.; Mori, T.; Sakaguchi, Y.; Mizui, M.; Ueda, Y.; Takahashi, A.; Doi, Y.; Shimada, K.; Yamaguchi, S.; et al. Severe Osteomalacia with Dent Disease Caused by a Novel Intronic Mutation of the CLCN5 gene. *Intern. Med.* **2018**, *57*, 3603–3610. [CrossRef] [PubMed]
45. Ye, Q.; Shen, Q.; Rao, J.; Zhang, A.; Zheng, B.; Liu, X.; Shen, Y.; Chen, Z.; Wu, Y.; Hou, L.; et al. Multicenter study of the clinical features and mutation gene spectrum of Chinese children with Dent disease. *Clin. Genet.* **2019**. [CrossRef]
46. Wu, F.; Roche, P.; Christie, P.T.; Loh, N.Y.; Reed, A.A.; Esnouf, R.M.; Thakker, R.V. Modeling study of human renal chloride channel (hCLC-5) mutations suggests a structural-functional relationship. *Kidney Int.* **2003**, *63*, 1426–1432. [CrossRef]
47. Meyer, S.; Savaresi, S.; Forster, I.C.; Dutzler, R. Nucleotide recognition by the cytoplasmic domain of the human chloride transporter ClC-5. *Nat. Struct. Mol. Biol.* **2007**, *14*, 60–67. [CrossRef]
48. Wellhauser, L.; Luna-Chavez, C.; D'Antonio, C.; Tainer, J.; Bear, C.E. ATP induces conformational changes in the carboxylterminal region of ClC-5. *J. Biol. Chem.* **2011**, *286*, 6733–6741. [CrossRef]
49. Zifarelli, G.; Pusch, M. Intracellular regulation of human ClC-5 by adenine nucleotides. *EMBO Rep.* **2009**, *10*, 1111–1116. [CrossRef]
50. Grand, T.; Mordasini, D.; L'Hoste, S.; Pennaforte, T.; Genete, M.; Biyeyeme, M.J.; Vargas-Poussou, R.; Blanchard, A.; Teulon, J.; Lourdel, S. Novel CLCN5 mutations in patients with Dent's disease result in altered ion currents or impaired exchanger processing. *Kidney Int.* **2009**, *76*, 999–1005. [CrossRef]
51. Pusch, M.; Ludewig, U.; Jentsch, T.J. Temperature dependence of fast and slow gating relaxations of CLC-0 chloride channels. *J. Gen. Physiol.* **1997**, *109*, 105–116. [CrossRef] [PubMed]
52. Igarashi, T.; Günther, W.; Sekine, T.; Inatomi, J.; Shiraga, H.; Takahashi, S.; Suzuki, J.; Tsuru, N.; Yanagihara, T.; Shimazu, M.; et al. Functional characterization of renal chloride channel, CLCN5, mutations associated with Dent's Japan disease. *Kidney Int.* **1998**, *54*, 1850–1856. [CrossRef] [PubMed]
53. Devuyst, O.; Christie, P.T.; Courtoy, P.J.; Beauwens, R.; Thakker, R.V. Intra-renal and subcellular distribution of the human chloride channel, CLC-5, reveals a pathophysiological basis for Dent's disease. *Hum. Mol. Genet.* **1999**, *8*, 247–257. [CrossRef] [PubMed]
54. Wang, Y.; Cai, H.; Cebotaru, L.; Hryciw, D.H.; Weinman, E.J.; Donowitz, M.; Guggino, S.E.; Guggino, W.B. ClC-5: Role in endocytosis in the proximal tubule. *Am. J. Physiol. Ren. Physiol.* **2005**, *289*, F850–F862. [CrossRef]
55. Hryciw, D.H.; Wang, Y.; Devuyst, O.; Pollock, C.A.; Poronnik, P.; Guggino, W.B. Cofilin interacts with ClC-5 and regulates albumin uptake in proximal tubule cell lines. *J. Biol. Chem.* **2003**, *278*, 40169–40176. [CrossRef]
56. Kellermayer, R. Translational readthrough induction of pathogenic nonsense mutations. *Eur. J. Med. Genet.* **2006**, *49*, 445–450. [CrossRef]
57. Oren, Y.S.; Pranke, I.M.; Kerem, B.; Sermet-Gaudelus, I. The suppression of premature termination codons and the repair of splicing mutations in CFTR. *Curr. Opin. Pharmacol.* **2017**, *34*, 125–131. [CrossRef]
58. Piwon, N.; Günther, W.; Schwake, M.; Bösl, M.R.; Jentsch, T.J. ClC-5 Cl$^-$-channel disruption impairs endocytosis in a mouse model for Dent's disease. *Nature* **2000**, *408*, 369–373. [CrossRef]

59. Norden, A.G.; Lapsley, M.; Igarashi, T.; Kelleher, C.L.; Lee, P.J.; Matsuyama, T.; Scheinman, S.J.; Shiraga, H.; Sundin, D.P.; Thakker, R.V.; et al. Urinary megalin deficiency implicates abnormal tubular endocytic function in Fanconi syndrome. *J. Am. Soc. Nephrol.* **2002**, *13*, 125–133.
60. Tanuma, A.; Sato, H.; Takeda, T.; Hosojima, M.; Obayashi, H.; Hama, H.; Iino, N.; Hosaka, K.; Kaseda, R.; Imai, N.; et al. Functional characterization of a novel missense CLCN5 mutation causing alterations in proximal tubular endocytic machinery in Dent's disease. *Nephron Physiol.* **2007**, *107*, p87–p97. [CrossRef]
61. Santo, Y.; Hirai, H.; Shima, M.; Yamagata, M.; Michigami, T.; Nakajima, S.; Ozono, K. Examination of megalin in renal tubular epithelium from patients with Dent disease. *Pediatr. Nephrol.* **2004**, *19*, 612–615. [CrossRef] [PubMed]
62. Gorvin, C.M.; Wilmer, M.J.; Piret, S.E.; Harding, B.; van den Heuvel, L.P.; Wrong, O.; Jat, P.S.; Lippiat, J.D.; Levtchenko, E.N.; Thakker, R.V. Receptor-mediated endocytosis and endosomal acidification is impaired in proximal tubule epithelial cells of Dent disease patients. *Proc. Natl. Acad. Sci. USA* **2013**, *110*, 7014–7019. [CrossRef] [PubMed]
63. Anglani, F.; D'Angelo, A.; Bertizzolo, L.M.; Tosetto, E.; Ceol, M.; Cremasco, D.; Bonfante, L.; Addis, M.A.; Del Prete, D. Dent Disease Italian Network. Nephrolithiasis; kidney failure and bone disorders in Dent disease patients with and without CLCN5 mutations. *SpringerPlus* **2015**, *4*, 492. [CrossRef]
64. Anglani, F.; Terrin, L.; Brugnara, M.; Battista, M.; Cantaluppi, V.; Ceol, M.; Bertoldi, L.; Valle, G.; Joy, M.P.; Pober, B.R.; et al. Hypercalciuria and nephrolithiasis: Expanding the renal phenotype of Donnai-Barrow syndrome. *Clin. Genet.* **2018**, *94*, 187–188. [CrossRef] [PubMed]
65. Köttgen, A.; Albrecht, E.; Teumer, A.; Vitart, V.; Krumsiek, J.; Hundertmark, C.; Pistis, G.; Ruggiero, D.; O'Seaghdha, C.M.; Haller, T.; et al. Genome-wide association analyses identify 18 new loci associated with serum urate concentrations. *Nat. Genet.* **2013**, *45*, 145–154. [CrossRef] [PubMed]
66. Phipps-Green, A.J.; Merriman, M.E.; Topless, R.; Altaf, S.; Montgomery, G.W.; Franklin, C.; Jones, G.T.; van Rij, A.M.; White, D.; Stamp, L.K.; et al. Twenty-eight loci that influence serum urate levels: Analysis of association with gout. *Ann. Rheum. Dis.* **2016**, *75*, 124–130. [CrossRef] [PubMed]
67. Ketharnathan, S.; Leask, M.; Boocock, J.; Phipps-Green, A.J.; Antony, J.; O'Sullivan, J.M.; Merriman, T.R.; Horsfield, J.A. A non-coding genetic variant maximally associated with serum urate levels is functionally linked to HNF4A-dependent PDZK1 expression. *Hum. Mol. Genet.* **2018**, *27*, 3964–3973. [CrossRef]
68. Gisler, S.M.; Pribanic, S.; Bacic, D.; Forrer, P.; Gantenbein, A.; Sabourin, L.A.; Tsuji, A.; Zhao, Z.S.; Manser, E.; Biber, J.; et al. PDZK1: I. a major scaffolder in brush borders of proximal tubular cells. *Kidney Int.* **2003**, *64*, 1733–1745. [CrossRef]
69. Capuano, P.; Bacic, D.; Stange, G.; Hernando, N.; Kaissling, B.; Pal, R.; Kocher, O.; Biber, J.; Wagner, C.A.; Murer, H. Expression and regulation of the renal Na/phosphate cotransporter NaPi-IIa in a mouse model deficient for the PDZ protein PDZK1. *Pflug. Arch.* **2005**, *449*, 392–402. [CrossRef]
70. Slattery, C.; Jenkin, K.A.; Lee, A.; Simcocks, A.C.; McAinch, A.J.; Poronnik, P.; Hryciw, D.H. Na+-H+ exchanger regulatory factor 1 (NHERF1) PDZ scaffold binds an internal binding site in the scavenger receptor megalin. *Cell. Physiol. Biochem.* **2011**, *27*, 171–178. [CrossRef]
71. Sakiyama, M.; Matsuo, H.; Nagamori, S.; Ling, W.; Kawamura, Y.; Nakayama, A.; Higashino, T.; Chiba, T.; Ichida, K.; Kanai, Y.; et al. Expression of a human NPT1/SLC17A1 missense variant which increases urate export. *Nucleosides Nucleotides Nucleic Acids* **2016**, *35*, 536–542. [CrossRef] [PubMed]
72. Böger, C.A.; Chen, M.H.; Tin, A.; Olden, M.; Köttgen, A.; de Boer, I.H.; Fuchsberger, C.; O'Seaghdha, C.M.; Pattaro, C.; Teumer, A.; et al. CUBN is a gene locus for albuminuria. *J. Am. Soc. Nephrol.* **2011**, *22*, 555–570. [CrossRef] [PubMed]
73. Ovunc, B.; Otto, E.A.; Vega-Warner, V.; Saisawat, P.; Ashraf, S.; Ramaswami, G.; Fathy, H.M.; Schoeb, D.; Chernin, G.; Lyons, R.H.; et al. Exome sequencing reveals cubilin mutation as a single-gene cause of proteinuria. *J. Am. Soc. Nephrol.* **2011**, *22*, 1815–1820. [CrossRef] [PubMed]
74. Tanner, S.M.; Sturm, A.C.; Baack, E.C.; Liyanarachchi, S.; de la Chapelle, A. Inherited cobalamin malabsorption. Mutations in three genes reveal functional and ethnic patterns. *Orphanet J. Rare Dis.* **2012**, *7*, 56. [CrossRef] [PubMed]
75. Schäffer, A.A. Digenic inheritance in medical genetics. *J. Med. Genet.* **2013**, *50*, 641–652. [CrossRef] [PubMed]
76. Deltas, C. Digenic inheritance and genetic modifiers. *Clin. Genet.* **2018**, *93*, 429–438. [CrossRef]

77. Janecke, A.R.; Heinz-Erian, P.; Yin, J.; Petersen, B.S.; Franke, A.; Lechner, S.; Fuchs, I.; Melancon, S.; Uhlig, H.H.; Travis, S.; et al. Reduced sodium/proton exchanger NHE3 activity causes congenital sodium diarrhea. *Hum. Mol. Genet.* **2015**, *24*, 6614–6623. [CrossRef]
78. Lin, Z.; Jin, S.; Duan, X.; Wang, T.; Martini, S.; Hulamm, P.; Cha, B.; Hubbard, A.; Donowitz, M.; Guggino, S.E. Chloride channel (Clc)-5 is necessary for exocytic trafficking of Na+/H+ exchanger 3 (NHE3). *J. Biol. Chem.* **2011**, *286*, 22833–22845. [CrossRef]
79. Pan, W.; Borovac, J.; Spicer, Z.; Hoenderop, J.G.; Bindels, R.J.; Shull, G.E.; Doschak, M.R.; Cordat, E.; Alexander, R.T. The epithelial sodium/proton exchanger; NHE3; is necessary for renal and intestinal calcium (re)absorption. *Am. J. Physiol. Ren. Physiol.* **2012**, *302*, F943–F956. [CrossRef]
80. Katsanis, N. The continuum of causality in human genetic disorders. *Genome Biol.* **2016**, *17*, 233. [CrossRef]
81. Cooper, D.N.; Krawczak, M.; Polychronakos, C.; Tyler-Smith, C.; Kehrer-Sawatzki, H. Where genotype is not predictive of phenotype: Towards an understanding of the molecular basis of reduced penetrance in human inherited disease. *Hum. Genet.* **2013**, *132*, 1077–1130. [CrossRef] [PubMed]
82. Tosetto, E.; Ghiggeri, G.M.; Emma, F.; Barbano, G.; Carrea, A.; Vezzoli, G.; Torregrossa, R.; Cara, M.; Ripanti, G.; Ammenti, A.; et al. Phenotypic and genetic heterogeneity in Dent's disease: The results of an Italian collaborative study. *Nephrol. Dial. Transplant.* **2006**, *21*, 2452–2463. [CrossRef] [PubMed]
83. Van Berkel, Y.; Ludwig, M.; van Wijk, J.A.E.; Bökenkamp, A. Proteinuria in Dent disease: A review of the literature. *Pediatr. Nephrol.* **2017**, *32*, 1851–1859. [CrossRef]
84. Schwarz, J.M.; Cooper, D.N.; Schuelke, M.; Seelow, D. MutationTaster2: Mutation prediction for the deep-sequencing age. *Nat. Methods* **2014**, *11*, 361–362. [CrossRef] [PubMed]
85. Bertoldi, L.; Forcato, C.; Vitulo, N.; Birolo, G.; De Pascale, F.; Feltrin, E.; Schiavon, R.; Anglani, F.; Negrisolo, S.; Zanetti, A.; et al. QueryOR: A comprehensive web platform for genetic variant analysis and prioritization. *BMC Bioinform.* **2017**, *18*, 225. [CrossRef] [PubMed]
86. Kumar, P.; Henikoff, S.; Ng, P.C. Predicting the effects of coding non-synonymous variants on protein function using the SIFT algorithm. *Nat. Protoc.* **2009**, *4*, 1073–1081. [CrossRef] [PubMed]
87. Adzhubei, I.; Jordan, D.M.; Sunyaev, S.R. Predicting functional effect of human missense mutations using PolyPhen-2. *Curr. Protoc. Hum. Genet.* **2013**, *7*, 7.20.1–7.20.41. [CrossRef]
88. Yongwook, C.; Agnes, P.C. PROVEAN web server: A tool to predict the functional effect of amino acid substitutions and indels. *Bioinformatics* **2015**, *31*, 2745–2747.
89. Kircher, M.; Witten, D.M.; Jain, P.; O'Roak, B.J.; Cooper, G.M.; Shendure, J. A general framework for estimating the relative pathogenicity of human genetic variants. *Nat. Genet.* **2014**, *46*, 310–315. [CrossRef]
90. Quang, D.; Chen, Y.; Xie, X. DANN: A deep learning approach for annotating the pathogenicity of genetic variants. *Bioinformatics* **2015**, *31*, 761–763. [CrossRef]
91. Ceol, M.; Tiralongo, E.; Baelde, H.J.; Vianello, D.; Betto, G.; Marangelli, A.; Bonfante, L.; Valente, M.; Della Barbera, M.; D'Angelo, A.; et al. Involvement of the tubular ClC-type exchanger ClC-5 in glomeruli of human proteinuric nephropathies. *PLoS ONE* **2012**, *7*, e45605. [CrossRef] [PubMed]
92. Gianesello, L.; Priante, G.; Ceol, M.; Radu, C.M.; Saleem, M.A.; Simioni, P.; Terrin, L.; Anglani, F.; Del Prete, D. Albumin uptake in human podocytes: A possible role for the cubilin-amnionless (CUBAM) complex. *Sci. Rep.* **2017**, *7*, 13705. [CrossRef] [PubMed]
93. R Development Core Team. *R: A Language and Environment for Statistical Computing*; R Foundation for Statistical Computing: Vienna, Austria, 2008; ISBN 3-900051-07-0.

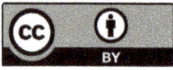

© 2020 by the authors. Licensee MDPI, Basel, Switzerland. This article is an open access article distributed under the terms and conditions of the Creative Commons Attribution (CC BY) license (http://creativecommons.org/licenses/by/4.0/).

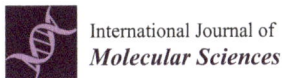

Article

Urinary NMR Profiling in Pediatric Acute Kidney Injury—A Pilot Study

Claudia Muhle-Goll [1,2,*], Philipp Eisenmann [2], Burkhard Luy [1,2], Stefan Kölker [3], Burkhard Tönshoff [4], Alexander Fichtner [4] and Jens H. Westhoff [4,*]

1. Karlsruhe Institute of Technology, Institute for Biological Interfaces 4, P.O. Box 3640, 76021 Karlsruhe, Germany; burkhard.luy@kit.edu
2. Karlsruhe Institute of Technology, Institute of Organic Chemistry, Fritz-Haber-Weg 6, 76131 Karlsruhe, Germany; philipp-michael.eisenmann@kit.edu
3. Division of Pediatric Neurology and Metabolic Medicine, University Children's Hospital Heidelberg, Im Neuenheimer Feld 430, 69120 Heidelberg, Germany; stefan.koelker@med.uni-heidelberg.de
4. Department of Pediatrics I, University Children's Hospital Heidelberg, Im Neuenheimer Feld 430, 69120 Heidelberg, Germany; burkhard.toenshoff@med.uni-heidelberg.de (B.T.); alexander.fichtner@med.uni-heidelberg.de (A.F.)
* Correspondence: claudia.muhle-goll@kit.edu (C.M.-G.); jens.westhoff@med.uni-heidelberg.de (J.H.W.)

Received: 17 December 2019; Accepted: 8 February 2020; Published: 11 February 2020

Abstract: Acute kidney injury (AKI) in critically ill children and adults is associated with significant short- and long-term morbidity and mortality. As serum creatinine- and urine output-based definitions of AKI have relevant limitations, there is a persistent need for better diagnostics of AKI. Nuclear magnetic resonance (NMR) spectroscopy allows for analysis of metabolic profiles without extensive sample manipulations. In the study reported here, we examined the diagnostic accuracy of NMR urine metabolite patterns for the diagnosis of neonatal and pediatric AKI according to the Kidney Disease: Improving Global Outcomes (KDIGO) definition. A cohort of 65 neonatal and pediatric patients (0–18 years) with established AKI of heterogeneous etiology was compared to both a group of apparently healthy children ($n = 53$) and a group of critically ill children without AKI ($n = 31$). Multivariate analysis identified a panel of four metabolites that allowed diagnosis of AKI with an area under the receiver operating characteristics curve (AUC-ROC) of 0.95 (95% confidence interval 0.86–1.00). Especially urinary citrate levels were significantly reduced whereas leucine and valine levels were elevated. Metabolomic differentiation of AKI causes appeared promising but these results need to be validated in larger studies. In conclusion, this study shows that NMR spectroscopy yields high diagnostic accuracy for AKI in pediatric patients.

Keywords: acute kidney injury; metabolomics; urine; NMR spectroscopy; multivariate analysis

1. Introduction

Acute kidney injury (AKI) is associated with poor outcomes, including increased morbidity (e.g., days on ventilator, length of hospital and intensive care unit stay) and mortality, and an increased risk for the development of chronic kidney disease [1–3]. The prevalence of neonatal and pediatric AKI among critically ill and high-risk cohorts is high, and AKI incidence is still increasing. Based on recent consensus definitions, AKI occurs in 27% and 29.9% of patients of the pediatric (PICU) and neonatal intensive care unit (NICU), respectively [4,5]. Remarkably, in non-critically ill hospitalized children and adolescents, AKI incidence is still as high as 5% [6]. The current gold standard for the diagnosis of AKI relies upon serum creatinine and urine output measurements, both of which, however, reveal relevant drawbacks. As such, serum creatinine is a late and indirect marker of reduced glomerular filtration rate that does not allow for differentiation of the specific cause of renal impairment. Urine output measurements, on the other hand, demand longer-term evaluations and are influenced, e.g., by diuretic medication. Of note, an earlier and more specific identification of patients with AKI and especially of those who are at highest risk for adverse outcome can influence physicians' decision-making and medical treatment and may ultimately improve patient outcome.

In recent years, several urinary proteins including neutrophil gelatinase-associated lipocalin (NGAL), kidney injury molecule-1 (KIM-1), tissue inhibitor of metalloprotease-2 (TIMP-2), insulin-like growth factor-binding protein 7 (IGFBP7), and others have been proposed as useful biomarkers for early diagnosis, differentiation, and/or prediction of patient outcome in adult and pediatric AKI [7–10]. Unfortunately, the specificity of the above protein biomarkers for kidney injury and their clinical performance are insufficient for clinical implementation [11,12]. Hence, there is an unmet need for novel markers of AKI alone or in combination that i) improve patient risk stratification, ii) optimize early and precise detection of renal damage, iii) enable an early etiological classification of AKI, iv) monitor and target clinical management, and v) predict clinical outcome following AKI.

Untargeted metabolomics provides a functional fingerprint of the physiological and pathophysiological state of an organism and can be used both for pattern recognition and metabolite identification [13]. Nuclear magnetic resonance (NMR) and gas chromatography or liquid chromatography, together with mass spectrometry, are generally used to separate and identify metabolites. Metabolic approaches, i.e., by mass spectrometry, have been adopted to uncover new small molecule biomarkers or biochemical mechanisms as well as signaling pathways in chronic kidney disease, diabetic nephropathy, AKI, renal cancer, kidney transplantation, and polycystic kidney diseases [14,15]. These studies were performed in either rodents or humans and investigated blood, urine, or kidney tissue samples. In an experimental pig model of sepsis-induced AKI, NMR-based metabolomics was a potentially useful tool for biomarker identification [16]. Characteristic urine NMR spectra were also demonstrated in murine renal ischemia-reperfusion injury models [17,18]. Archdekin et al. using mass spectrometry of urine samples demonstrated the potential of a urine metabolite classifier to detect non-rejection kidney injury in pediatric kidney transplant patients and non-invasively discriminated non-rejection kidney injury from rejection [19]. While metabolomic profiles have been investigated in prematurity, low birth weight neonates, perinatal asphyxia, pediatric respiratory and neurological diseases, gastrointestinal diseases and inborn errors of metabolism, only very few clinical studies have been published that investigated the application of a metabolomic approach in pediatric AKI [20,21].

This prompted us to investigate the accuracy of NMR-based urine metabolomics for the diagnosis of AKI in a pilot cohort study of neonates and children with established Kidney Disease: Improving Global Outcomes (KDIGO) AKI of heterogeneous etiology. We further aimed to investigate if metabolomic fingerprints and biomarkers allow for a differentiation of specific AKI subtypes.

2. Results

2.1. Characteristics of the Study Population

Subject characteristics are shown in Table 1. As the urine heavily reflects environmental influences, two different control groups were included into the study in order to reduce the risk of a selection bias. While the first control group consisted of apparently healthy children ("healthy controls"), the second control group comprised neonatal and pediatric ICU patients without AKI ("non-AKI patients"). In brief, there was no significant difference regarding age, gender, proportion of neonates, and body mass index (BMI) standard deviation score (SDS) between AKI patients, non-AKI patients, and healthy controls. The etiology of AKI was heterogeneous including both prerenal and intrinsic causes. The more frequent AKI etiologies included dehydration ($n = 15$), hemolytic uremic syndrome ($n = 13$), septic shock ($n = 12$), perinatal asphyxia ($n = 7$), hemodynamic instability ($n = 4$), and interstitial nephritis ($n = 4$). Serum creatinine on study enrollment was significantly ($p < 0.001$) higher in AKI patients compared to non-AKI patients and, accordingly, estimated creatinine clearance (eCCl) was significantly reduced ($p < 0.001$).

Table 1. Characteristics of the study population. Numeric data are presented as median with interquartile range (IQR) in parenthesis. Categorical data are presented as a number with the percentage in parenthesis. Statistical tests used for the individual parameters are described in the section Statistical Analysis. $p < 0.05$ was regarded as statistically significant. Abbreviations: AKI, acute kidney injury; BMI, body mass index; eCCl, estimated creatinine clearance; KDIGO, Kidney Disease: Improving Global Outcomes; SDS, standard deviation score.

Characteristic	AKI Patients ($n = 65$)	Non-AKI Patients ($n = 31$)	Healthy Controls ($n = 53$)	p-Value
Age (years)	3.0 (0.6 to 13.5)	1.0 (0.4 to 7.4)	6.0 (1.0 to 10.0)	0.21
Male	30 (46.2%)	15 (48.4%)	26 (49.1%)	0.57
Female	35 (53.8%)	16 (51.6%)	27 (50.9%)	
Neonates	12 (18.5%)	6 (19.4%)	11 (20.8%)	0.95
BMI SDS	−0.5 (−1.2 to 0.5)	−0.8 (−1.9 to 0.6)		0.25
AKI etiology				
Dehydration	15 (23.0%)			
Hemolytic uremic syndrome	13 (20.0%)			
Septic shock	12 (18.5%)			
Perinatal asphyxia	7 (10.8%)			
Hemodynamic	4 (6.2%)			
Interstitial nephritis	4 (6.2%)			
Other	10 (15.4%)			
Serum creatinine on study enrollment (mg/dL)	1.60 (0.9 to 3.5)	0.3 (0.2 to 0.5)		<0.001
eCCl on study enrollment (mL/min per 1.73 m^2)	19.2 (11.0 to 42.0)	123.0 (80.9 to 170)		<0.001
KDIGO staging of AKI				
Stage 1	5 (7.7%)			
Stage 2	9 (13.8%)			
Stage 3	51 (78.5%)			
Proteinuria (g/L)	0.6 (0.2 to 1.5)	0.1 (0.0 to 0.1)		<0.001
Urinary protein-to-creatinine ratio (mg/g)	239 (48.6 to 955)	34.6 (24.6 to 49.3)		<0.001
Urinary leukocytes (per µL)	22.0 (4.5 to 93.0)	5.0 (0.0 to 26.5)		<0.01
Urinary erythrocytes (per µL)	15.0 (2.0 to 136.0)	5.0 (2.0 to 37.3)		<0.05
Squamous epithelium (per µL)	0.0 (0.0 to 1.5)	0.0 (0.0 to 0.0)		0.074
C-reactive protein (mg/L)	30.9 (7.5 to 98.8)	2.4 (0.0 to 19.0)		0.001
Renal replacement therapy	27 (41.5%)	0 (0%)	0 (0%)	<0.001
3-month mortality	11 (16.9%)	0 (0%)	0 (0%)	<0.05

Maximum KDIGO stage during the clinical course was Stage 3 in 51 patients (78,5%), Stage 2 in nine patients (13.8%), and Stage 1 in five patients (7.7%). Proteinuria ($p < 0.001$), urinary protein-to-creatinine-ratio ($p < 0.001$), urinary leukocytes ($p = 0.002$), urinary erythrocytes ($p < 0.05$), and C-reactive protein ($p = 0.001$) were significantly increased in AKI patients compared to non-AKI patients. Twenty-seven AKI patients (41.5%) required renal replacement therapy during the clinical course, 11 AKI patients (16.9%) deceased within 3 months following study enrollment.

2.2. Nuclear Magnetic Resonance (NMR) Spectroscopy Analysis

Ten typical spectra of the urines of AKI patients, non-AKI patients, and healthy controls, respectively, are shown in Supplemental Figure S1. Whereas spectra of healthy children had a uniform appearance, corresponding to the typical urine spectra of healthy people [22], AKI spectra revealed a different picture. Not only did the spectra show increased intensities due to the reduced urine volume, but metabolite composition varied between the different individuals. In addition, some AKI spectra revealed a background of broad unresolved resonances most likely originating from large protein or lipid/steroid signals. Non-AKI patient spectra were in-between the two other groups, showing variation in their metabolite composition, but not to the same extent as the AKI spectra. Because of the observed spectral diversity, we performed variable bucketing and selected preferably those peaks that were common among all three groups.

2.3. Multivariate Analysis

When performing a principle component analysis (PCA), the AKI group could be clearly separated from the healthy control group (Figure 1A). However, the separation between the AKI and the non-AKI group was less apparent. Principal components 1 (PC1) and 2 (PC2) explained 13.4% and 12.4% of the variation. Quality control (QC) samples clustered tightly within the healthy control group and showed that measurements were highly reproducible. Neonatal spectra appeared to have more negative PC1 values. Especially among the healthy control group, neonatal spectra clustered in the upper left corner. Thus, the subsequent analyses were performed twice, with neonates either included or excluded. When neonates were excluded from the analysis (12 AKI patients, 11 healthy control subjects, six non-AKI control patients), separation was more pronounced (Figure 1B).

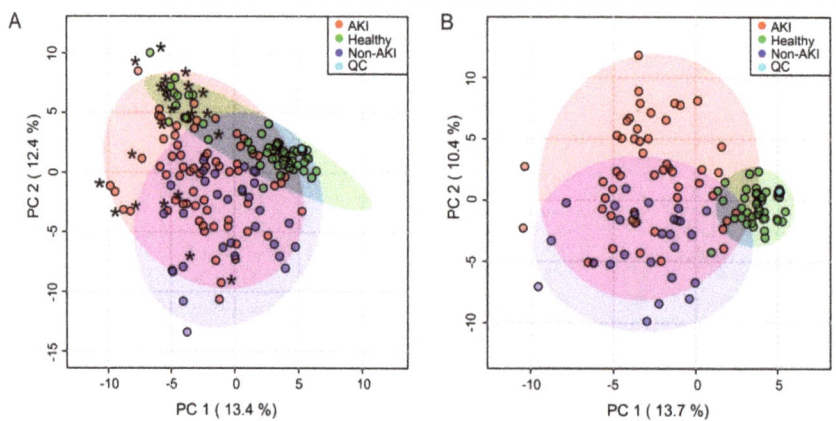

Figure 1. Principle component analysis of the urine spectral bucket table. Variable bucketing was employed leading to 129 buckets. Metabolites were assigned, whenever possible, based on comparison with database entries or literature and were confirmed by spiking experiments. (**A**) All spectra (AKI patients, $n = 65$; healthy controls, $n = 53$; non-AKI patients, $n = 31$; QC, $n = 15$), * denotes neonatal spectra, (**B**) neonatal spectra excluded (AKI patients, $n = 53$; healthy controls, $n = 42$; non-AKI patients, $n = 25$; QC, $n = 15$). Outliers were not detectable. AKI, acute kidney injury; QC, quality control.

Partial least squares discriminant analysis (PLS-DA) was performed to separate within group variation from class-related differentiation (Figure 2A). Quality control parameters showed that AKI patients could be reliably separated from the control group (quality of prediction Q^2: 0.55, explained variance R^2: 0.76). Omitting neonatal samples (Figure 2B) only slightly improved the separation and predictive power (Q^2: 0.64, R^2: 0.82). A 1000-fold permutation analysis confirmed that this result was not fortuitous in both cases ($p < 0.001$). Separation into prerenal and intrinsic causes of AKI based on previously published criteria [23] was explored, but did not lead to improved clustering in the PCA or PLS-DA (Supplemental Figure S2) and was consequently abandoned.

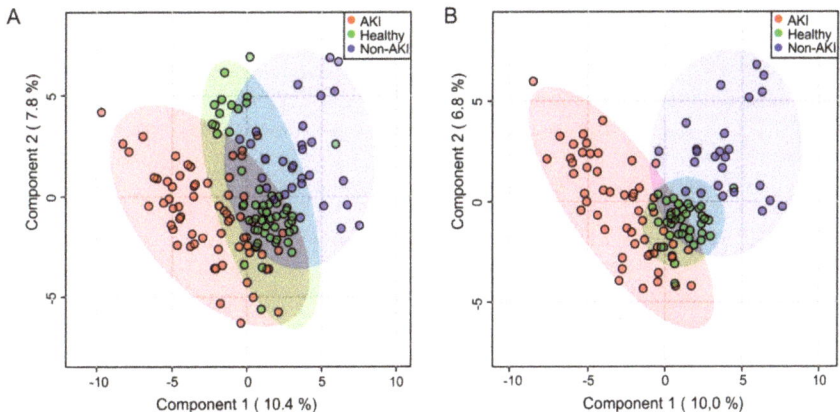

Figure 2. Partial least squares discriminant analysis of the urine spectral bucket table. Neonatal spectra (**A**) included (AKI patients, $n = 65$; healthy controls, $n = 53$; non-AKI patients, $n = 31$), (**B**) excluded (AKI patients, $n = 53$; healthy controls, $n = 42$; non-AKI patients, $n = 25$). AKI, acute kidney injury.

As mentioned before, non-AKI patient spectra separated less well from AKI spectra than healthy control spectra. We questioned whether the analysis preferentially selected general traits of morbidity like markers of increased catabolic pathways or drug metabolism. To rule out this argument, we performed both PCA and PLS-DA in healthy controls and non-AKI controls (Supplemental Figure S3). Metabolites that separated the two groups were identified in a PLS-DA (Supplemental Table S1) and those with variable importance in projection (VIP) values higher than 1.5 were excluded in the following analyses. For further analyses, the healthy control group and the non-AKI patient group were combined. This led to a visibly better separation already in a PCA (Supplemental Figure S4A). A PLS-DA model could be obtained with three components and quality parameters Q^2 of 0.66 and R^2 of 0.79 (Supplemental Figure S4B, Table 2). Omitting neonates further improved the separation between the groups to a Q^2 value of 0.73 and a R^2 value of 0.89 (Supplemental Figure S5A and S5B, Table 2). The VIP plot (Supplemental Figures S4C and S5C) revealed that citrate, bile acid signals, leucine, valine, general lipid signals, cis-aconitic acid, formate, as well as non-assigned aliphatic (unk_al/x) compounds were mainly responsible for the separation.

Table 2. Explained variance and predictability for AKI and subgroups when compared to the combined control group (non-AKI patients plus healthy control subjects).

Group	No. of Components	PLS-DA Parameters		Permutation *: Empirical p-Value
		Q^2	R^2	
AKI (total)	3	0.63	0.78	< 0.001
AKI (neonates excluded in AKI and CTL)	4	0.73	0.89	< 0.001
Dehydration	3	0.44	0.80	< 0.001
Perinatal asphyxia	2	0.26	0.61	0.159
Septic shock	4	0.73	0.95	< 0.001
Hemolytic uremic syndrome	4	0.69	0.90	< 0.001

* resulting from 1000 times permutation analysis.

2.4. Biomarker Analysis

To analyze whether the spectral information or a combination of several metabolites could be used as biomarker, 20% of randomly selected spectra (11 AKI, six non-AKI, and eight healthy control spectra) were not used for initial analysis and served as validation cohort. Neonates were excluded as the previous analysis had shown that their spectral characteristics differ to a certain degree. We developed a diagnostic model based on the metabolites with the highest VIP values in the PLS-DA analysis (Supplemental Figure S5C, Table 3). They all demonstrated AUC-ROC values > 0.70 and confidence intervals that did not cross 0.5. Yet a logistic regression model with these 15 markers did not converge. Thus, we successively reduced the number of potential markers based on the calculated z values and Pr(>|z|) to a set of four markers: Citrate with its resonance at 2.69 ppm, leucine (0.96 ppm), valine with its resonance at 1.00 ppm, and bile acid (0.69–0.81 ppm).

Table 3. Top 15 metabolites according to PLS-DA of AKI compared to the combined control group (non-AKI patients plus healthy control subjects), neonatal spectra excluded. AKI, acute kidney injury; PLS-DA, partial least squares discriminant analysis.

Metabolite Importance Number	Metabolite	VIP Score	AUC *	95% CI **
1	Citrate1 ***	2.73	0.94	0.88–0.98
2	Bile acid	2.52	0.91	0.84–0.97
3	Citrate2 ***	2.50	0.92	0.85–0.96
4	Unk_al1	2.49	0.90	0.83–0.96
5	unk_al28	2.19	0.84	0.75–0.91
6	Leucine	2.13	0.83	0.73–0.90
7	unk_al24	2.07	0.83	0.74–0.92
8	unk_al26	2.07	0.82	0.73–0.91
9	Valine	1.89	0.79	0.70–0.89
10	unk_al10	1.86	0.80	0.70–0.89
11	cis-Aconitic acid	1.86	0.79	0.69–0.88
12	Formate	1.80	0.84	0.75–0.91
13	LipidCH$_2$	1.65	0.82	0.72–0.90
14	Glycine	1.50	0.71	0.61–0.81
15	Asparagine	1.48	0.76	0.65–0.85

* ROC AUC values from univariate testing. ** 95% confidence interval was calculated using 500 bootstrappings. *** Citrate is characterized by two separate buckets, one for each proton of the degenerate CH$_2$ group.

We obtained a regression equation with a best threshold (or cut-off) for the predicted p (= Pr(y=1|x)) of 0.34 (Table 4A).

Table 4. Logistic regression model—summary of each feature: (**A**) With four, (**B**) with six features.

(A) logit(p) = log(p/(1 − P)) = −0.667 − 2.723 citrate + 2.538 leucine − 3.42 valine + 3.164 bile acid					
	Estimate	Std. Error	z Value	Pr(>|z|)	Odds
(Intercept)	−0.667	0.571	−1.167	0.243	-
citrate (2.69 ppm)	−2.723	0.83	−3.281	0.001	0.07
leucine	2.538	1.089	2.33	0.02	12.65
valine	−3.42	1.374	−2.489	0.013	0.03
bile acid	3.164	1.096	2.887	0.004	23.67

(B) logit(P) = log(P/(1 − P)) = 0.034 − 3.193 citrate + 4.859 leucine − 6.191 valine + 4.207 bile acid - 2.694 unk_al1 − 2.489 unk_al28					
	Estimate	Std. Error	z value	Pr(>|z|)	Odds
(Intercept)	0.034	0.998	0.034	0.973	-
citrate (2.69 ppm)	−3.193	1.682	−1.898	0.058	0.04
leucine	4.859	2.182	2.227	0.026	128.88
valine	−6.191	2.617	−2.366	0.018	0
bile acid	4.207	1.774	2.372	0.018	67.18
unk_al1/3.16 ppm	2.694	1.414	−1.906	0.057	0.07
unk_al28/2.15 ppm	−2.489	1.093	−2.278	0.023	0.08

p-values above this threshold classified samples as AKI. The area under the receiver operating characteristics curve (AUC-ROC) was 0.95 with a 95% confidence interval of 0.86–1.00 (Figure 3A). When the classification performance was tested on the validation cohort, one AKI test sample (out of 11) was wrongly classified, but no control spectra. A modified marker set including two additional unidentified aliphatic compounds, one with a resonance at 3.16 ppm (unk_al1) and one overlapping with glutamine (2.12–2.17 ppm, unk_al28), classified all spectra of the validation set correctly, but had a slightly lower AUC-ROC value of 0.93 (95% CI: 0.82–0.99) (Table 4B and Figure 3B). Details about each feature are listed in Table 4A,B.

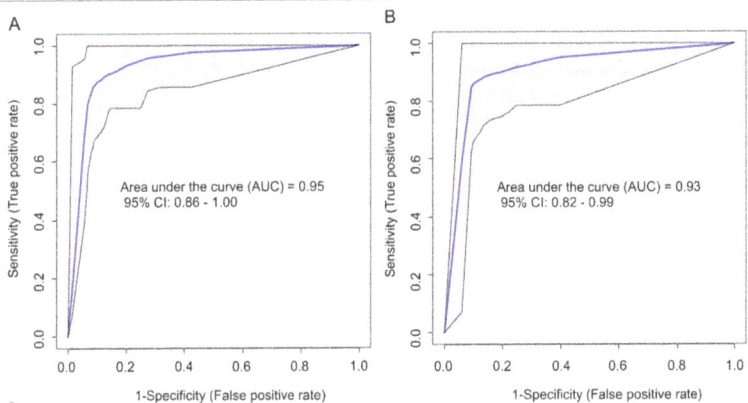

Figure 3. ROC curve for the diagnostic accuracy of selected metabolites from NMR spectroscopy for the diagnosis of KDIGO AKI obtained from a linear regression analysis using (**A**) four selected features (citrate (2.69 ppm), leucine (0.96 ppm), valine (1.00 ppm), and bile acid (0.69–0.81 ppm)) and (**B**) six selected features (citrate (2.69 ppm), leucine (0.96 ppm), valine (1.00 ppm), bile acid (0.69–0.81 ppm), unk_al1 (3.16 ppm), and unk_al28 (2.12–2.17 ppm)). AKI, acute kidney injury; KDIGO, Kidney Disease: Improving Global Outcomes; NMR, nuclear magnetic resonance; ROC, receiver operating characteristic.

2.5. Differentiation of Acute Kidney Injury (AKI) Etiologies

We next analyzed whether NMR spectroscopy allows for etiologic differentiation of underlying AKI causes (Figure 4). Four AKI subgroups had sufficient patient numbers for statistical analysis ($n > 5$). Here we used a reduced set of buckets and excluded all buckets of the original set that had variable importance in projection (VIP) values < 1.1 when the AKI group was compared against the combined control group. This led to a reduced set of 48 buckets. The logic behind this choice was to remove potential noise as the number of variables by far exceeded the number of spectra.

We performed PLS-DA with each of the subgroups (i.e., dehydration, hemolytic uremic syndrome, septic shock, perinatal asphyxia) against the combined control group to search for distinct group specific patterns. Quality control values were good for two subgroups (septic shock and hemolytic uremic syndrome) and acceptable for the dehydration subgroup (Table 2). A moderate Q^2-value and a high empirical *p*-value for a 1000-fold permutation test showed that the subgroup perinatal asphyxia was less well identifiable with the employed metabolite set.

Figure 4 displays the VIP values of the most important metabolites (VIP > 1.1 in at least one group) together with their fold change calculated for each subgroup. The VIP patterns (Figure 4A) showed that in addition to metabolite buckets that were important for general AKI identification in all AKI subjects, AKI subtype-specific metabolite buckets appeared to be identifiable. Fold changes analysis displayed an even more distinct picture (Figure 4B). A fold change in citrate was common in all groups. Others seemed to be specific for the underlying AKI etiology. For example, gluconate and lactate-to-threonine ratio had large fold changes in perinatal asphyxia and septic shock, but were less informative for dehydration and hemolytic uremic syndrome.

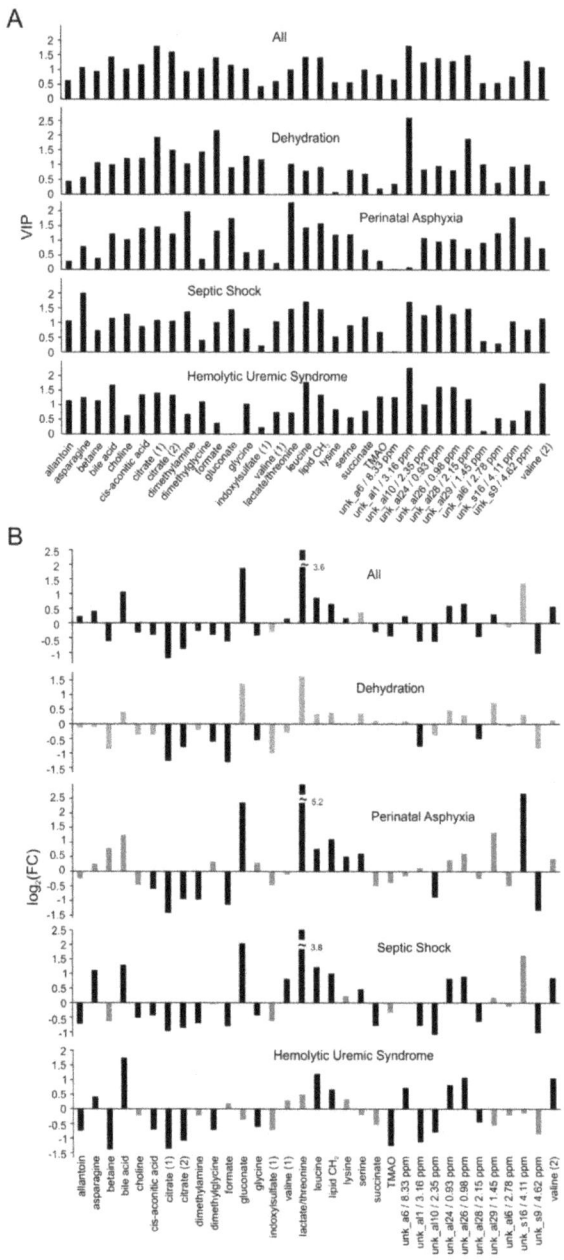

Figure 4. (**A**) Overview of discriminant identified metabolites according to variable importance in projection (VIP) values analyzed separately for each etiology. VIP values were obtained from a PLS-DA analysis. Only metabolite buckets are shown that had VIP values > 1.1 for at least one of the different groups. (**B**) The respective fold changes ($\log_2(FC)$) for the same metabolites are given for comparison. Black bars denote fold changes with an associated p-value < 0.01, grey bars those with a p-value > 0.01. PLS-DA, partial least squares discriminant analysis.

3. Discussion

Several metabolomic studies investigating various renal diseases have been published in the past decade, however, metabolomics data on pediatric AKI is scarce (for an overview see [14,15,24]). In the present study, ^{1}H-NMR profiling was applied to urinary samples of neonatal and pediatric patients with established AKI and compared to healthy children and to hospitalized children without AKI. By multivariate analysis, we identified a panel of metabolites that enabled AKI diagnosis by yielding an AUC-ROC of 0.95. The identified metabolites that enabled the diagnosis of AKI (KDIGO) included, among several unknown compounds, increases in leucine, valine, bile acid and decreases in citrate (Figure 4B). In addition, in our rather small pilot study population NMR-fingerprints seemed to allow for differentiation between different AKI etiologies.

A crucial point in our analysis was the selection of the control group. The AKI cohort was very heterogeneous with respect to the underlying cause of AKI, and patients were treated with a variety of medications. As urine reflects all these impacts as well as nutritional influences, comparing the AKI children only to a healthy control cohort would enhance the risk for the selection of markers not related to AKI but rather to general morbidity. Creatinine may be such an example, as it is not only used to determine renal clearance but is also a marker of muscle mass. For that reason, we decided to further include a control group of critically ill ICU patients without AKI that were also exposed to diverse medical treatments. PCA and PLS-DA analysis proved that this grouping was possible and that AKI spectra showed their own distinct pattern. Moreover, in this way we identified metabolites like mannitol, lactose, and creatinine as crucial for the general distinction between healthy children and hospitalized patients without AKI. Mannitol and lactose are applied as additive drug components, whereas creatinine may be a common sign of catabolic metabolism or a sign of a minor reduction in renal clearance (Supplemental Table S1). By omitting these metabolites, we are confident that the distinction of AKI from non-AKI patients was not based on common medication or general signs of morbidity. Strikingly, some markers that were excluded from analysis after comparison of healthy control and non-AKI patient control spectra (hippurate, indoxylsulfate, creatinine) were among those that were previously classified as markers for AKI in animal models [25–27]. However, in animal models, only healthy untreated animals served as control. This does not allow a distinction between general signs of morbidity and specific ones for AKI.

Previous human AKI studies resulted in the identification of a variety of potential metabolite biomarkers [14,24]. Interestingly, almost no overlap exists between the respective metabolites [28–34] and the metabolites identified in our study. For example, Beger et al. identified homovanillinic acid sulfate, a dopamine metabolite as the most important marker in the urine of children who developed AKI after cardiac surgery [21]. This finding was confirmed by Mercier et al. investigating the urine of neonates with AKI [29]. By contrast, aromatic compounds other than 3-indoxylsulfate and hippurate are not among the important metabolites in our study.

Animal studies present a somewhat more homogeneous picture of putative biomarkers. In the majority, AKI was induced in healthy animals through application of drugs or surgery [25–27,34–38]. Although the identified biomarkers rarely fully matched between the different studies, metabolites of the citric acid cycle (TCA) cycle, branched-chain amino acids, creatinine, hippurate, and 3-indoxylsulfate emerged as common markers of drug-induced AKI [25–27,34–38]. Some prospective markers in rodent models of drug-induced AKI (e.g., by cisplatin or gentamicin) were already altered in early phases of drug-induced nephrotoxicity [25]. Strikingly though, the metabolite selection mentioned above overlaps with the markers identified in our study. Especially citrate, leucine, and valine were among the most relevant metabolites responsible for AKI diagnosis and were main components of our developed logistic regression model.

Why do our results match better to studies on animals than on humans? Previous human studies generally examined very homogeneous groups of patients with respect to AKI etiology. In our study, AKI patients comprised a broad etiologic spectrum of AKI which is reflected by the diverse peak patterns in the aromatic area (Figure 1). This diversity may have helped in identifying a robust common denominator. Enhanced branched-chain amino acids and a reduction in citrate excretion has been reported previously, but for other nephropathies including chronic kidney disease, [39,40], diabetic nephropathy [41] and polycystic kidney disease [42]. They may be signs of early kidney damage, as a reduction of citrate can be a sign for mitochondrial dysfunction of the proximal tubular cell [24].

In fact, a reduction of TCA cycle metabolites as reflected in our study presumably mirrors tubular dysfunction due to inadequate energy supply. This dysfunction might originate from missing driving forces of the tubular cell membrane due to a lack of adenosine triphosphate (ATP) that ultimately impairs transcellular transport of dicarbonic acids by organic anion transporters (OAT), i.e., OAT4 [43]. The reason for the reduction of urinary formic acid in pediatric AKI patients can only be speculated on. Energy deficiency might cause a reduced outwardly directed electrochemical gradient for formate, a metabolite that was also significantly reduced in AKI patients. This, in consequence, is a driving force for tertiary active Cl- absorption via the Cl-/formate anion exchange transporter [44].

In our study, the percentage of spectra originating from neonates was 18.5% in the AKI group, 19.4% in the non-AKI patient group, and 20.8% in the healthy control group. Omitting these from the statistical analyses further improved the separation between the AKI group and the combined control group comprising both healthy children and critically ill ICU patients without AKI. Similar observations were made previously when investigating novel protein biomarkers of renal damage in mixed neonatal and pediatric cohorts [23]. This observation might be attributed, at least in part, to the relatively high percentage of low KDIGO AKI stages in neonates. As such, four neonates (33.3%) were classified as Stage 1 KDIGO AKI, three neonates (25%) were classified as Stage 2 and only five patients (41.7%) were classified as Stage 3 AKI. By contrast, 46 (86.8%) pediatric AKI patients fulfilled Stage 3 KDIGO AKI criteria, six (11.3%) fulfilled Stage 2 criteria and only one pediatric AKI patient (1.9%) fulfilled Stage 1 criteria. In addition, several metabolomics studies demonstrated that the urine of neonates shows characteristic differences compared to older children. Scalabre et al. stressed the differential impact of age, height, and weight in metabolomic studies on urinary metabolic profiles in children aged < 1 year [45]. Among the metabolites identified as markers of age, they also identified citrate as an important marker. In that study, it was correlated with an increase in weight and height, and showed a negative correlation with age like succinate, which was confirmed in two other studies [20,46,47]. In comparison, in our study AKI patients of all ages showed a decrease of citrate levels compared to non-AKI subjects. Other age-related metabolites identified in these studies showed no significant effect in our analysis. Thus, we are confident that in our study age-related effects were marginal compared to the metabolic changes caused by AKI.

There are several limitations to our study. First, the number of patients participating in our single-center pilot study was low, hence requiring larger population studies. Nevertheless, robust identification of AKI patients by ^{1}H-NMR spectroscopy was feasible despite the wide variety of AKI etiologies. Second, due to the low number of study participants investigated, this study was not appropriate for analyzing the impact of AKI severity as reflected by KDIGO stage on NMR spectra. Third, the presented study primarily focuses on the diagnosis of established AKI using the serum creatinine- and urine output-based KDIGO AKI criteria as gold standard. However, due to a variety of reasons both parameters can be problematic for AKI diagnosis, especially in children. Future studies will have to deal with the implementation of ^{1}H-NMR spectroscopy for early detection of imminent AKI, for differentiation of varying AKI subtypes and for therapy monitoring and prognosis of AKI outcome. In fact, early identification of patients at highest risk for AKI and for adverse outcome can help physicians in early decision-making, e.g., with respect to the timely insertion of dialysis catheters and initiation of renal replacement therapy.

4. Materials and Methods

4.1. Ethics Statement

The study was conducted in accordance with the Declaration of Helsinki and approved by the ethics committee of the Heidelberg Medical Faculty (Protocol S-133/2011, permission: 15 July 2011, amendment: 13 June 2016). Legal guardian of each patient gave written informed consent and, when appropriate, assent from the patient was obtained as well.

4.2. Study Design and Participants

A prospective pilot cohort study was conducted at the University Children's Hospital Heidelberg. Patients aged 0 to 18 years who developed AKI during their hospital stay and patients who were referred to our Children's Hospital with established AKI were enrolled in the study from October 2011 to March 2019. Of note, the study population has partly been published before [23,48,49]. Criteria for study exclusion were (i) prematurity, (ii) postrenal AKI as examined by initial renal ultrasound, and (iii) children undergoing cardiac surgery. AKI was classified either according to the Kidney Disease: Improving Global Outcomes (KDIGO) AKI definition [50] for pediatric patients or according to the modified KDIGO definition for neonatal patients aged $\leq$ 28 days of life [51]. When serum creatinine and urine output criteria resulted in different KDIGO stages, the higher stage was chosen. The revised Schwartz formula ($k = 0.413 \times$ height / serum creatinine) was used for calculation of eCCl [52]. Baseline serum creatinine was defined as last value within the previous three months before study enrollment. In the case of missing baseline data, the eCCl was assumed to be 120 mL per minute per 1.73 m^2 in pediatric patients and 40 mL per minute per 1.73 m^2 in neonates [4,48]. Control subjects without AKI were taken from two different cohorts [23]. While the "non-AKI patients" group ($n = 31$) consisted of neonatal and pediatric ICU patients without AKI, the "healthy controls" group ($n = 53$) comprised apparently healthy neonates, children, and adolescents aged 0–18 years. Diagnoses of inpatients without AKI were postoperative care ($n = 25$ including neurosurgery, $n = 11$; pediatric surgery, $n = 6$; maxillofacial surgery, $n = 6$; orthopedics, $n = 1$; otorhinolaryngology, $n = 1$), seizures ($n = 1$), respiratory diseases ($n = 1$), perinatal asphyxia ($n = 1$), infectious diseases ($n = 2$), and cardiovascular diseases ($n = 1$). Exclusion criteria for the healthy control group have been previously published [48]. Patients' characteristics are given in Table 1.

4.3. Sample and Data Collection

Urine samples were collected immediately following KDIGO AKI diagnosis or after admission to our hospital. In case of anuria, urine samples were obtained after restoration of diuresis. Following centrifugation, the supernatants of the urine samples were frozen, stored at −80 °C and thawed prior to analysis. After thawing urine samples were centrifuged for 10 min at 15,871 g. A total of 500 μL of samples were mixed with 100 μL sodium phosphate buffer (150 mM final concentration in D_2O, pH 7.2) containing 2 mM trimethylsilylpropanoic acid for spectral referencing. D_2O was used as lock substance. Measurement of SCr was performed using an IDMS-traceable enzymatic method.

4.4. ^{1}H-NMR Spectroscopy of Urine Samples

A 600 MHz Avance II spectrometer (Bruker Biospin, Rheinstetten, Germany) with a double resonance 5-mm BBI probe was used to acquire the ^{1}H NMR spectra at 300 K. Temperature calibration was performed on a daily basis. Quality control (QC) samples consisting of urine aliquots of a healthy male volunteer were included every 10 h of measurement. One-dimensional spectra were acquired with the Bruker pulse sequence noesygppr1D using a relaxation delay of 10 s, 32 transients of 64 K data points, and a spectral width of 20 ppm. Water suppression was achieved through presaturation with a bandwidth of 25 Hz. Automatic phase- and baseline-correction was employed. Spectra were calibrated to the signal of TSP. Prior to Fourier transformation, spectra were multiplied with an exponential function with a 0.3 Hz line broadening factor. Topspin3.2 (Bruker Biospin, Rheinstetten, Germany) was used for data acquisition and processing.

Variable bucketing was employed leading to 129 buckets. Metabolites were assigned on the basis of comparison with data bases entries or literature whenever possible. Spiking experiments, where specific metabolites were added to a representative, already measured sample, were used to confirm the assignments in cases of doubt. Two windows were excluded: 4.74–4.84 ppm and 6.0–5.56 ppm, where water or urea resonances, respectively, appear. Missing values did not occur.

4.5. Statistical Analysis

As clinical data was non-normally distributed, median and interquartile range are presented. For statistical analysis of intergroup differences of numeric parameters, the Kruskal–Wallis test with post hoc Dunn's test or the Mann–Whitney U-test were used. Categorical parameters were compared by Pearson's Chi-squared test. For age-independent estimates, BMI was converted to SDS values, related to age- and gender-specific means and SD of European reference populations.

PCA and PLS-DA were performed with R (version 3.5.3) using the package MetaboanalystR and default parameters [53]. Probabilistic quotient normalization [54] was employed prior to statistical analysis using the healthy control samples as reference to take into account that the urine of AKI patients is as such more often concentrated leading to higher peak intensities. Data distribution showed that the data were skewed. To take this into account, data were log transformed and scaled to unit variance. To assess the quality of the resulting statistical models, 10-fold internal cross-validation as well as permutation tests were performed. To judge the predictive power of PLS-DA, quality parameters Q^2 (quality of prediction) and R^2 (explained variance) were calculated. In a second round, metabolites that separated healthy controls and non-AKI controls were identified in a PLS-DA (Supplemental Table S1) and those with VIP values higher than 1.5 (18 buckets) were excluded from the subsequent analyses.

Biomarker analysis was performed with the respective module of MetaboanalystR using PLS-DA for identification of a set of marker peaks, support vector machines, and logistic regression to assess the suitability of a reduced set for class prediction of unknown spectra and univariate ROC curve analysis for the calculation of individual metabolite AUC values.

For etiological analysis a reduced set of metabolites was used. All buckets were taken out that had variable importance in projection (VIP) values < 1.1 when the AKI group was compared against the combined control group. This led to a reduced set of 48 buckets. Metabolite fold changes between the groups were assessed with the non-parametric Mann-Whitney U-test using the Fold-Change Analysis Module of MetaboanalystR.

5. Conclusions

In conclusion, the present study underlines the value of 1H-NMR spectroscopy for the identification of novel biomarkers of renal damage in pediatric AKI. By use of this elegant technique, we were able to identify a panel of four metabolites that in linear regression analysis yielded an excellent accuracy for the diagnosis of AKI. In addition, detailed breakdown of signaling pathways being involved in the AKI cascade might further pave the way for the development of new therapeutic options for AKI.

Supplementary Materials: The following are available online at http://www.mdpi.com/1422-0067/21/4/1187/s1, Figure S1: Ten representative spectra of each group, Figure S2: PCA of AKI classified into prerenal (AKI-pre) and intrinsic (AKI-intrin), Figure S3: PCA and PLS-DA of healthy control group vs. hospitalized patients without AKI (Non-AKI), Figure S4: PCA and PLS-DA after taking out buckets separating healthy control group from hospitalized patients without AKI, Figure S5: Same as Figure S4, with neonatal spectra excluded. Table S1: Variable importance in projection (VIP) –Values from PLS-DA of healthy control group vs. hospitalized patients without AKI (Non-AKI).

Author Contributions: All authors have read and agreed to the published version of the manuscript. Conceptualization, C.M.-G., P.E., B.T. and J.H.W.; methodology, C.M.-G., P.E., A.F. and J.H.W.; validation, C.M.-G. and J.H.W.; formal analysis, C.M.-G., P.E. and J.H.W.; data curation, C.M.-G., P.E. and J.H.W.; writing—original draft preparation, C.M.-G. and J.H.W.; writing—review and editing, B.L., S.K., B.T., A.F.

Funding: This research received no external funding.

Acknowledgments: The authors would like to thank Miriam Himmelsbach and Anne Mayer for help with spectra acquisition and spiking of metabolites. Pavleta Tzvetkova has been invaluable in help with spectrometer and many discussions. C.M.-G. acknowledges support by the Helmholtz-Gesellschaft. We are indebted to all children and their parents who participated in the study.

Conflicts of Interest: The authors declare no conflict of interest.

Abbreviations

AKI	acute kidney injury
AUC	area under the curve
BMI	body mass index
eCCl	estimated creatinine clearance
KDIGO	Kidney Disease: Improving Global Outcomes
NICU	neonatal intensive care unit
NMR	nuclear magnetic resonance
PCA	principle component analysis
PICU	pediatric intensive care unit
PLS-DA	partial least squares discriminant analysis
QC	quality control
ROC	receiver operating characteristic
SDS	standard deviation score
VIP	variable importance in projection

References

1. Mammen, C.; Al Abbas, A.; Skippen, P.; Nadel, H.; Levine, D.; Collet, J.P.; Matsell, D.G. Long-term risk of CKD in children surviving episodes of acute kidney injury in the intensive care unit: A prospective cohort study. *Am. J. Kidney Dis.* **2012**, *59*, 523–530. [CrossRef]
2. Menon, S.; Kirkendall, E.S.; Nguyen, H.; Goldstein, S.L. Acute kidney injury associated with high nephrotoxic medication exposure leads to chronic kidney disease after 6 months. *J. Pediatr.* **2014**, *165*, 522–527 e2. [CrossRef] [PubMed]
3. Askenazi, D.J.; Feig, D.I.; Graham, N.M.; Hui-Stickle, S.; Goldstein, S.L. 3–5 year longitudinal follow-up of pediatric patients after acute renal failure. *Kidney Int.* **2006**, *69*, 184–189. [CrossRef] [PubMed]
4. Kaddourah, A.; Basu, R.K.; Bagshaw, S.M.; Goldstein, S.L. Investigators, A., Epidemiology of Acute Kidney Injury in Critically Ill Children and Young Adults. *N. Engl. J. Med.* **2017**, *376*, 11–20. [CrossRef] [PubMed]
5. Jetton, J.G.; Boohaker, L.J.; Sethi, S.K.; Wazir, S.; Rohatgi, S.; Soranno, D.E.; Chishti, A.S.; Woroniecki, R.; Mammen, C.; Swanson, J.R.; et al. Incidence and outcomes of neonatal acute kidney injury (AWAKEN): A multicentre, multinational, observational cohort study. *Lancet Child. Adolesc. Health* **2017**, *1*, 184–194. [CrossRef]
6. McGregor, T.L.; Jones, D.P.; Wang, L.; Danciu, I.; Bridges, B.C.; Fleming, G.M.; Shirey-Rice, J.; Chen, L.; Byrne, D.W.; Van Driest, S.L. Acute Kidney Injury Incidence in Noncritically Ill Hospitalized Children, Adolescents, and Young Adults: A Retrospective Observational Study. *Am. J. Kidney Dis.* **2016**, *67*, 384–390. [CrossRef]
7. Schrezenmeier, E.V.; Barasch, J.; Budde, K.; Westhoff, T.; Schmidt-Ott, K.M. Biomarkers in acute kidney injury - pathophysiological basis and clinical performance. *Acta Physiol. (Oxf)* **2017**, *219*, 554–572. [CrossRef]
8. Malhotra, R.; Siew, E.D. Biomarkers for the Early Detection and Prognosis of Acute Kidney Injury. *Clin. J. Am. Soc. Nephrol.* **2017**, *12*, 149–173. [CrossRef]
9. Waldherr, S.; Fichtner, A.; Beedgen, B.; Bruckner, T.; Schaefer, F.; Tonshoff, B.; Poschl, J.; Westhoff, T.H.; Westhoff, J.H. Urinary acute kidney injury biomarkers in very low-birth-weight infants on indomethacin for patent ductus arteriosus. *Pediatr. Res.* **2019**, *85*, 678–686. [CrossRef]
10. Greenberg, J.H.; Parikh, C.R. Biomarkers for Diagnosis and Prognosis of AKI in Children: One Size Does Not Fit All. *Clin. J. Am. Soc Nephrol.* **2017**, *12*, 1551–1557. [CrossRef]

11. van Duijl, T.T.; Ruhaak, L.R.; de Fijter, J.W.; Cobbaert, C.M. Kidney Injury Biomarkers in an Academic Hospital Setting: Where Are We Now? *Clin. Biochem. Rev.* **2019**, *40*, 79–97. [PubMed]
12. Cerda, J. A biomarker able to predict acute kidney injury before it occurs? *Lancet* **2019**, *394*, 448–450. [CrossRef]
13. Weiss, R.H.; Kim, K. Metabolomics in the study of kidney diseases. *Nat. Rev. Nephrol.* **2011**, *8*, 22–33. [CrossRef] [PubMed]
14. Abbiss, H.; Maker, G.L.; Trengove, R.D. Metabolomics Approaches for the Diagnosis and Understanding of Kidney Diseases. *Metabolites* **2019**, *9*, 34. [CrossRef]
15. Kalim, S.; Rhee, E.P. An overview of renal metabolomics. *Kidney Int.* **2017**, *91*, 61–69. [CrossRef]
16. Izquierdo-Garcia, J.L.; Nin, N.; Cardinal-Fernandez, P.; Rojas, Y.; de Paula, M.; Granados, R.; Martinez-Caro, L.; Ruiz-Cabello, J.; Lorente, J.A. Identification of novel metabolomic biomarkers in an experimental model of septic acute kidney injury. *Am. J. Physiol. Renal. Physiol.* **2019**, *316*, F54–F62. [CrossRef] [PubMed]
17. Chihanga, T.; Ma, Q.; Nicholson, J.D.; Ruby, H.N.; Edelmann, R.E.; Devarajan, P.; Kennedy, M.A. NMR spectroscopy and electron microscopy identification of metabolic and ultrastructural changes to the kidney following ischemia-reperfusion injury. *Am. J. Physiol. Renal. Physiol.* **2018**, *314*, F154–F166. [CrossRef]
18. Jouret, F.; Leenders, J.; Poma, L.; Defraigne, J.O.; Krzesinski, J.M.; de Tullio, P. Nuclear Magnetic Resonance Metabolomic Profiling of Mouse Kidney, Urine and Serum Following Renal Ischemia/Reperfusion Injury. *PLoS ONE* **2016**, *11*, e0163021. [CrossRef]
19. Archdekin, B.; Sharma, A.; Gibson, I.W.; Rush, D.; Wishart, D.S.; Blydt-Hansen, T.D. Non-invasive differentiation of non-rejection kidney injury from acute rejection in pediatric renal transplant recipients. *Pediatr. Transplant.* **2019**, *23*, e13364. [CrossRef]
20. Mussap, M.; Antonucci, R.; Noto, A.; Fanos, V. The role of metabolomics in neonatal and pediatric laboratory medicine. *Clin. Chim. Acta* **2013**, *426*, 127–138. [CrossRef]
21. Beger, R.D.; Holland, R.D.; Sun, J.; Schnackenberg, L.K.; Moore, P.C.; Dent, C.L.; Devarajan, P.; Portilla, D. Metabonomics of acute kidney injury in children after cardiac surgery. *Pediatr. Nephrol.* **2008**, *23*, 977–984. [CrossRef] [PubMed]
22. Bouatra, S.; Aziat, F.; Mandal, R.; Guo, A.C.; Wilson, M.R.; Knox, C.; Bjorndahl, T.C.; Krishnamurthy, R.; Saleem, F.; Liu, P.; et al. The human urine metabolome. *PLoS ONE* **2013**, *8*, e73076. [CrossRef] [PubMed]
23. Westhoff, J.H.; Fichtner, A.; Waldherr, S.; Pagonas, N.; Seibert, F.S.; Babel, N.; Tonshoff, B.; Bauer, F.; Westhoff, T.H. Urinary biomarkers for the differentiation of prerenal and intrinsic pediatric acute kidney injury. *Pediatr. Nephrol.* **2016**, *31*, 2353–2363. [CrossRef] [PubMed]
24. Fanos, V.; Fanni, C.; Ottonello, G.; Noto, A.; Dessi, A.; Mussap, M. Metabolomics in adult and pediatric nephrology. *Molecules* **2013**, *18*, 4844–4857. [CrossRef]
25. Boudonck, K.J.; Mitchell, M.W.; Nemet, L.; Keresztes, L.; Nyska, A.; Shinar, D.; Rosenstock, M. Discovery of metabolomics biomarkers for early detection of nephrotoxicity. *Toxicol. Pathol.* **2009**, *37*, 280–292. [CrossRef]
26. Won, A.J.; Kim, S.; Kim, Y.G.; Kim, K.B.; Choi, W.S.; Kacew, S.; Kim, K.S.; Jung, J.H.; Lee, B.M.; Kim, S.; et al. Discovery of urinary metabolomic biomarkers for early detection of acute kidney injury. *Mol. Biosyst.* **2016**, *12*, 133–144. [CrossRef]
27. Sieber, M.; Hoffmann, D.; Adler, M.; Vaidya, V.S.; Clement, M.; Bonventre, J.V.; Zidek, N.; Rached, E.; Amberg, A.; Callanan, J.J.; et al. Comparative analysis of novel noninvasive renal biomarkers and metabonomic changes in a rat model of gentamicin nephrotoxicity. *Toxicol. Sci.* **2009**, *109*, 336–349. [CrossRef]
28. Martin-Lorenzo, M.; Gonzalez-Calero, L.; Ramos-Barron, A.; Sanchez-Nino, M.D.; Gomez-Alamillo, C.; Garcia-Segura, J.M.; Ortiz, A.; Arias, M.; Vivanco, F.; Alvarez-Llamas, G. Urine metabolomics insight into acute kidney injury point to oxidative stress disruptions in energy generation and H2S availability. *J. Mol. Med. (Berl)* **2017**, *95*, 1399–1409. [CrossRef]
29. Mercier, K.; McRitchie, S.; Pathmasiri, W.; Novokhatny, A.; Koralkar, R.; Askenazi, D.; Brophy, P.D.; Sumner, S. Preterm neonatal urinary renal developmental and acute kidney injury metabolomic profiling: An exploratory study. *Pediatr. Nephrol.* **2017**, *32*, 151–161. [CrossRef]
30. Elmariah, S.; Farrell, L.A.; Daher, M.; Shi, X.; Keyes, M.J.; Cain, C.H.; Pomerantsev, E.; Vlahakes, G.J.; Inglessis, I.; Passeri, J.J.; et al. Metabolite Profiles Predict Acute Kidney Injury and Mortality in Patients Undergoing Transcatheter Aortic Valve Replacement. *J. Am. Heart Assoc.* **2016**, *5*, e002712. [CrossRef]

31. Doskocz, M.; Marchewka, Z.; Jez, M.; Passowicz-Muszynska, E.; Dlugosz, A. Preliminary Study on J-Resolved NMR Method Usability for Toxic Kidney's Injury Assessment. *Adv. Clin. Exp. Med.* **2015**, *24*, 629–635. [CrossRef] [PubMed]
32. Zacharias, H.U.; Hochrein, J.; Vogl, F.C.; Schley, G.; Mayer, F.; Jeleazcov, C.; Eckardt, K.U.; Willam, C.; Oefner, P.J.; Gronwald, W. Identification of Plasma Metabolites Prognostic of Acute Kidney Injury after Cardiac Surgery with Cardiopulmonary Bypass. *J. Proteome Res.* **2015**, *14*, 2897–2905. [CrossRef] [PubMed]
33. Sun, J.; Shannon, M.; Ando, Y.; Schnackenberg, L.K.; Khan, N.A.; Portilla, D.; Beger, R.D. Serum metabolomic profiles from patients with acute kidney injury: A pilot study. *J. Chromatogr B Analyt Technol. Biomed. Life Sci.* **2012**, *893*, 107–113. [CrossRef] [PubMed]
34. Portilla, D.; Schnackenberg, L.; Beger, R.D. Metabolomics as an extension of proteomic analysis: Study of acute kidney injury. *Semin. Nephrol.* **2007**, *27*, 609–620. [CrossRef]
35. Zgoda-Pols, J.R.; Chowdhury, S.; Wirth, M.; Milburn, M.V.; Alexander, D.C.; Alton, K.B. Metabolomics analysis reveals elevation of 3-indoxyl sulfate in plasma and brain during chemically-induced acute kidney injury in mice: Investigation of nicotinic acid receptor agonists. *Toxicol. Appl. Pharmacol.* **2011**, *255*, 48–56. [CrossRef]
36. Hauet, T.; Baumert, H.; Gibelin, H.; Hameury, F.; Goujon, J.M.; Carretier, M.; Eugene, M. Noninvasive monitoring of citrate, acetate, lactate, and renal medullary osmolyte excretion in urine as biomarkers of exposure to ischemic reperfusion injury. *Cryobiology* **2000**, *41*, 280–291. [CrossRef]
37. Xu, E.Y.; Perlina, A.; Vu, H.; Troth, S.P.; Brennan, R.J.; Aslamkhan, A.G.; Xu, Q. Integrated pathway analysis of rat urine metabolic profiles and kidney transcriptomic profiles to elucidate the systems toxicology of model nephrotoxicants. *Chem. Res. Toxicol.* **2008**, *21*, 1548–1561. [CrossRef]
38. Portilla, D.; Li, S.; Nagothu, K.K.; Megyesi, J.; Kaissling, B.; Schnackenberg, L.; Safirstein, R.L.; Beger, R.D. Metabolomic study of cisplatin-induced nephrotoxicity. *Kidney Int.* **2006**, *69*, 2194–2204. [CrossRef]
39. Shah, V.O.; Townsend, R.R.; Feldman, H.I.; Pappan, K.L.; Kensicki, E.; Vander Jagt, D.L. Plasma metabolomic profiles in different stages of CKD. *Clin. J. Am. Soc. Nephrol.* **2013**, *8*, 363–370. [CrossRef]
40. Luck, M.; Bertho, G.; Bateson, M.; Karras, A.; Yartseva, A.; Thervet, E.; Damon, C.; Pallet, N. Rule-Mining for the Early Prediction of Chronic Kidney Disease Based on Metabolomics and Multi-Source Data. *PLoS ONE* **2016**, *11*, e0166905. [CrossRef]
41. Sharma, K.; Karl, B.; Mathew, A.V.; Gangoiti, J.A.; Wassel, C.L.; Saito, R.; Pu, M.; Sharma, S.; You, Y.H.; Wang, L.; et al. Metabolomics reveals signature of mitochondrial dysfunction in diabetic kidney disease. *J. Am. Soc. Nephrol.* **2013**, *24*, 1901–1912. [CrossRef]
42. Gronwald, W.; Klein, M.S.; Zeltner, R.; Schulze, B.D.; Reinhold, S.W.; Deutschmann, M.; Immervoll, A.K.; Boger, C.A.; Banas, B.; Eckardt, K.U.; et al. Detection of autosomal dominant polycystic kidney disease by NMR spectroscopic fingerprinting of urine. *Kidney Int.* **2011**, *79*, 1244–1253. [CrossRef]
43. Dantzler, W.H. Renal organic anion transport: A comparative and cellular perspective. *Biochim Biophys Acta* **2002**, *1566*, 169–181. [CrossRef]
44. Karniski, L.P.; Aronson, P.S. Chloride/formate exchange with formic acid recycling: A mechanism of active chloride transport across epithelial membranes. *Proc. Natl. Acad Sci. USA* **1985**, *82*, 6362–6365. [CrossRef]
45. Scalabre, A.; Jobard, E.; Demede, D.; Gaillard, S.; Pontoizeau, C.; Mouriquand, P.; Elena-Herrmann, B.; Mure, P.Y. Evolution of Newborns' Urinary Metabolomic Profiles According to Age and Growth. *J. Proteome Res.* **2017**, *16*, 3732–3740. [CrossRef]
46. Gu, H.; Pan, Z.; Xi, B.; Hainline, B.E.; Shanaiah, N.; Asiago, V.; Gowda, G.A.; Raftery, D. 1H NMR metabolomics study of age profiling in children. *NMR Biomed.* **2009**, *22*, 826–833. [CrossRef]
47. Chiu, C.Y.; Yeh, K.W.; Lin, G.; Chiang, M.H.; Yang, S.C.; Chao, W.J.; Yao, T.C.; Tsai, M.H.; Hua, M.C.; Liao, S.L.; et al. Metabolomics Reveals Dynamic Metabolic Changes Associated with Age in Early Childhood. *PLoS ONE* **2016**, *11*, e0149823. [CrossRef]
48. Westhoff, J.H.; Seibert, F.S.; Waldherr, S.; Bauer, F.; Tonshoff, B.; Fichtner, A.; Westhoff, T.H. Urinary calprotectin, kidney injury molecule-1, and neutrophil gelatinase-associated lipocalin for the prediction of adverse outcome in pediatric acute kidney injury. *Eur. J. Pediatr.* **2017**, *176*, 745–755. [CrossRef]
49. Westhoff, J.H.; Tonshoff, B.; Waldherr, S.; Poschl, J.; Teufel, U.; Westhoff, T.H.; Fichtner, A. Urinary Tissue Inhibitor of Metalloproteinase-2 (TIMP-2) * Insulin-Like Growth Factor-Binding Protein 7 (IGFBP7) Predicts Adverse Outcome in Pediatric Acute Kidney Injury. *PLoS ONE* **2015**, *10*, e0143628. [CrossRef]

50. Kellum, J.A.; Lameire, N.; Group, K.A.G.W. Diagnosis, evaluation, and management of acute kidney injury: A KDIGO summary (Part 1). *Crit. Care.* **2013**, *17*, 204. [CrossRef]
51. Selewski, D.T.; Charlton, J.R.; Jetton, J.G.; Guillet, R.; Mhanna, M.J.; Askenazi, D.J.; Kent, A.L. Neonatal Acute Kidney Injury. *Pediatrics* **2015**, *136*, e463–e473. [CrossRef]
52. Schwartz, G.J.; Munoz, A.; Schneider, M.F.; Mak, R.H.; Kaskel, F.; Warady, B.A.; Furth, S.L. New equations to estimate GFR in children with CKD. *J. Am. Soc. Nephrol.* **2009**, *20*, 629–637. [CrossRef]
53. Chong, J.; Xia, J. MetaboAnalystR: An R package for flexible and reproducible analysis of metabolomics data. *Bioinformatics* **2018**, *34*, 4313–4314. [CrossRef]
54. Dieterle, F.; Ross, A.; Schlotterbeck, G.; Senn, H. Probabilistic quotient normalization as robust method to account for dilution of complex biological mixtures. Application in 1H NMR metabonomics. *Anal. Chem.* **2006**, *78*, 4281–4290. [CrossRef]

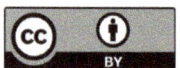

© 2020 by the authors. Licensee MDPI, Basel, Switzerland. This article is an open access article distributed under the terms and conditions of the Creative Commons Attribution (CC BY) license (http://creativecommons.org/licenses/by/4.0/).

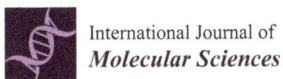

Article

Mitochondrial Dynamics of Proximal Tubular Epithelial Cells in Nephropathic Cystinosis

Domenico De Rasmo [1,*,†], Anna Signorile [2,†], Ester De Leo [3], Elena V. Polishchuk [4], Anna Ferretta [1], Roberto Raso [3], Silvia Russo [2], Roman Polishchuk [4], Francesco Emma [5] and Francesco Bellomo [3,*]

1. Institute of Biomembranes, Bioenergetics and Molecular Biotechnology (IBIOM), National Research Council (CNR), 70124 Bari, Italy; a.ferretta@ibiom.cnr.it
2. Department of Basic Medical Sciences, Neurosciences and Sense Organs, University of Bari "Aldo Moro", 70124 Bari, Italy; anna.signorile@uniba.it (A.S.); silvia.russo92@gmail.com (S.R.)
3. Renal Diseases Research Unit, Genetics and Rare Diseases Research Division, Bambino Gesù Children's Hospital—IRCCS, 00146 Rome, Italy; ester.deleo@opbg.net (E.D.L.); roberto.raso@opbg.net (R.R.)
4. Telethon Institute of Genetics and Medicine, 80078 Pozzuoli, Italy; epolish@tigem.it (E.V.P.); polishchuk@tigem.it (R.P.)
5. Division of Nephrology, Department of Pediatric Subspecialties, Bambino Gesù Children's Hospital—IRCCS, 00165 Rome, Italy; francesco.emma@opbg.net
* Correspondence: d.derasmo@ibiom.cnr.it (D.D.R.); francesco.bellomo@opbg.net (F.B.); Tel.: +39-080-5448516 (D.D.R.); +39-06-68592997 (F.B)
† These authors contribute equally to this work.

Received: 29 November 2019; Accepted: 24 December 2019; Published: 26 December 2019

Abstract: Nephropathic cystinosis is a rare lysosomal storage disorder caused by mutations in *CTNS* gene leading to Fanconi syndrome. Independent studies reported defective clearance of damaged mitochondria and mitochondrial fragmentation in cystinosis. Proteins involved in the mitochondrial dynamics and the mitochondrial ultrastructure were analyzed in *CTNS*−/− cells treated with cysteamine, the only drug currently used in the therapy for cystinosis but ineffective to treat Fanconi syndrome. *CTNS*−/− cells showed an overexpression of parkin associated with deregulation of ubiquitination of mitofusin 2 and fission 1 proteins, an altered proteolytic processing of optic atrophy 1 (OPA1), and a decreased OPA1 oligomerization. According to molecular findings, the analysis of electron microscopy images showed a decrease of mitochondrial cristae number and an increase of cristae lumen and cristae junction width. Cysteamine treatment restored the fission 1 ubiquitination, the mitochondrial size, number and lumen of cristae, but had no effect on cristae junction width, making *CTNS*−/− tubular cells more susceptible to apoptotic stimuli.

Keywords: Fanconi syndrome; nephropathic cystinosis; mitochondrial dynamics; cysteamine; mitochondrial fusion; mitochondrial fission; mitochondrial cristae

1. Introduction

Nephropathic cystinosis (MIM 219800) is a rare inherited metabolic disease characterized by an impaired transport of the amino acid cystine out of lysosomes due to reduced or absent function of the specific carrier cystinosin, which is encoded by *CTNS* gene [1–3]. Kidneys are affected at the initial stage of the disease, leading to early onset Fanconi syndrome, which is characterized by polyuria, glycosuria, phosphaturia, aminoaciduria, and urinary loss of electrolytes and low-molecular-weight proteins [4]. The cystine-depleting agent, cysteamine (MEA), significantly delays symptoms [5,6], but does not treat Fanconi syndrome and is ineffective to prevent the progression of kidney disease. Fanconi syndrome has also been reported in children with specific mitochondrial syndromes [7]. Renal tubular cells are very rich in mitochondria due to the intense reabsorption and excretion processes that occur in this district. We recently reported, in *CTNS−/−* cells derived from proximal tubules, mitochondrial fragmentation associated with respiratory chain dysfunction and low mitochondrial 3′,5′-cyclic adenosine monophosphate (cAMP) levels [8]. Furthermore, enhanced apoptosis [9,10], defect of autophagic flux [11,12], and endo-lysosomal dysfunction [13,14] were observed.

Communication between mitochondria and the endo-lysosomal system is complex. Increasing evidences show close relationship between these two cellular compartments [15,16]. Mitochondria constantly undergo fission and fusion processes to adapt to environmental changes in a continuous and balanced way, in order to maintain morphology and regulate cellular ATP levels. Mitochondrial fission regulates the production of new mitochondria and the segregation of damaged mitochondria. In this process, receptor proteins such as mitochondrial fission factor (Mff), mitochondrial fission 1 protein (Fis1), mitochondrial dynamics protein of 49 kDa (MiD49), and mitochondrial dynamics protein of 51 kDa (MiD51) recruit the large GTPase dynamin-related protein 1 (Drp1) from the cytosol to the outer mitochondrial membrane (OMM), which forms a multimeric complex with mitochondrial membrane adaptors [17,18]. Mitochondrial fusion is mediated by three key regulatory fusion proteins: the dynamin-related GTPases mitofusin 1 (MFN1) and mitofusin 2 (MFN2), responsible for the fusion of OMM and the dynamin-related GTPases optic atrophy 1 (OPA1), which mediates fusion of the inner mitochondrial membrane (IMM) and contributes to the maintenance of mitochondrial potential, to control respiratory chain activity and apoptosis [19,20]. When mitochondrial dynamics are impaired, dysfunctional mitochondria are selectively eliminated through mitophagy, which is initiated by ubiquitin-dependent or ubiquitin-independent signals [21]. The lysosomal alterations in cystinosis lead to defective autophagic clearance of damaged mitochondria [12], therefore the purpose of our study was to investigate mitochondrial dynamics in *CTNS−/−* conditionally immortalized proximal tubular epithelial cells (ciPTEC) carrying the classical homozygous 57-kb deletion in the intent of identifying new therapeutic targets and biomarkers for treatment follow-up.

2. Results

2.1. CTNS−/− ciPTEC Showed Deregulation of Proteins Involved in Mitochondrial Fission/Fusion Processes

Recruitment of the GTPase dynamin-related protein 1 (Drp1) to mitochondria is a key step required for mitochondrial fission and its reversible phosphorylation was implicated in the regulation of this process. The analysis of phosphorylated Drp1 at Ser-637 (Drp1^{pS637}) showed high variability of protein phosphorylation with no significant differences in wild type and *CTNS−/−* ciPTEC, also 24 h treatment with 100 μM cysteamine (MEA) did not affect Drp1^{pS637} phosphorylation (Figure 1). The western blotting of the pro-fission mitochondrial protein Fis1 revealed the ubiquitinated and not-ubiquitinated forms of protein. *CTNS−/−* ciPTEC showed increased level of Fis1 (2.47 ± 0.27 vs. 1.08 ± 0.08, $p = 0.0027$). Treatment with 100 μM MEA for 24 h further increased total Fis1 protein level (2.47 ± 0.27 vs. 3.59 ± 0.15, $p = 0.011$) but almost completely reduced the ubiquitinated counterpart by 96.3% ($p < 0.001$) (Figure 1). Third key regulatory protein analyzed was mitochondrial fission factor (Mff), which localizes on OMM and promotes the recruitment of DRP1 to the mitochondrial surface. This protein, shown in its four isoforms, was not modified in *CTNS−/−* ciPTEC and the expression was unchanged after MEA treatment (Figure 1).

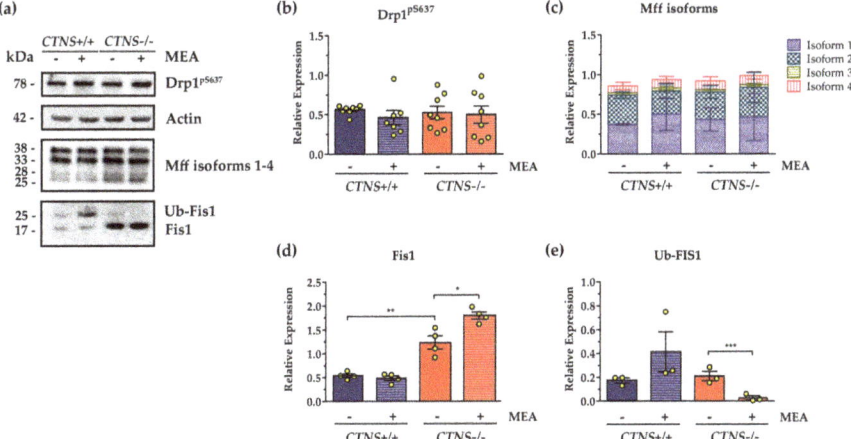

Figure 1. Analysis of proteins involved in fission process of mitochondrial dynamics in untreated and cysteamine (MEA)-treated *CTNS−/−* compared to *CTNS+/+*. Cell cultures were treated with 100 µM cysteamine (MEA) or DMSO (vehicle) for 24 h as specified in the figure. (**a**) Representative immunoblotting analysis in cellular lysate of conditionally immortalized proximal tubular epithelial cells (ciPTEC) from a healthy subject (*CTNS+/+*) and cystinotic patient (*CTNS−/−*). (**b–e**) The histograms (Drp1^{pS637}, panel (**b**), $n = 8$; mitochondrial fission factor (Mff), panel (**c**), $n = 3$; mitochondrial fission 1 protein (Fis1), panel (**d**), $n = 4$; ubiquitinated Fis1 (Ub-Fis1), panel (**e**), $n = 3$) represent the means values ± SEM of the relative expression normalized on actin level. Densitometric analysis was performed by Versa-Doc imaging system BioRad, using Quantity One software. *p*-value less than 0.05 was considered as statistically significant, (Student's *t* test, *** $p < 0.001$; ** $p < 0.01$; * $p < 0.05$). For further details see under "materials and methods" section.

The inner mitochondrial membrane GTPase OPA1 undergoes constitutive processing leading to the conversion of the un-cleaved long OPA1 (L-OPA1) in cleaved short variants (S-OPA1). Various stress conditions, including apoptotic stimuli, trigger the complete conversion of L-OPA1 into S-OPA1. In this regard, *CTNS−/−* ciPTEC were characterized by a significant increase of short variants (52.4%, $p < 0.05$), but 24 h treatment with 100 µM MEA did not show significant effects (Figure 2). In agreement with higher S-OPA1 levels, we found that the active form of mitochondrial metallo-endopetidase OMA1, which catalyze conversion of OPA1 into short isoforms and triggers mitochondrial fragmentation, was increased by 79.8% in *CTNS−/−* ciPTEC ($p < 0.001$), and not rescued by MEA treatment (Figure 2). OPA1 can oligomerize at the inner mitochondrial membrane to keep the cristae junction tight, therefore cell fresh pellets were treated with the cross-linker bis-maleimidohexane (BMH) 1 mM or with vehicle to test the oligomeric state of OPA1. The OPA1 oligomer, immune-revealed as a high molecular-weight band (≈250 kDa), decreased in *CTNS−/−* cells by 23.5% compared to *CTNS+/+* cells and was not affected by MEA treatment. The absence of OPA1 oligomerization in cells treated with vehicle (DMSO) confirmed the specificity of cross-linking (Figure 2).

The expression of MFN2, an outer mitochondrial membrane GTPase involved in fusion processes, was not changed in *CTNS−/−* ciPTEC with respect to control cells (Figure 3). However, the higher molecular weight band, corresponding to ubiquitinated MFN2, indicated an increase of ubiquitination in *CTNS−/−* ciPTEC by 70.8% ($p < 0.001$). Treatment with MEA showed 37.8% reduction of ubiquitination but the effect was not statistically significant (Figure 3).

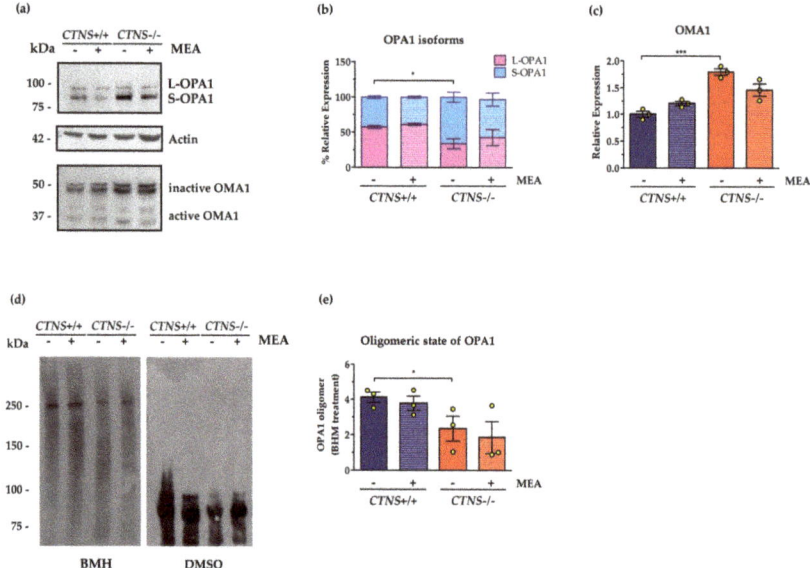

Figure 2. Processing and oligomerization of optic atrophy 1 (OPA1) fusion protein in untreated and MEA-treated *CTNS−/−* compared to *CTNS+/+*. (**a**) Representative immunoblotting analysis of ciPTEC obtained from *CTNS+/+* and *CTNS−/−*. Where indicated, the cells were treated with MEA or DMSO (vehicle) for 24 h. The histograms of OPA1 (**b**) represent the percentage of relative expression of L and S forms of OPA1 in each lane ($n = 3$). The histograms of OMA1 (**c**) represent the means values ± SEM of the relative expression normalized on actin level ($n = 3$). (**d**) The fresh collected cells were treated with the cross-linker 1,6-bismaleimidohexane (BMH) 1 mM or with vehicle (DMSO) for 30 min at 37 °C, then centrifuged and resuspended in sodium dodecyl sulfate (SDS) lysis buffer for western blotting analysis with the antibody against OPA1. (**e**) The histograms represent the means values ± SEM of the relative expression of OPA1 oligomers ($n = 3$). Densitometric analysis was performed by Versa-Doc imaging system BioRad, using Quantity One software. Student's *t* test, *** $p < 0.001$; * $p < 0.05$. For further details see under "materials and methods" section.

Numerous mitochondrial outer membrane proteins are modified with K48- and K63-linked ubiquitin chains, including the mitochondrial fusion factors MFN1 and MFN2 and fission factors Fis1 and Drp1, triggering a cascade of events that result in mitophagy. According with previous results, we found in *CTNS−/−* ciPTEC a significant increase in protein levels of the E3 ubiquitin ligase parkin (2.92 ± 0.22 in *CTNS−/−* vs. 1.0 ± 0.04 in *CTNS+/+*, $p = 0.001$). MEA treatment did not change parkin expression (Figure 4A). Ubiquitin carboxyl-terminal hydrolase 30 (USP30) mediates the removal of the ubiquitin chains added by parkin to ubiquitilated forms of mitofusins, such as MFN2, therefore we analyzed the expression of this deubiquitinating enzyme tethered to the OMM and showed in *CTNS−/−* ciPTEC 62.9% decreasing compared to wild type cells ($p < 0.001$). Treatment with MEA rescued USP30 expression in *CTNS−/−* ciPTEC by 87.9% ($p = 0.037$) (Figure 4B).

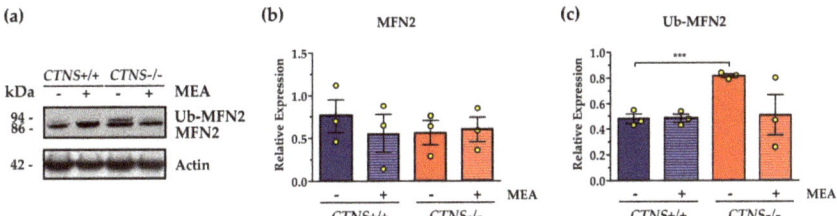

Figure 3. Expression and ubiquitination of mitofusin 2 (MFN2) in untreated and MEA-treated *CTNS*+/+ and *CTNS*−/−. (**a**) Representative immunoblotting analysis of untreated and MEA-treated ciPTEC *CTNS*+/+ and *CTNS*−/−. (**b**) The histogram of MFN2, *n* = 3, and (**c**) the histogram of ubiquitinated MFN2 Ub-MFN2, *n* = 3, represent the mean values ± SEM of the relative expression normalized on actin level. Densitometric analysis was performed by Versa-Doc imaging system BioRad, using Quantity One software. Student's *t* test, *** $p < 0.001$.

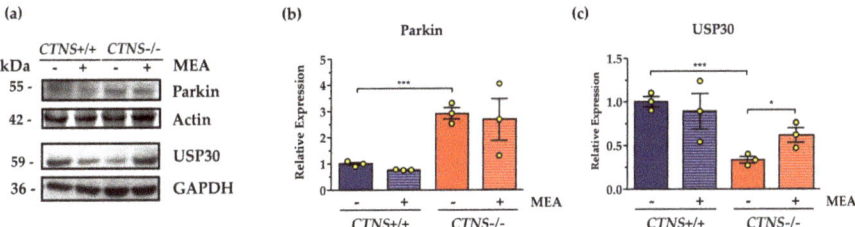

Figure 4. Parkin and ubiquitin carboxyl-terminal hydrolase 30 (USP30) proteins levels and MEA effect in *CTNS*+/+ and *CTNS*−/−. (**a**) Immunoblotting analysis of untreated and MEA-treated ciPTEC *CTNS*+/+ and *CTNS*−/−. (**b**) The histogram represents the means values ± SEM of the relative expression of Parkin normalized on actin level (*n* = 3). (**c**) The histogram represents the means values ± SEM of the relative expression of USP30 normalized on actin level (*n* = 3). Densitometric analysis was performed by Versa-Doc imaging system BioRad, using Quantity One software. Student's *t* test, *** $p < 0.001$; * $p < 0.05$.

2.2. Mitochondrial Cristae Organization Was Impaired in CTNS−/− ciPTEC

Comparative ultrastructural analysis of mitochondria in ciPTEC, by transmission electron microscopy (TEM), showed the presence of smaller mitochondria in *CTNS*−/− ciPTEC compared to *CTNS*+/+ ciPTEC (0.12 ± 0.01 µm² in *CTNS*−/− vs. 0.26 ± 0.01 µm² in *CTNS*+/+, $p < 0.0001$). Mitochondrial area was completely recovered by MEA treatment (0.32 ± 0.04 µm² in *CTNS*−/− + MEA vs. 0.12 ± 0.01 µm² in *CTNS*−/−, $p < 0.0001$). Moreover, TEM showed a substantial reduction in number of cristae per mitochondrial section in *CTNS*−/− (5.1 ± 0.6 in *CTNS*+/+ vs. 1.6 ± 0.2 in *CTNS*−/−, $p < 0.0001$). This parameter was rescued by MEA by 167.5% ($p < 0.0001$). Because evidences underlined a critical role of cristae junction in mitochondrial function and organization, we measured them. It was found an increase in cristae junction width (39.65 ± 4.83 nm in *CTNS*+/+ vs. 53.21 ± 10.05 nm in *CTNS*−/−, $p < 0.0001$) and cristae lumen width (29.68 ± 3.53 nm in *CTNS*+/+ vs. 37.04 ± 6.13 nm in *CTNS*−/−, $p < 0.0003$) partially rescued by cysteamine (Figure 5).

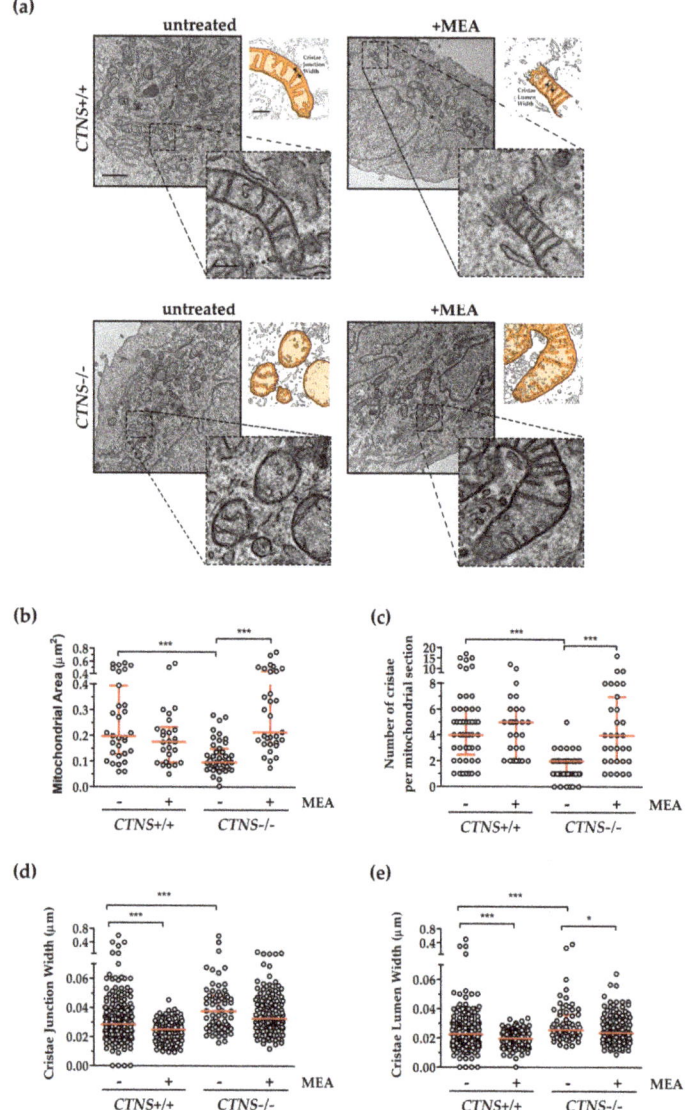

Figure 5. Comparative ultrastructural analysis of mitochondria in ciPTEC. (**a**) Representative images of TEM with magnification 16,000× of untreated and MEA-treated ciPTEC *CTNS+/+* and *CTNS−/−*; scale bar = 1 µm. As shown in high magnification cropped micrographs and in ad hoc schematic reconstruction, mitochondria kept preserved ultrastructure in ciPTEC *CTNS+/+* and in MEA-treated ciPTEC *CTNS+/+* and *CTNS−/−*, whereas ciPTEC *CTNS−/−* showed disruption of mitochondrial cristae and the disarrangement of the internal structures; scale bar = 200 nm. (**b**–**e**) Quantitative analysis was performed with ImageJ v.1.52p in $n \geq 5$ double-blind acquisitions for each experimental condition, red lines represent median with interquartile range. (**b**) Evaluation of relative mitochondrial size measured as area of $n \geq 27$ mitochondrial sections. (**c**) Average number of cristae per mitochondrion in each cell ($n \geq 27$ mitochondrial sections). (**d**) The measure of distance of cristae junction near the inner membrane boundary and (**e**) the measure of cristae lumen, assessed on cristae membranes that outline the lumen boundary, were assessed in $n \geq 100$ cristae. Non-parametric Mann-Whitney test was applied, *** $p < 0.001$; * $p < 0.05$.

3. Discussion

Nephropathic cystinosis is a rare inherited metabolic disorder, belonging to the group of lysosomal storage diseases (LSD). The disease is the first cause of Fanconi syndrome in children, characterized by loss of electrolytes, glucose, amino acid, low-molecular weight proteins in urine caused by proximal tubule dysfunction [4,22]. The molecular mechanism at the basis of Fanconi syndrome in cystinosis is not completely understood. Several mechanisms have been suggested to contribute to the pathogenesis of cystinosis, including lysosomal overload, endo-lysosomal transport defect, altered chaperone-mediated autophagy, mTOR signaling, transcription factor EB (TFEB) expression [11,13,23–27]. Cysteamine, a cystine-depleting agent, which allows clearance of cystine from lysosomes, represents the only specific treatment for cystinosis. However, cysteamine does not correct the above cited cellular alterations and does not stop the progress of the Fanconi syndrome. Our recent studies have shown in CTNS−/− ciPTEC a higher mitochondrial fragmentation index associated with lower mitochondrial potential and mitochondrial cyclic AMP levels, rescued by 24 h treatment with 100 µM cysteamine or with the cell-permeant analogue of cyclic AMP, 8-Br-cAMP [8]. cAMP, in fact, is one of the major regulators of mitochondrial function [28–30] and dynamics [31]. In this contest, it should be noted that MEA has been found to improve mitochondrial function in mitochondrial respiratory chain diseases [32]. Mitochondrial dynamics is balanced between rates of fusion and fission that respond to pathophysiologic signals. This finely regulated equilibrium is closely related to the quality control system, which is mainly ascribed to the ubiquitin protease system (UPS) and to the intra-mitochondrial proteolytic systems [33]. In our experimental model, no significant differences were observed on protein levels of phosphorylated Drp1 at Ser-637. The PKA-dependent phosphorylation of Drp1 at Ser-637 is generally recognized to block Drp1 GTPase activity and to suppress mitochondrial fission. However, and in agreement with data previously reported by Yu et al., Drp1^{PS637} did not contribute substantially to mitochondrial fission regulation in CTNS−/− ciPTEC [18]. Several key effector proteins of mitochondrial fusion (MFN1 and MFN2) and fission (Fis1, Mff) are located at the OMM with their domains exposed at the cytosolic side of the membrane. This peculiar topology allows selective removing of fusion or fission components exposed by the UPS, providing fine tuning of this high-level regulatory processes. In mammalian cells, Fis1 accumulates in the mitochondrial outer membrane during the fission process, whereas MFN1 and MFN2 are ubiquitinated and degraded by the proteasome [34]. In this respect, we observed an increase in Fis1, ubiquitinated MFN2 and of the E3 ubiquitin ligase Parkin in CTNS−/− ciPTEC, indicating the tendency to mitochondrial fragmentation. The effect of MEA on the reduction of ubiquitilated MFN2 could be ascribed to the modulation of USP30, a mitochondrion-localized deubiquitilase, which counteracts Parkin by deubiquitilating OMM proteins and regulate mitophagy [35]. These findings are consistent with data showing that an increase of parkin expression results in mitochondrial fragmentation [36] and is associated with MFN2 ubiquitination [37]. In addition, the increase of FIS1, in cystinotic cell, might be due to Sirt3 protein [38] that was found downregulated in the same cystinotic cell line [8]. OPA1, an inner mitochondrial membrane GTPase protein, has gained attention because it regulates important mitochondrial functions, including the balance between mitochondrial fusion and fission processes, the stability of the mitochondrial respiratory chain complexes, the proapoptotic release of cytochrome c molecules sequestered within the mitochondrial cristae and the maintenance of mitochondrial cristae architecture [39]. The protein expression levels of OPA1 were not significantly changed in mutated cells, compared to control ciPTEC cells (data not shown). However, the activity of OPA1 is also controlled at the post-translational level by proteolytic and acetylation changes [31]. Various stress conditions, including apoptotic stimulation, trigger the complete conversion of L-OPA1 into S-OPA1. The pro-fusion activity of OPA1 depends on the balanced formation of L-OPA1 and S-OPA1 [40]. In this respect, we observed an alteration of OPA1 processing in CTNS−/− ciPTEC cells. In particular, cystinotic cells were characterized by a significant increase of S-OPA1, associated with an increase in the protease OMA1 activity, that was not prevented by MEA. In addition to its role as a fusion protein, OPA1 controls the remodeling of mitochondrial cristae. Specifically, OPA1 forms oligomers in the inner mitochondrial membrane that keep the cristae junctions tight. During apoptosis, oligomers are destabilized causing the opening of cristae and release of cytochrome c out of the mitochondria. OPA1 oligomers were decreased in cystinotic cells. MEA did not rescue this phenotype. This defect correlates with increased cristae junction width that we observed in our TEM ultrastructural analyses.

In summary, our study shows deregulation of several proteins involved in mitochondrial dynamics in *CTNS*−/− cells. We observed mitochondrial fragmentation in cystinotic cells associated with altered proteolytic processing of OPA1, increased Fis1 and parkin protein levels. The deregulation of parkin could result in increase of ubiquitination of MFN2. The cristae number was decreased while the cristae lumen was increased in cystinotic cells, which parallels the previously reported bioenergetic defects in these cells. The cristae junction width was increased in *CTNS*−/− cells, which is most likely secondary to low OPA1 oligomerization levels. MEA treatment restored mitochondrial size, cristae number, and lumen, but had no effect on cristae junction width, making tubular cells more susceptible to apoptotic stimuli. In this contest, we highlight several cellular mediators of mitochondrial dynamics that could be useful to develop new therapeutic interventions [41].

4. Materials and Methods

4.1. Cell Culture

Conditionally immortalized proximal tubular epithelial cells (ciPTEC), from healthy donor and cystinotic patients were obtained from Radboud University Medical Center, Nijmegen, The Netherlands and cultured as described in [42]. Cells were grown in a humidified atmosphere with 5% CO_2 at 37 °C. Where indicated, the cells were treated with 100 μM MEA or water (vehicle) for 24 h.

4.2. SDS-PAGE and Western Blotting

Monolayer cell cultures were harvested with 0.05% trypsin, 0.02% EDTA. After trypsinization, cells were centrifuged at 500× g and resuspended in RIPA buffer (150 mM NaCl, 5 mM EDTA, 50 mM Tris/HCl, 0.1% SDS, 1% Triton X-100, pH 7.4), in the presence of a protease inhibitor (0.25 mM PMSF). Cell lysate proteins were subjected to SDS-polyacrylamide gel electrophoresis (PAGE), transferred to a nitrocellulose membrane and immunoblotted with antibodies against OPA1 (Thermo scientific, Waltham, MA, USA; Pierce Antibodies); Fis1; Mfn2 (Merck Millipore, Burlington, MA, USA); parkin, USP30 (Santa Cruz Biotechnology, Dallas, TX, USA); OMA1 (Abcam, Cambridge, UK); Drp1, Mff (Cell Signaling, Danvers, MA, USA) and actin (Merck, Kenilworth, NJ, USA). After being washed in TTBS, the membranes were incubated for 1 h with anti-mouse or anti-rabbit IgG peroxidase-conjugate antibody. Immunodetection was performed with the enhanced chemiluminescence (ECL) (Thermo scientific, Waltham, MA, USA). VersaDoc imaging system (BioRad, Milan, Italy) was used for densitometric analysis.

4.3. Analysis of OPA1 Oligomers

To investigate on OPA1 oligomerization, cell fresh pellets were treated with the cross-linker bismaleimidohexane (BMH) 1 mM or with vehicle (DMSO) for 30 min at 37 °C. After incubation, the samples were centrifuged, resuspended in SDS lysis buffer and then subjected to SDS-PAGE and western blotting analysis with the antibody against OPA1.

4.4. Electron Microscopy

For routine EM the cells were grown in 12 well plates as a monolayer. At the end of the experiment the cells were fixed with 1% Glutaraldehyde prepared in 0.2 M Hepes buffer. Then the cells were scraped, pelleted, post-fixed in OsO4 and uranyl acetate and embedded in Epon as described previously [43]. From each sample, thin 60 nm sections were cut using Leica EM UC7 (Leica Microsystems, Vienna, Austria). EM images were acquired from thin sections using a FEI Tecnai-12 electron microscope

(FEI, Eindhoven, Netherlands) equipped with a VELETTA CCD digital camera (Soft Imaging Systems GmbH, Munster, Germany).

Author Contributions: F.B. and D.D.R. conceptualization; A.S., E.D.L., E.V.P., A.F., R.R., and S.R. investigation; F.B. and D.D.R. writing—original draft preparation; F.B., D.D.R., A.S., R.P., and F.E. writing—review and editing; F.B. and D.D.R. funding acquisition. All authors have read and agreed to the published version of the manuscript.

Funding: This research was funded by Cystinosis Research Foundation, grant number CRFF-2017-001 and by Ricerca Corrente of the Italian Ministry of Health.

Acknowledgments: We thank Paolo Lattanzio for technical assistance and Manuela Colucci for statistical analysis contribution.

Conflicts of Interest: The authors declare no conflict of interest.

Abbreviations

cAMP	3′,5′-cyclic adenosine monophosphate
Fis1	Mitochondrial fission 1 protein
IMM	Inner Mitochondrial Membrane
MEA	β-Mercaptoethylamine (cysteamine)
Mff	Mitochondrial fission factor
OMM	Outer Mitochondrial Membrane
OPA1	Dynamin-related GTPases Optic Atrophy 1
TEMTFEB	Transmission Electron MicroscopyTranscription factor EB
UPS	Ubiquitin Protease System
USP30	Ubiquitin carboxyl-terminal hydrolase 30

References

1. Cherqui, S.; Sevin, C.; Hamard, G.; Kalatzis, V.; Sich, M.; Pequignot, M.O.; Gogat, K.; Abitbol, M.; Broyer, M.; Gubler, M.C.; et al. Intralysosomal Cystine Accumulation in Mice Lacking Cystinosin, the Protein Defective in Cystinosis. *Mol. Cell. Biol.* **2002**, *22*, 7622–7632. [CrossRef] [PubMed]
2. Gahl, W.A.; Bashan, N.; Tietze, F.; Bernardini, I.; Schulman, J.D. Cystine Transport is Defective in Isolated Leukocyte Lysosomes from Patients with Cystinosis. *Science* **1982**, *217*, 1263–1265. [CrossRef] [PubMed]
3. Town, M.; Jean, G.; Cherqui, S.; Attard, M.; Forestier, L.; Whitmore, S.A.; Callen, D.F.; Gribouval, O.; Broyer, M.; Bates, G.P.; et al. A Novel Gene Encoding an Integral Membrane Protein is Mutated in Nephropathic Cystinosis. *Nat. Genet.* **1998**, *18*, 319–324. [CrossRef] [PubMed]
4. Cherqui, S.; Courtoy, P.J. The Renal Fanconi Syndrome in Cystinosis: Pathogenic Insights and Therapeutic Perspectives. *Nat. Rev. Nephrol.* **2017**, *13*, 115–131. [CrossRef] [PubMed]
5. Conforti, A.; Taranta, A.; Biagini, S.; Starc, N.; Pitisci, A.; Bellomo, F.; Cirillo, V.; Locatelli, F.; Bernardo, M.E.; Emma, F. Cysteamine Treatment Restores the in Vitro Ability to Differentiate Along the Osteoblastic Lineage of Mesenchymal Stromal Cells Isolated from Bone Marrow of a Cystinotic Patient. *J. Transl. Med.* **2015**, *13*, 143. [CrossRef] [PubMed]
6. Medic, G.; van der Weijden, M.; Karabis, A.; Hemels, M. A Systematic Literature Review of Cysteamine Bitartrate in the Treatment of Nephropathic Cystinosis. *Curr. Med. Res. Opin.* **2017**, *33*, 2065–2076. [CrossRef] [PubMed]
7. Emma, F.; Montini, G.; Parikh, S.M.; Salviati, L. Mitochondrial Dysfunction in Inherited Renal Disease and Acute Kidney Injury. *Nat. Rev. Nephrol.* **2016**, *12*, 267–280. [CrossRef]
8. Bellomo, F.; Signorile, A.; Tamma, G.; Ranieri, M.; Emma, F.; De Rasmo, D. Impact of Atypical Mitochondrial Cyclic-AMP Level in Nephropathic Cystinosis. *Cell Mol. Life Sci.* **2018**, *75*, 3411–3422. [CrossRef]
9. Park, M.; Helip-Wooley, A.; Thoene, J. Lysosomal Cystine Storage Augments Apoptosis in Cultured Human Fibroblasts and Renal Tubular Epithelial Cells. *J. Am. Soc. Nephrol.* **2002**, *13*, 2878–2887. [CrossRef]
10. Taranta, A.; Bellomo, F.; Petrini, S.; Polishchuk, E.; De Leo, E.; Rega, L.R.; Pastore, A.; Polishchuk, R.; De Matteis, M.A.; Emma, F. Cystinosin-LKG Rescues Cystine Accumulation and Decreases Apoptosis Rate in Cystinotic Proximal Tubular Epithelial Cells. *Pediatr. Res.* **2016**, *81*, 113. [CrossRef]

11. Napolitano, G.; Johnson, J.L.; He, J.; Rocca, C.J.; Monfregola, J.; Pestonjamasp, K.; Cherqui, S.; Catz, S.D. Impairment of Chaperone-Mediated Autophagy Leads to Selective Lysosomal Degradation Defects in the Lysosomal Storage Disease Cystinosis. *EMBO Mol. Med.* **2015**, *7*, 158–174. [CrossRef] [PubMed]
12. Festa, B.P.; Chen, Z.; Berquez, M.; Debaix, H.; Tokonami, N.; Prange, J.A.; Hoek, G.V.; Alessio, C.; Raimondi, A.; Nevo, N.; et al. Impaired Autophagy Bridges Lysosomal Storage Disease and Epithelial Dysfunction in the Kidney. *Nat. Commun.* **2018**, *9*, 161. [CrossRef] [PubMed]
13. Raggi, C.; Luciani, A.; Nevo, N.; Antignac, C.; Terryn, S.; Devuyst, O. Dedifferentiation and Aberrations of the Endolysosomal Compartment Characterize the Early Stage of Nephropathic Cystinosis. *Hum. Mol. Genet.* **2014**, *23*, 2266–2278. [CrossRef] [PubMed]
14. Ivanova, E.A.; De Leo, M.G.; Van Den Heuvel, L.; Pastore, A.; Dijkman, H.; De Matteis, M.A.; Levtchenko, E.N. Endo-Lysosomal Dysfunction in Human Proximal Tubular Epithelial Cells Deficient for Lysosomal Cystine Transporter Cystinosin. *PLoS ONE* **2015**, *10*, 120998. [CrossRef]
15. Soto-Heredero, G.; Baixauli, F.; Mittelbrunn, M. Interorganelle Communication between Mitochondria and the Endolysosomal System. *Front. Cell. Dev. Biol.* **2017**, *5*, 95. [CrossRef]
16. Wong, Y.C.; Ysselstein, D.; Krainc, D. Mitochondria-Lysosome Contacts Regulate Mitochondrial Fission via RAB7 GTP Hydrolysis. *Nature* **2018**, *554*, 382–386. [CrossRef]
17. Koirala, S.; Guo, Q.; Kalia, R.; Bui, H.T.; Eckert, D.M.; Frost, A.; Shaw, J.M. Interchangeable Adaptors Regulate Mitochondrial Dynamin Assembly for Membrane Scission. *Proc. Natl. Acad. Sci. USA* **2013**, *110*, 1342–1351. [CrossRef]
18. Yu, R.; Liu, T.; Ning, C.; Tan, F.; Jin, S.B.; Lendahl, U.; Zhao, J.; Nister, M. The Phosphorylation Status of Ser-637 in Dynamin-Related Protein 1 (Drp1) does Not Determine Drp1 Recruitment to Mitochondria. *J. Biol. Chem.* **2019**, *294*, 17262–17277. [CrossRef]
19. Pernas, L.; Scorrano, L. Mito-Morphosis: Mitochondrial Fusion, Fission, and Cristae Remodeling as Key Mediators of Cellular Function. *Annu. Rev. Physiol.* **2016**, *78*, 505–531. [CrossRef]
20. Zhang, J.; Liu, X.; Liang, X.; Lu, Y.; Zhu, L.; Fu, R.; Ji, Y.; Fan, W.; Chen, J.; Lin, B.; et al. A Novel ADOA-Associated OPA1 Mutation Alters the Mitochondrial Function, Membrane Potential, ROS Production and Apoptosis. *Sci. Rep.* **2017**, *7*, 5704. [CrossRef]
21. Khaminets, A.; Behl, C.; Dikic, I. Ubiquitin-Dependent and Independent Signals in Selective Autophagy. *Trends Cell Biol.* **2016**, *26*, 6–16. [CrossRef] [PubMed]
22. Emma, F.; Nesterova, G.; Langman, C.; Labbe, A.; Cherqui, S.; Goodyer, P.; Janssen, M.C.; Greco, M.; Topaloglu, R.; Elenberg, E.; et al. Nephropathic Cystinosis: An International Consensus Document. *Nephrol. Dial. Transplant.* **2014**, *29*, 87–94. [CrossRef] [PubMed]
23. Gaide Chevronnay, H.P.; Janssens, V.; Van Der Smissen, P.; N'Kuli, F.; Nevo, N.; Guiot, Y.; Levtchenko, E.; Marbaix, E.; Pierreux, C.E.; Cherqui, S.; et al. Time Course of Pathogenic and Adaptation Mechanisms in Cystinotic Mouse Kidneys. *J. Am. Soc. Nephrol.* **2014**, *25*, 1256–1269. [CrossRef] [PubMed]
24. Johnson, J.L.; Napolitano, G.; Monfregola, J.; Rocca, C.J.; Cherqui, S.; Catz, S.D. Upregulation of the Rab27a-Dependent Trafficking and Secretory Mechanisms Improves Lysosomal Transport, Alleviates Endoplasmic Reticulum Stress, and Reduces Lysosome Overload in Cystinosis. *Mol. Cell. Biol.* **2013**, *33*, 2950–2962. [CrossRef] [PubMed]
25. Ivanova, E.A.; van den Heuvel, L.P.; Elmonem, M.A.; De Smedt, H.; Missiaen, L.; Pastore, A.; Mekahli, D.; Bultynck, G.; Levtchenko, E.N. Altered mTOR Signalling in Nephropathic Cystinosis. *J. Inherit. Metab. Dis.* **2016**, *39*, 457–464. [CrossRef]
26. Andrzejewska, Z.; Nevo, N.; Thomas, L.; Chhuon, C.; Bailleux, A.; Chauvet, V.; Courtoy, P.J.; Chol, M.; Guerrera, I.C.; Antignac, C. Cystinosin is a Component of the Vacuolar H+-ATPase-Ragulator-Rag Complex Controlling Mammalian Target of Rapamycin Complex 1 Signaling. *J. Am. Soc. Nephrol.* **2016**, *27*, 1678–1688. [CrossRef]
27. Rega, L.R.; Polishchuk, E.; Montefusco, S.; Napolitano, G.; Tozzi, G.; Zhang, J.; Bellomo, F.; Taranta, A.; Pastore, A.; Polishchuk, R.; et al. Activation of the Transcription Factor EB Rescues Lysosomal Abnormalities in Cystinotic Kidney Cells. *Kidney Int.* **2016**, *89*, 862–873. [CrossRef]
28. De Rasmo, D.; Signorile, A.; Santeramo, A.; Larizza, M.; Lattanzio, P.; Capitanio, G.; Papa, S. Intramitochondrial Adenylyl Cyclase Controls the Turnover of Nuclear-Encoded Subunits and Activity of Mammalian Complex I of the Respiratory Chain. *Biochim. Biophys. Acta* **2015**, *1853*, 183–191. [CrossRef]

29. Papa, S.; Scacco, S.; De Rasmo, D.; Signorile, A.; Papa, F.; Panelli, D.; Nicastro, A.; Scaringi, R.; Santeramo, A.; Roca, E. cAMP-Dependent Protein Kinase Regulates Post-Translational Processing and Expression of Complex I Subunits in Mammalian Cells. *Biochim. Biophys. Acta* **2010**, *1797*, 649–658. [CrossRef]
30. Signorile, A.; Micelli, L.; De Rasmo, D.; Santeramo, A.; Papa, F.; Ficarella, R.; Gattoni, G.; Scacco, S.; Papa, S. Regulation of the Biogenesis of OXPHOS Complexes in Cell Transition from Replicating to Quiescent State: Involvement of PKA and Effect of Hydroxytyrosol. *Biochim. Biophys. Acta* **2014**, *1843*, 675–684. [CrossRef]
31. Signorile, A.; Santeramo, A.; Tamma, G.; Pellegrino, T.; D'Oria, S.; Lattanzio, P.; De Rasmo, D. Mitochondrial cAMP Prevents Apoptosis Modulating Sirt3 Protein Level and OPA1 Processing in Cardiac Myoblast Cells. *Biochim. Biophys. Acta* **2017**, *1864*, 355–366. [CrossRef] [PubMed]
32. Guha, S.; Konkwo, C.; Lavorato, M.; Mathew, N.D.; Peng, M.; Ostrovsky, J.; Kwon, Y.J.; Polyak, E.; Lightfoot, R.; Seiler, C.; et al. Pre-Clinical Evaluation of Cysteamine Bitartrate as a Therapeutic Agent for Mitochondrial Respiratory Chain Disease. *Hum. Mol. Genet.* **2019**, *28*, 1837–1852. [CrossRef]
33. Ali, S.; McStay, G.P. Regulation of Mitochondrial Dynamics by Proteolytic Processing and Protein Turnover. *Antioxidants* **2018**, *7*, 15.
34. Bragoszewski, P.; Turek, M.; Chacinska, A. Control of Mitochondrial Biogenesis and Function by the Ubiquitin-Proteasome System. *Open Biol.* **2017**, *7*, 170007. [CrossRef] [PubMed]
35. Liang, J.R.; Martinez, A.; Lane, J.D.; Mayor, U.; Clague, M.J.; Urbe, S. USP30 Deubiquitylates Mitochondrial Parkin Substrates and Restricts Apoptotic Cell Death. *EMBO Rep.* **2015**, *16*, 618–627. [CrossRef] [PubMed]
36. Yu, W.; Sun, Y.; Guo, S.; Lu, B. The PINK1/Parkin Pathway Regulates Mitochondrial Dynamics and Function in Mammalian Hippocampal and Dopaminergic Neurons. *Hum. Mol. Genet.* **2011**, *20*, 3227–3240. [CrossRef] [PubMed]
37. Tanaka, A.; Cleland, M.M.; Xu, S.; Narendra, D.P.; Suen, D.F.; Karbowski, M.; Youle, R.J. Proteasome and p97 Mediate Mitophagy and Degradation of Mitofusins Induced by Parkin. *J. Cell Biol.* **2010**, *191*, 1367–1380. [CrossRef]
38. Zhou, J.; Shi, M.; Li, M.; Cheng, L.; Yang, J.; Huang, X. Sirtuin 3 Inhibition Induces Mitochondrial Stress in Tongue Cancer by Targeting Mitochondrial Fission and the JNK-Fis1 Biological Axis. *Cell Stress Chaperones* **2019**, *24*, 369–383. [CrossRef]
39. Burte, F.; Carelli, V.; Chinnery, P.F.; Yu-Wai-Man, P. Disturbed Mitochondrial Dynamics and Neurodegenerative Disorders. *Nat. Rev. Neurol.* **2015**, *11*, 11–24. [CrossRef]
40. Lee, H.; Smith, S.B.; Yoon, Y. The Short Variant of the Mitochondrial Dynamin OPA1 Maintains Mitochondrial Energetics and Cristae Structure. *J. Biol. Chem.* **2017**, *292*, 7115–7130. [CrossRef]
41. Bellomo, F.; Medina, D.L.; De Leo, E.; Panarella, A.; Emma, F. High-Content Drug Screening for Rare Diseases. *J. Inherit. Metab. Dis.* **2017**, *40*, 601–607. [CrossRef] [PubMed]
42. Wilmer, M.J.; Emma, F.; Levtchenko, E.N. The Pathogenesis of Cystinosis: Mechanisms beyond Cystine Accumulation. *Am. J. Physiol. Renal Physiol.* **2010**, *299*, 905–916. [CrossRef] [PubMed]
43. Polishchuk, E.V.; Polishchuk, R.S. Pre-Embedding Labeling for Subcellular Detection of Molecules with Electron Microscopy. *Tissue Cell* **2019**, *57*, 103–110. [CrossRef] [PubMed]

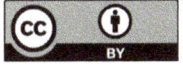

© 2019 by the authors. Licensee MDPI, Basel, Switzerland. This article is an open access article distributed under the terms and conditions of the Creative Commons Attribution (CC BY) license (http://creativecommons.org/licenses/by/4.0/).

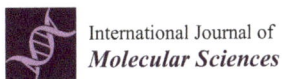

Article

Plasma Oxalate as a Predictor of Kidney Function Decline in a Primary Hyperoxaluria Cohort

Ronak Jagdeep Shah [1], Lisa E. Vaughan [2], Felicity T. Enders [2], Dawn S. Milliner [1,3] and John C. Lieske [1,4,*]

1. Division of Nephrology and Hypertension, Mayo Clinic, Rochester, MN 55905, USA; dr.ronakjagshah@gmail.com (R.J.S.); Milliner.Dawn@mayo.edu (D.S.M.)
2. Division of Biomedical Statistics and Informatics, Mayo Clinic, Rochester, MN 55905, USA; Vaughan.Lisa@mayo.edu (L.E.V.); Enders.Felicity@mayo.edu (F.T.E.)
3. Division of Pediatric Nephrology, Mayo Clinic, Rochester, MN 55905, USA
4. Division of Laboratory Medicine and Pathology, Mayo Clinic, Rochester, MN 55905, USA
* Correspondence: lieske.john@mayo.edu; Tel.: +1-507-266-7960; Fax: +1-507-266-9315

Received: 1 April 2020; Accepted: 16 May 2020; Published: 20 May 2020

Abstract: This retrospective analysis investigated plasma oxalate (POx) as a potential predictor of end-stage kidney disease (ESKD) among primary hyperoxaluria (PH) patients. PH patients with type 1, 2, and 3, age 2 or older, were identified in the Rare Kidney Stone Consortium (RKSC) PH Registry. Since POx increased with falling estimated glomerular filtration rate (eGFR), patients were stratified by chronic kidney disease (CKD) subgroups (stages 1, 2, 3a, and 3b). POx values were categorized into quartiles for analysis. Hazard ratios (HRs) and 95% confidence intervals (95% CIs) for risk of ESKD were estimated using the Cox proportional hazards model with a time-dependent covariate. There were 118 patients in the CKD1 group (nine ESKD events during follow-up), 135 in the CKD 2 (29 events), 72 in CKD3a (34 events), and 45 patients in CKD 3b (31 events). During follow-up, POx Q4 was a significant predictor of ESKD compared to Q1 across CKD2 (HR 14.2, 95% CI 1.8–115), 3a (HR 13.7, 95% CI 3.0–62), and 3b stages (HR 5.2, 95% CI 1.1–25), $p < 0.05$ for all. Within each POx quartile, the ESKD rate was higher in Q4 compared to Q1–Q3. In conclusion, among patients with PH, higher POx concentration was a risk factor for ESKD, particularly in advanced CKD stages.

Keywords: plasma oxalate; primary hyperoxaluria; estimated glomerular filtration rate; chronic kidney disease; Urine Oxalate; end-stage renal disease

1. Introduction

Primary hyperoxaluria (PH) is a rare inherited autosomal recessive genetic disease caused by defects in genes that encode proteins important for glyoxylate metabolism [1]. Currently, three distinct forms are known—PH1 results from mutations in the enzyme alanine-glyoxylate aminotransferase (AGT) which is encoded the *AGXT* gene, PH2 is caused by a deficiency of the glyoxylate reductase/hydroxypyruvate reductase (GRHPR) enzyme encoded by *GRHPR*, and PH3 occurs when the mitochondrial enzyme, 4-hydroxy-2-oxoglutarate aldolase (HOGA) is deficient due to mutations in the *HOGA1* gene. Based upon current numbers in the Rare Kidney Stone Consortium (RKSC) PH registry, approximately 70% of diagnosed patients are PH1, 10% are PH2, 10% PH3, and 10% do not have an identified genetic cause [2].

The metabolic consequence of each of these enzyme deficiencies is a marked increase in hepatic oxalate production. Since oxalate cannot be metabolized by humans, the excess released into the plasma must be excreted by the kidneys, with less than 10% eliminated through the gastrointestinal tract. Calcium oxalate stones and nephrocalcinosis can result from high urinary oxalate (UOx) excretion; the latter can be associated with interstitial inflammation and fibrosis and may contribute to progressive chronic kidney disease (CKD) and end-stage kidney disease (ESKD) [3]. Once patients approach ESKD, excess oxalate can no longer be eliminated by the kidneys, and it accumulates in the body, potentially leading to systemic oxalosis. Among PH patients, there is wide variability in clinical course, with some progressing to ESKD in early childhood, while other PH patients retain kidney function into their fifth or sixth decade. Prediction of long-term outcomes using biomarkers is an important tool for clinical management, particularly now that novel treatment strategies with the potential to reduce hepatic oxalate production in PH are ready for clinical trials [4]. Patients with PH typically excrete >0.7 mmol/1.73 m^2/day [5], and we previously reported that higher UOx predicts future ESKD risk within the PH patient group [2]. We also recently reported that plasma oxalate (POx) concentration correlates with UOx excretion [6].

Since 24 h urine collections can be difficult to obtain, especially on a repeated basis or in younger children, a blood biomarker that predicts UOx and other clinical features of PH could be clinically valuable. Furthermore, in patients with advanced CKD, UOx may no longer reflect systemic oxalate burden; in such cases, POx may represent a more accurate biomarker [7]. Therefore, we examined data in the RKSC PH registry in order to determine whether POx represents a viable biomarker that predicts the future loss of kidney function among patients with confirmed PH and at varying CKD stages.

2. Results

2.1. Baseline Characteristics

There were 227 patients who met the criteria for this study (Figure 1). During follow-up, ESKD developed in nine of the 118 patients (7.6%) in the CKD 1 group, 29 of 135 (21.5%) of the CKD 2 patients, 34 of 72 (47.2%) in the CKD3a, and 31 of 45 (68.8%) in the CKD 3b. There was one death in the CKD 1 group, nine deaths each in the CKD 2 and 3a groups, and 10 deaths in the CKD 3b group. The proportion of patients with PH1 increased by CKD stage (Table 1), representing 56.8% with CKD1, 73.3% with CKD2, 86.1% with CKD3a, and 84.4% with CKD3b. Due to the analysis plan, the median age at PH diagnosis also differed according to which patients experienced each CKD stage, from 5.4 years (CKD1) to 16.0 years (CKD3b). Median follow-up time was 5.3, 8.8, 6.6, and 1.8 years for CKD stages 1–3b, respectively.

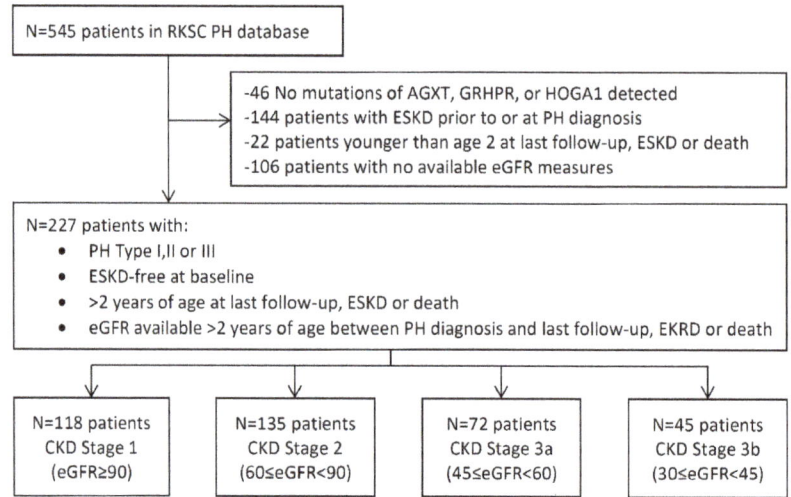

Figure 1. Flowchart of inclusion criteria for analysis cohort. From a total of 545 PH1 patients in the Registry, 227 were eligible for this analysis.

Table 1. Clinical characteristics of patients with primary hyperoxaluria who did not have ESKD at or before diagnosis.

	CKD Stage			
	Stage 1 (≥90)	Stage 2 (60–89)	Stage 3a (45–59)	Stage 3b (30–44)
Characteristics	n = 118	n = 135	n = 72	n = 45
Type of PH, % (n)				
PH1	67 (56.8%)	99 (73.3%)	62 (86.1%)	38 (84.4%)
PH2	23 (19.5%)	16 (11.9%)	6 (8.3%)	5 (11.1%)
PH3	28 (23.7%)	20 (14.8%)	4 (5.6%)	2 (4.4%)
Sex, % (n)				
Male	68 (57.6%)	76 (56.3%)	39 (54.2%)	23 (51.1%)
Female	50 (42.4%)	59 (43.7%)	33 (45.8%)	22 (48.9%)
Age at diagnosis, y	5.4 (2.7, 11.1)	7.9 (4.0, 23.9)	10.7 (4.6, 26.4)	16.0 (7.0, 41.7)
Follow-up time, y	5.3 (2.9, 10.0)	8.8 (3.1, 15.2)	6.6 (3.4, 12.8)	1.8 (1.0, 3.8)
Patients with follow-up Pox labs	n = 50	n = 69	n = 37	n = 17
No. follow-up labs	2.5 (1,5)	3 (1,6)	3 (1,5)	1 (1,3)

Continuous variables are expressed as median with 25th, 75th percentiles. n, number; PH, primary hyperoxaluria; PH1, primary hyperoxaluria type 1; PH2, primary hyperoxaluria type 2; PH3, primary hyperoxaluria type 3; y, years.

Baseline POx increased by CKD stage from (3.1 (2.1, 5.7) µmol/L in CKD1 (n = 38) to 14.4 (10.5, 20.0) µmol/L in CKD3b (n = 17) (Table 2). The results were similar within the PH1 subset, increasing from 3.9 [2.4, 6.8] µmol/L in CKD1 (n = 24) to 14.9 (11.6, 21.5) µmol/L in CKD3b (n = 16). The numbers were not sufficient for a similar sub-analysis in PH2 and PH3. The risk of incident ESKD was higher in patients with PH1 compared to PH2 and PH3 in CKD2 and CKD3b; the results were similar albeit non-significant in CKD1 (HR 7.45; 95% CI 0.92–60.2; p = 0.06) and CKD3a (HR 5.74; 95% CI 0.78–42.1; p = 0.085) (Table 3).

Table 2. Baseline and follow-up POx quartiles, by CKD stage.

Oxalate Measure	n	Q1	Median	Q3
Baseline				
POx, umol/L				
CKD stage 1	38	2.1	3.1	5.7
CKD stage 2	44	1.9	4.1	7.2
CKD stage 3a	25	2.9	4.8	8.2
CKD stage 3b	17	10.5	14.4	20.0
Follow-up				
POx, umol/L				
CKD stage 1	171	1.9	3.0	4.8
CKD stage 2	288	2.1	4.1	7.1
CKD stage 3a	165	4.2	7.0	12.9
CKD stage 3b	38	9.9	15.2	18.0

2.2. POx and ESKD

When treated as a continuous predictor, higher baseline POx values were significantly associated with a higher risk of ESKD in CKD2 (HR 1.17; 95% CI 1.01–1.35; p = 0.033), CKD3a (HR 1.29; 95% CI 1.09–1.53; p = 0.004) and CKD3b (HR 1.24; 95% CI 1.08–1.42; p = 0.003) (Table 3). Baseline POx values in Q4 compared to POx in Q1 were also associated with a higher risk of ESKD in CKD3a (HR 13.88; 95% CI 1.41–137; p = 0.024) and CKD3b (HR 42.1; 95% CI 3.29–539; p = 0.004) (Table 3).

During follow-up (Table 4), POx was significantly associated with ESKD risk across all CKD stages: CKD1 (HR 1.12; 95% CI 1.02–1.24, p = 0.018), CKD2 (HR 1.17; 95% CI 1.08–1.25; p < 0.001), CKD3a (HR 1.19; 95% CI 1.11–1.27; p < 0.001), and CKD3b (HR 1.12; 95% CI 1.04–1.21; p = 0.003). When POx was considered by quartile, Q4 was a significant predictor of ESKD compared to Q1 across the CKD stages as well: CKD 2 (HR 14.2; 95% CI 1.76–115; $p = 0.013$), CKD3a (HR 13.7; 95% CI 3.02–62; $p < 0.001$), and CKD3b (HR 5.19; 95% CI 1.10–24.5; $p = 0.038$). Within each POx quartile, the ESKD rate was higher for the later CKD stages. Within each CKD stage, the ESKD rate was also higher in the fourth POx quartile compared to the first three (Table S1 and Figure 2). Thus, the greatest ESKD rate was for the CKD 3b subjects in the highest POx quartile (Figure 2).

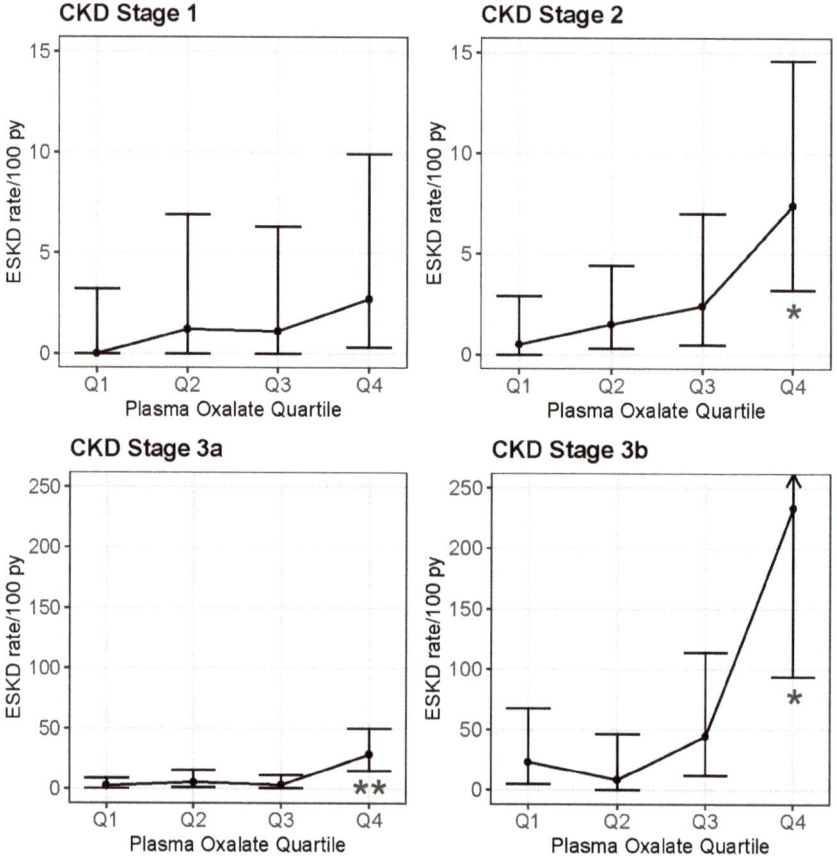

Figure 2. ESKD rate by POx quartile during follow-up by CKD stage. ESKD rates were estimated for each CKD stage group by dividing individual patient follow-up times into intervals based on the time between the POx measures or last follow-up. Person-time and ESKD events were summed within POx quartiles with the rate = [100 × (events/person-time)]; error bars represent 95% CI of the ESKD rate (see Supplemental Table S1 for numerical values). ESKD rates were similar for the lower three quartiles (Q) but increased for the highest POx quartile across CKD stages 2–3b (Q4 vs. Q1 HR 14.21; 95% CI 1.76–114.7; * $p < 0.05$ for CKD stage 2, HR 13.66; 95% CI 3.02–61.91; ** $p < 0.001$ for CKD stage 3a, and HR 5.19; 95% CI 1.10–24.5; * $p < 0.05$ for CKD stage 3b).

Table 3. Factors univariately associated with incident ESKD among patients with primary hyperoxaluria without ESKD at baseline.

	Stage 1 (≥90)				Stage 2 (60–89)				Stage 3a (45–59)				Stage 3b (30–44)			
Variable	n; E	HR (95% CI)	p	C-Index	n; E	HR (95% CI)	p	C-Index	n; E	HR (95% CI)	p	C-Index	n; E	HR (95% CI)	p	C-Index
Demographics																
PH1	118; 9	7.45 (0.92–60.2)	0.06	0.677	135; 29	23.9 (3.06–186)	**0.003**	0.630	72; 34	5.74 (0.78–42.1)	0.085	0.544	45; 31	9.45 (1.28–69.8)	**0.028**	0.607
Male	118; 9	1.31 (0.32–5.34)	0.71	0.535	135; 29	1.73 (0.80–3.74)	0.17	0.577	72; 34	1.10 (0.56–2.18)	0.78	0.517	45; 31	1.07 (0.51–2.23)	0.86	0.520
Age at diagnosis	118; 9	0.98 (0.90–1.08)	0.69	0.500	135; 29	1.00 (0.98–1.03)	0.78	0.577	72; 34	1.01 (0.98–1.03)	0.70	0.550	45; 31	0.98 (0.96–1.01)	0.13	0.612
Plasma Oxalate																
POx, umol/l	38; 2	NE[†]	NE[†]	NE[†]	44; 9	1.17 (1.01–1.35)	**0.033**	0.623	25; 10	1.29 (1.09–1.53)	**0.004**	0.727	17; 14	1.24 (1.08–1.42)	**0.003**	0.810
POx, quartile	38; 2	-	-	NE[†]	44; 9	-	-	0.610	25; 10	-	-	0.698	17; 14	-	-	0.791
Q1	-	REF	REF	-	-	REF	REF	-	-	REF	REF	-	-	REF	REF	-
Q2	-	NE[†]	NE[†]	-	-	0.41 (0.04–4.52)	0.47	-	-	2.40 (0.14–40.0)	0.54	-	-	7.85 (0.82–75.0)	0.074	-
Q3	-	NE[†]	NE[†]	-	-	1.68 (0.27–10.52)	0.58	-	-	4.39 (0.49–39.5)	0.19	-	-	10.1 (1.11–91.5)	**0.040**	-
Q4	-	NE[†]	NE[†]	-	-	1.57 (0.25–9.75)	0.63	-	-	13.88 (1.41–136.5)	**0.024**	-	-	42.1 (3.29–539)	**0.004**	-

PH1, primary hyperoxaluria type 1; n: number available for analysis; E: = ESKD events; 95% CI, 95% confidence interval. p-values in bold denote significance at the 0.05 level. Harrell's c index is provided. The proportional hazards assumption was met for all models with reported HRs. [†] Not estimable, sample size, and no. of events too small for a variable with four levels.

Table 4. Plasma oxalate excretion on follow-up (>6 months after entry into the CKD group) and risk of ESKD.

	Stage 1 (≥90)				Stage 2 (60–89)				Stage 3a (45–59)				Stage 3b (30–44)			
Follow-up Plasma Oxalate	n; E	HR (95% CI)	p	C-Index	n; E	HR (95% CI)	p	C-Index	n; E	HR (95% CI)	p	C-Index	n; E	HR (95% CI)	p	C-Index
POx, umol/L	171; 4	1.12 (1.02–1.24)	**0.018**	0.854	288; 15	1.17 (1.08–1.25)	**<0.001**	0.806	165; 19	1.19 (1.11–1.27)	**<0.001**	0.795	38; 15	1.12 (1.04–1.21)	**0.003**	0.729
POx, quartile	171; 4	-	-	0.818	288; 15	-	-	0.772	165; 19	-	-	0.757	38; 15	-	-	0.752
Q1	-	REF	REF	-	-	REF	REF	-	-	REF	REF	-	-	REF	REF	-
Q2	-	NE[†]	NE[†]	-	-	2.70 (0.28–26.03)	0.39	-	-	2.10 (0.35–12.65)	0.42	-	-	0.39 (0.04–4.40)	0.45	-
Q3	-	NE[†]	NE[†]	-	-	3.98 (0.41–38.82)	0.24	-	-	1.28 (0.18–9.17)	0.80	-	-	0.98 (0.19–5.04)	0.98	-
Q4	-	NE[†]	NE[†]	-	-	14.21 (1.76–114.7)	**0.013**	-	-	13.66 (3.02–61.91)	**<0.001**	-	-	5.19 (1.10–24.5)	**0.038**	-

[†] Not estimable, sample size, and no. events, too small for a variable with four levels. p-values in bold denote significance at the 0.05 level. Harrell's c index is provided. n = Follow-up intervals; E = ESKD events.

2.3. UOx and ESKD

Risk of ESKD increased at higher UOx levels when follow-up UOx was employed as a continuous time-dependent covariate, yielding an HR of 1.8 (95% CI 1.35–2.5) per each UOx increased of 1 mmol/1.73 m^2/24 h ($p < 0.001$). When examined by follow-up UOx quartile (cut-off points of 0.77, 1.21, and 1.84 mmol/1.73 m^2 h), UOx Q4 had a higher ESKD risk than Q1 (HR, 3.7; 95% CI 1.5–9.55) ($p < 0.01$).

2.4. ESKD or 40% Sustained Reduction in eGFR

Results were similar when the combined endpoint of ESKD and a 40% sustained eGFR reduction in eGFR were used for CKD progression. A higher baseline POx remained a significant predictor of incident CKD progression at CKD3b (HR 1.27; 95% CI 1.09–1.48; $p = 0.002$). Higher POx values during follow-up also remained a significant predictor of CKD progression in CKD2 (HR 1.15, 95% CI 1.07–1.23; $p < 0.001$) and CKD3a (HR 1.17, 95% CI 1.08–1.27; $p < 0.001$) when treated both as a continuous predictor and when comparing POx Q4 to POx Q1 (HR 10.71; 95% CI 1.34–85.4; $p = 0.025$ and HR 8.15; 95% CI 1.74–38.2; $p = 0.008$; respectively). Follow-up time was shorter, and there were fewer laboratory parameters available when considering this composite endpoint.

2.5. eGFR Slope

There were 59 patients with a total of 369 POx and eGFR laboratory measures obtained within three months of each other throughout follow-up. The number of lab values per patient ranged from 1 to 20. After adjusting for follow-up time, eGFR was significantly lower among those with higher POx (eGFR reduced by 1.27 mL/min/1.73 m^2 per 1 µmol/L increase in POx; ($p < 0.001$).

3. Discussion

In the current study, we analyzed the predictive value of POx for the subsequent decline in eGFR in PH patients, stratified by CKD stage. These data suggest that POx is a useful predictor of ESKD risk across CKD stages 2–3b (Figure 2), with the effect most pronounced in CKD3b. These data and our previous study [2] suggest that the use of POx and UOx could be complimentary, with UOx being particularly informative across CKD stages 1–3b, and POx particularly informative in CKD stages 3a and 3b.

The clinical management of PH is challenging due to the lifelong nature of the disease and the risk for ESKD observed in a vast majority of PH1 patients, although this can occur at markedly variable ages. The ability to predict long term outcomes using biomarkers facilitates the most effective use of current treatments and also has the potential to provide an important outcome measure for clinical trials of novel therapeutics. Newer treatment options, including the potential use of small inhibitory RNA (siRNA) therapeutics to impact oxalate generating pathways in the liver are under current development [8]. These newer approaches make it important to better understand the prognostic features of PH, which could both identify patients who could be eligible candidates for clinical trials and also potentially be used as surrogate endpoints in future studies.

In the current study, we examined whether POx is a useful prognostic marker for the future of loss of kidney function. The data demonstrate that higher POx levels both at baseline and during follow-up were significantly associated with loss of kidney function over time. When stratified by quartile, those in POx Q4 were at increased risk of ESKD compared to POx Q1 across CKD stages 2–3b. As expected, based upon previous prevalence data, patients that progressed to later CKD stages tended to be older and more likely to have PH1. The current study also confirms our previous observation that baseline UOx and UOx over follow-up predict ESKD, with those in the highest quartile at the greatest additional risk [2]. Furthermore, the HRs for the subsequent ESKD of the highest UOx quartile at baseline (2.5) and during follow-up (3.7) were similar to our previous work [2].

Much as the serum creatinine concentration is a net result of creatinine generation from muscle and elimination by the kidneys, POx is the net result of oxalate generated in the liver and absorbed from the GI tract and its elimination by the kidneys. Thus, higher POx can reflect higher hepatic oxalate generation, greater gastrointestinal absorption, lower GFR, or some combination of these. Indeed, our previous publications demonstrated that UOx excretion could be used to predict POx and eGFR [6]. Recent studies also suggest that higher UOx excretion predicts a higher renal tubular fluid oxalate concentration at the S3 segment of the proximal tubule, the anatomic site of nephrocalcinosis in PH [9]. Thus, the results from our current study demonstrating the predictive value of POx across the CKD stage 2–3b spectrum may reflect the fact that POx provides integration of oxalate generation and elimination, and thus becomes a sensitive marker of oxalate burden at the level of the proximal tubule.

One issue with the widespread use of POx is the challenging nature of the available laboratory assays [10]. Under normal circumstances, POx is present in micro-molar concentrations in blood. Thus, sample handling, including prevention of ascorbate conversion to oxalate, is quite important. In addition, methods for measuring oxalate, including sample type, preparation, and analysis, are not interchangeable [10–12]. Our study benefitted from use of a single clinical laboratory over many decades with data to support that POx results could be compared over that time period. However, because of the barriers for analysis in routine laboratories, the POx measurement is not widely available. Additionally, when GFR is normal or near-normal, POx concentrations typically are near or below the limit of quantification in the general population [10]. However, due to a markedly increased oxalate generation, POx is typically above the limit of quantification in most PH patients, even with preserved eGFR [6], suggesting that with a consistent and sensitive assay, POx could be a useful biomarker. Moreover, as GFR declines, POx values rise well within the quantification range with good reproducibility in all PH patients.

The current study has several limitations. Due to the retrospective nature of this analysis based on registry data, laboratory measures and follow-up were limited by availability, and variability in the diagnosis and ability to recruit patients with this rare disease may have introduced bias. There was also no controlled intervention to change POx values. Nevertheless, we were able to analyze a relatively large cohort of over 200 PH patients with available POx values. Furthermore, comorbidities such as obesity, dyslipidemia, hypertension, and albuminuria, which are important CKD risk factors, were not available for multivariate analysis. However, many PH patients progress to ESKD at a very young age, and thus these comorbidities likely play a relatively minimal role in CKD progression, in comparison to common causes of CKD such as diabetic nephropathy in which vascular/microvascular injury and dysfunction play a major role.

In conclusion, there is a need for improved knowledge regarding the utility of biomarkers to predict ESKD risk in PH patients at various stages of CKD. The current study suggests that POx, perhaps in combination with other risk factors, is a useful marker for this purpose.

4. Materials and Methods

Natural history and laboratory data from PH patients enrolled in the RKSC PH Registry were used for analysis [13]. PH1, PH2, and PH3 patients were confirmed by mutations in the AGXT, GRHPR, or HOGA1 genes, respectively. POx was measured in the Mayo Clinic Renal Testing Laboratory (Rochester, MN, USA) by an oxalate oxidase (1991–6/2016) or ion chromatography (6/2016–2019) based-assay per the standard Mayo Renal Testing Laboratory Protocol [10]. Detailed validation data was available to determine that assay results could be compared over the course of this time period. UOx was measured by oxalate oxidase also in the Mayo Renal Testing Laboratory or another accredited clinical laboratory [10,14]. Data for subjects <2 years old were excluded from this analysis due to potential confounding effects of renal maturation in very young children on GFR (and thus POx).

This project was approved by the Mayo Clinic Institutional Review Board (IRB 11-001702; initial approval 16 August 2011). A total of 545 PH patients were identified in the Registry as of March 31, 2019 (Figure 1). After excluding patients who met clinical criteria but had no detectable mutations of AGXT, GRHPR, or HOGA1, ($n = 46$), those with ESKD at diagnosis ($n = 144$), patients less than two years old at ESKD or last follow-up ($n = 22$), and those patients without eGFR data after diagnosis and older than two years before ESKD or death ($n = 106$), a total of 227 patients remained in the final cohort for analysis. Since our previous study suggested an association between POx and CKD stage [6], patients were then divided into four groups based on CKD stage (1, 2, 3a, 3b) in a landmark-style analysis, such that a patient started in a given CKD stage subgroup on their first eGFR observed in that range, while also remaining in any prior groups through all available follow-ups. For instance, a patient whose eGFR measurements were 64, 72, 43, 47, 38, 29, and 21 mL/min/1.73 m^2 would never be included in the CKD stage 1 group, would enter the eGFR 60–89 group with the date of the eGFR = 64 mL/min/1.73 m^2 measurement and be followed until kidney progression or censoring, would enter the eGFR 30–44 group with the date of the eGFR = 43 mL/min/1.73 m^2 measurement and be followed until kidney progression or censoring, and would enter the eGFR 45–59 group with the date of the eGFR = 47 mL/min/1.73 m^2 measurement and be followed until kidney progression or censoring.

Laboratory results were extracted from the registry data, and were from baseline (defined as within one year prior to or within six months of entry into the CKD stage group and prior to kidney progression) or follow-up (defined from six months after the entry into the CKD stage group and prior to kidney progression). None of this patient cohort experienced acute kidney injury events during follow-up. GFR was estimated via the CKD-EPI creatinine equation for adults greater than 18 years old [15] and the Schwartz equation for those less than 18 years old [16]. POx values were manually examined, and outlying transient results not fitting the clinical picture were removed from the analysis.

4.1. Statistical Methods

Plasma Oxalate

Progression to ESKD (eGFR < 15 mL/min/1.73 m^2 or the start of dialysis or renal transplantation) was selected as the primary endpoint. Sensitivity analyses were also performed using a combined endpoint of ESKD or sustained 40% reduction in eGFR from baseline. The results were expressed in terms of the median (25th, 75th percentiles) for continuous variables and as percentages for categorical variables. To maximize available data, the diagnosis/baseline labs were defined as the closest reading between one year before entry and up to six months after entry into a CKD stage group.

The percentage of patients who were free of renal progression (ESKD and > 40% decline in eGFR) after entry into each CKD stage was estimated using the Kaplan–Meier method. The effects of baseline clinical characteristics, as well as Pox on renal progression, were estimated by univariate analyses using the Cox proportional hazard model with log-rank tests. The primary outcome of interest was time to ESKD and was censored on death or loss to follow-up. Hazard ratios (HRs) and 95% confidence intervals (95% CIs) are presented. A time-dependent Cox model was used to explore the effect of POx concentration on renal outcome during follow-up. Times to ESKD by POx quartile during follow-up were estimated for each CKD stage group by dividing individual-patient follow-up time into intervals based on the time between POx measures or last follow-up. Person-time and ESKD events were summed within the POx quartile with the rate = 100 × (Events/Person-time). The proportional hazards assumption was checked for all models using martingale residuals. Generalized estimating equations (GEE) adjusting for time were used to evaluate the association between POx and eGFR throughout follow-up. The effect of follow-up UOx concentration on the risk of renal outcomes were also assessed using a time-dependent Cox model.

Supplementary Materials: Supplementary materials can be found at http://www.mdpi.com/1422-0067/21/10/3608/s1.

Author Contributions: Conceptualization, L.E.V., F.T.E., D.S.M. and J.C.L.; Methodology, L.E.V., F.T.E., D.S.M. and J.C.L.; Formal Analysis, L.E.V. and F.T.E.; Investigation, R.J.S., L.E.V., F.T.E., D.S.M. and J.C.L.; Resources, F.T.E., D.S.M., and J.C.L.; Data Curation, R.J.S. and L.E.V.; Writing—Original Draft Preparation, R.J.S.; Writing—Review & Editing, L.E.V., F.T.E., D.S.M., and J.C.L.; Visualization, L.E.V.; Supervision, J.C.L.; Project Administration, J.C.L.; Funding Acquisition, F.T.E., D.S.M., and J.C.L. All authors have read and agreed to the published version of the manuscript.

Funding: This study was supported by the Rare Kidney Stone Consortium (U54KD083908), a part of the Rare Diseases Clinical Research Network (RDCRN), an initiative of the Office of Rare Diseases Research (ORDR), National Center for Advancing Translational Sciences' (NCATS). This consortium is funded through a collaboration between NCATS and the National Institute of Diabetes and Digestive and Kidney Diseases (NIDDK) and the Oxalosis and Hyperoxaluria Foundation and the Mayo Foundation. Investigators of the RKSC coordinating sites with contributions to the PH Registry include Dean Assimos (University of Alabama, Birmingham), Michelle Baum and Michael Somers (Children's Hospital, Harvard Medical School), Lawrence Copelovitch (Children's Hospital of Philadelphia), Prasad Devarajan (Cincinnati Children's Hospital Medical Center), David Goldfarb (New York University), Elizabeth Harvey and Lisa Robinson (The Hospital for Sick Children [Sickkids], Toronto), William Haley (Mayo Clinic, Jacksonville), Mini Michael (University of Texas) and Craig Langman (Ann & Robert H. Lurie Children's Memorial Hospital, Chicago).

Acknowledgments: We thank the patients and their families for their gracious participation. We are grateful to the investigators of the RKSC coordinating sites and many additional individual contributors to the PH Registry for generously providing clinical data.

Conflicts of Interest: The authors declare no conflicts of interest. The funders had no role in the design of the study; in the collection, analyses, or interpretation of data; in the writing of the manuscript, or in the decision to publish the results.

References

1. Cochat, P.; Rumsby, G. Primary hyperoxaluria. *N. Engl. J. Med.* **2013**, *369*, 649–658. [CrossRef] [PubMed]
2. Zhao, F.; Bergstralh, E.J.; Mehta, R.A.; Vaughan, L.E.; Olson, J.B.; Seide, B.M.; Meek, A.M.; Cogal, A.G.; Lieske, J.C.; Milliner, D.S. Predictors of incident ESRD among patients with primary hyperoxaluria presenting prior to kidney failure. *Clin. J. Am. Soc. Nephrol.* **2016**, *11*, 119–126. [CrossRef] [PubMed]
3. Hoppe, B.; Beck, B.B.; Milliner, D.S. The primary hyperoxalurias. *Kidney Int.* **2009**, *75*, 1264–1271. [CrossRef] [PubMed]
4. Dutta, C.; Avitahl-Curtis, N.; Pursell, N.; Larsson Cohen, M.; Holmes, B.; Diwanji, R.; Zhou, W.; Apponi, L.; Koser, M.; Ying, B.; et al. Inhibition of Glycolate Oxidase with Dicer-substrate siRNA Reduces Calcium Oxalate Deposition in a Mouse Model of Primary Hyperoxaluria Type 1. *Mol. Ther.* **2016**, *24*, 770–778. [CrossRef] [PubMed]
5. Edvardsson, V.O.; Goldfarb, D.S.; Lieske, J.C.; Beara-Lasic, L.; Anglani, F.; Milliner, D.S.; Palsson, R. Hereditary causes of kidney stones and chronic kidney disease. *Pediatr. Nephrol.* **2013**. [CrossRef] [PubMed]
6. Perinpam, M.; Enders, F.T.; Mara, K.C.; Vaughan, L.E.; Mehta, R.A.; Voskoboev, N.; Milliner, D.S.; Lieske, J.C. Plasma oxalate in relation to eGFR in patients with primary hyperoxaluria, enteric hyperoxaluria and urinary stone disease. *Clin. Biochem.* **2017**, *50*, 1014–1019. [CrossRef] [PubMed]
7. Elgstoen, K.B.; Johnsen, L.F.; Woldseth, B.; Morkrid, L.; Hartmann, A. Plasma oxalate following kidney transplantation in patients without primary hyperoxaluria. *Nephrol. Dial. Transplant.* **2010**, *25*, 2341–2345. [CrossRef] [PubMed]
8. Bhasin, B.; Ürekli, H.M.; Atta, M.G. Primary and secondary hyperoxaluria: Understanding the enigma. *World J. Nephrol.* **2015**, *4*, 235. [CrossRef] [PubMed]
9. Worcester, E.M.; Evan, A.P.; Coe, F.L.; Lingeman, J.E.; Krambeck, A.; Sommers, A.; Philips, C.L.; Milliner, D. A test of the hypothesis that oxalate secretion produces proximal tubule crystallization in primary hyperoxaluria type I. *Am. J. Physiol.-Ren. Physiol.* **2013**, *305*, F1574–F1584. [CrossRef] [PubMed]
10. Ladwig, P.M.; Liedtke, R.R.; Larson, T.S.; Lieske, J.C. Sensitive spectrophotometric assay for plasma oxalate. *Clin. Chem.* **2005**, *51*, 2377–2380. [CrossRef] [PubMed]
11. Hoppe, B.; Kemper, M.J.; Hvizd, M.G.; Sailer, D.E.; Langman, C.B. Simultaneous determination of oxalate, citrate and sulfate in children's plasma with ion chromatography. *Kidney Int.* **1998**, *53*, 1348–1352. [CrossRef] [PubMed]

12. Elgstoen, K.B. Liquid chromatography-tandem mass spectrometry method for routine measurement of oxalic acid in human plasma. *J. Chromatogr. B Analyt. Technol. Biomed. Life Sci.* **2008**, *873*, 31–36. [CrossRef] [PubMed]
13. Lieske, J.C.; Monico, C.G.; Holmes, W.S.; Bergstralh, E.J.; Slezak, J.M.; Rohlinger, A.L.; Olson, J.B.; Milliner, D.S. International registry for primary hyperoxaluria. *Am. J. Nephrol.* **2005**, *25*, 290–296. [CrossRef] [PubMed]
14. Wilson, D.M.; Liedtke, R.R. Modified enzyme-based colorimetric assay of urinary and plasma oxalate with improved sensitivity and no ascorbate interference: Reference values and specimen handling procedures. *Clin. Chem.* **1991**, *37*, 1229–1235. [CrossRef] [PubMed]
15. Inker, L.A.; Schmid, C.H.; Tighiouart, H.; Eckfeldt, J.H.; Feldman, H.I.; Greene, T.; Kusek, J.W.; Manzi, J.; Van Lente, F.; Zhang, Y.L. Estimating glomerular filtration rate from serum creatinine and cystatin C. *N. Engl. J. Med.* **2012**, *367*, 20–29. [CrossRef] [PubMed]
16. Schwartz, G.J.; Munoz, A.; Schneider, M.F.; Mak, R.H.; Kaskel, F.; Warady, B.A.; Furth, S.L. New equations to estimate GFR in children with CKD. *J. Am. Soc. Nephrol.* **2009**, *20*, 629–637. [CrossRef] [PubMed]

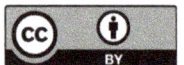

© 2020 by the authors. Licensee MDPI, Basel, Switzerland. This article is an open access article distributed under the terms and conditions of the Creative Commons Attribution (CC BY) license (http://creativecommons.org/licenses/by/4.0/).

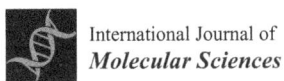

Review

Complement and Complement Targeting Therapies in Glomerular Diseases

Sofia Andrighetto [1,2], Jeremy Leventhal [1], Gianluigi Zaza [2] and Paolo Cravedi [1,*]

[1] Department of Medicine, Division of Nephrology, Icahn School of Medicine at Mount Sinai, 1 Levy Place, New York, NY 10029, USA; sofia.andrighetto@gmail.com (S.A.); jeremy.leventhal@mssm.edu (J.L.)
[2] Renal Unit, Department of Medicine, University/Hospital of Verona, 37126 Verona, Italy; gianluigi.zaza@univr.it
* Correspondence: paolo.cravedi@mssm.edu; Tel.: +1-212-241-3349; Fax: +1-212-987-0389

Received: 14 November 2019; Accepted: 10 December 2019; Published: 16 December 2019

Abstract: The complement cascade is part of the innate immune system whose actions protect hosts from pathogens. Recent research shows complement involvement in a wide spectrum of renal disease pathogenesis including antibody-related glomerulopathies and non-antibody-mediated kidney diseases, such as C3 glomerular disease, atypical hemolytic uremic syndrome, and focal segmental glomerulosclerosis. A pivotal role in renal pathogenesis makes targeting complement activation an attractive therapeutic strategy. Over the last decade, a growing number of anti-complement agents have been developed; some are approved for clinical use and many others are in the pipeline. Herein, we review the pathways of complement activation and regulation, illustrate its role instigating or amplifying glomerular injury, and discuss the most promising novel complement-targeting therapies.

Keywords: complement; alternative complement pathway; complement-targeting therapies; C3 glomerulopathy; hemolytic uremic syndrome; focal segmental glomerulosclerosis

---

1. Complement Cascade

The complement system consists of soluble or membrane-bound molecules, mostly zymogens, activated through a tightly regulated proteolytic cascade [1,2]. Current understanding of complement immune mechanisms include (1) functioning as opsonins; (2) producing chemoattractants to recruit immune cells thereby enhancing site specific angiogenesis, vasodilation and coagulation cascade regulator; and (3) functioning as an enhancing bridge to adaptive T and B lymphocyte responses [3]. Current research suggests that abnormal complement activation plays a role in autoimmune inflammatory diseases and particularly in those targeting the kidney.

2. Complement Cascade Activation and Regulation

Complement activation proceeds via three pathways: the classical, alternative, and mannitol-binding lectin (MBL). The pathways have both unique and overlapping proteins, activated by a proteolytic cascade, that respond to pathogenic insults [3,4] (Figure 1). The classical and MBL pathways are initiated by antibodies and bacterial mannose motifs binding to C1q and mannose-associated serine proteases (MASPs), respectively [5,6]. Conversely, spontaneous hydrolysis of C3 on cell surfaces produces constitutive alternative pathway (AP) activation [7], and is tightly controlled by a number of regulators [8]. Decay accelerating factor (DAF) and membrane cofactor protein (MCP) (CD46, murine homolog Crry) are cell surface-expressed complement regulators that accelerate the decay of surface-assembled C3 convertases, thereby limiting amplification of the downstream cascade. DAF restrains convertase-mediated C3 cleavage; MCP and factor H (fH) also have a cofactor activity: together with soluble factor I (fI), they irreversibly cleave C3b into iC3b, thereby preventing reformation of the C3 convertase.

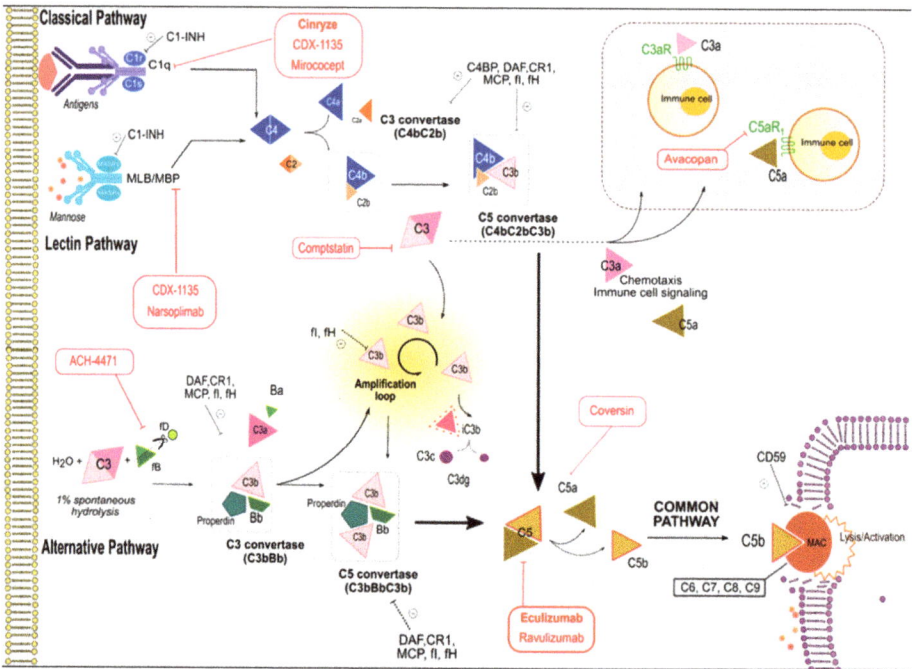

Figure 1. Overview of the complement cascade and principal complement targeting molecules. Three pathways can initiate complement cascade: (1) The classical, (2) the mannose-binding lectin (MBL), and (3) the alternative pathway. They all converge on C3 convertases formation which continuously cleave C3; after they are activated, the C3 convertase from alternative pathway dominates within an amplification loop that sustains the production of C3b (circular arrow). The three C3 convertases associate with an additional C3b to form the C5 convertases, which cleave C5 into C5a + C5b. C5b fragments recruits C6, C7, C8, and multiple C9 molecules to generate the terminal membrane attack complex (MAC); MAC inserts pores into cell membranes to induce cell lysis or activation. Anaphilotoxins C3a and C5a through their G protein-coupled receptors C3aR and C5aR, respectively, can promote signaling, inflammation, chemotaxis of leukocytes, vasodilation, cytokine and chemokine release, and activation of adaptive immunity. Dotted black arrows: inhibitor function of a complement effector on its target. Red arrows emerging from balloons: inhibitor function of anti complement drug on its target (bold drugs' names are the FDA approved ones). Full arrow: consequential interaction between complement fractions leads to the subsequent cascade step. Full bold arrow: final convergence of the three complement pathways on same final target. MBL: Mannose binding lectin; MASP: Mannose-binding lectin-associated serine protease; C4BP: C4 binding protein; C1-INH: C1 inhibitor; DAF: Decay accelerating factor; CR1: Surface complement receptor 1; MCP: Membrane cofactor protein; CD59: Protectin; fD: Factor D; fB: Factor B; fI: Factor I; fH: Factor H. Red balloons highlights complement target drugs' points of action (see Table 1).

Table 1. Summary of complement blocking agents.

Name.	Class	Pharmacodinamics	Disease	Status	Additional Info
Eculizumab	Humanized monoclonal antibody	Binds C5 preventing MAC generation	aHUS, DDD, C3GN	Available for use in PHN and aHUS	First USA FDA-approved among anti-complement drugs
Ravulizumab ALXN1210	Humanized monoclonal antibody	Binds C5 preventing MAC generation	aHUS	Phase III for PHN	Induces prolonged decease of C5 plasmatic levels allowing longer dosing intervals compared to Eculizumab
Coversin	Small dimension recombinant protein	Prevents cleavage of C5 into C5a/C5b by C5 convertase	aHUS	Phase II for PHN	Valid alternative for patients bearer of C5 molecule polymorphisms which interferes with correct binding of Eculizumab
Azacopan CCX168	Small dimension anti-inflammatory molecule	Inhibits selectively C5aR	aHUS ANCA-vasculitides	Phanse III for ANCA vasculitides. Phase II for aHUS	Effective replacing high-dose glucocorticoids in treating vasculitis
CDX-1135	C1R-based molecule	Inhibits CR1	DDD	Phase I for DDD	
Mirococept APT070	CR1-based molecule	Inhibits CR1	IRI in Tx	Phase I for DDD, C3GN	
Cinryze	C1 estarase	Inhibits CR1	Antibody-mediated rejection in renal transplant	Available for use in HAE. Phase III for prevention of DGF in cadaveric allograft	FDA approved for hereditary angioedema
Narsoplimab OMS721	Humanized monoclonal antibody	Binds the mannan-binding lectin-associated serinprotease-2	aHUS, TTP IgAN	Phase II for aHUS, IgA, LES, MN, C3G	Multi-dose administration is needed
ACH-4471	Small dimension molecule	Inhibits factor D	aHUS	Phase II for IC-MPGN, DDD, C3GN	Oral assumption with delivery advantage over intravenously infused agents

aHUS: Atypical hemolytic uremic syndrome, DDD: Dense deposit disease, C3GN: C3 glomerular disease, MAC: Membrane attack complex, ANCA: Antineutrophilic cystoplasmic antibody, IRI: Ischemia riper fusion injury, TTP: Thrombotic thrombocytopenia, IgAN: IgA Nephropathy, HAE: Hereditary angioedema, DGF: Delayed graft function.

The three activation pathways converge in C3 convertases that continuously cleave C3 into C3a and C3b. C3a signals on cell surface G protein-coupled receptor (GPCR) C3aR, while C3b forms additional alternative pathways C3 convertases (even if initiated via the other pathways), as well as C5 convertases. C5 convertases produce the split products C5a and C5b. While C5a functions similarly to C3a (but signals via C5aR) C5b, in conjunction with C6–C9, forms the membrane attack complex (MAC) leading to cell lysis/activation [9]. Countering distal complement MAC formation is CD59, a circulating complement inhibitor.

3. Effector Functions

Complement proteins promote inflammation and immune cell activity in multiple ways. C3a and C5a ligate their transmembrane-spanning receptors, C3aR and C5aR, on immune cells, leading to the production of proinflammatory cytokines and chemokines and promoting vasodilation. They also mediate neutrophil and macrophage chemoattraction, activate macrophages to promote intracellular killing of engulfed organisms, and contribute to T-cell and antigen-presenting cell (APC) activation, expansion, and survival [10–13]. The more distal complement proteins (C5b-9) form MAC complexes on cell membranes, promoting lysis of non-nucleated cells, such as red blood cells, or pathogens lacking cell surface complement inhibitors, such as bacteria. MAC insertion into nucleated eukaryotic cells generally does not result in lysis, but rather induces immune activation [14] and/or promotes tissue injury [15]. C3b and other bound cleavage products function as opsonins binding to specific surface-expressed receptors (complement receptors CR1, CR2, CR3, and CR4).

4. Complement in Glomerular Diseases

4.1. Diseases with Antibody-Mediated Complement Activation

The majority of circulating, or fluid-phase, complement components are produced by the liver. Liver produced complement components are involved in auto-antibody initiated glomerulonephritis (GN) through the classical and/or MBL pathways. Inadequate regulation of alternative pathway activity, due to inherited and/or acquired abnormalities of complement regulators, can result in glomerular injury from persistent C3 convertase activity with consequent excessive MAC activity. Complement can also be produced by parenchymal (e.g., tubular cells in the kidney [16] and resident/infiltrating immune cells, (e.g., T cells and APCs) [17–19]. The relative contributions of systemic or locally produced complement in GN pathogenesis remains unclear.

4.2. IgA Nephropathy

IgA nephropathy (IgAN) is the most common form of GN worldwide [20,21]; its clinical presentation varies, but it often includes proteinuria and hematuria. The disease is associated with aberrant O-glycosylation of mucosal IgA1 with galactose-deficient IgA1 (Gd-IgA1) which plays a pivotal role in the progression of IgAN [22]. They deposit in glomeruli and, subsequently, development of circulating/in situ immunoglobulins (IgA or IgG) targeting glycosylated IgA takes place [23,24]. Mesangial IgA and immune complexes deposits are often observed and initiate glomerular injury.

In vitro and in vivo studies showed that polymeric mucosal IgA activates the complement system through the alternative or MBL pathway [25], and glomerular MBL correlates with greater disease severity and a worse prognosis [26]. Although C3 levels in plasma are usually normal, glomerular C3 deposits can be detected in approximately 85% of biopsies, with C5b-9 also often present along with C3 during infections [27]. MAC generated from complement activation attack on mesangial cells inducing them to proliferate and over-produce oxidants, proteases, cytokines, growth factors (e.g., transforming growth factor β and platelet-derived growth factor) and extracellular matrix material that together result in the typical focal proliferative GN with mesangial matrix expansion characteristic of IgA nephropathy [28].

A genomic wide association study (GWAS) of IgAN in a cohort of 3144 cases of Chinese and European ancestry, linked allele deletion polymorphisms of complement factor H-related proteins one and three (*CFHR1* and *CFHR3*) with less severe IgA nephropathy [29,30]. Since CFHR proteins interfere with factor H complement regulation (Figure 1) their deficiency might reduce complement activation and lessen IgAN. CFHR1, CFHR3, and CFHR5 especially have been studied for their role in IgAN [29,31]; another study of 1126 Chinese patients concluded that circulating CFHR5 levels are an independent risk factor for the disease: levels were higher in IgAN subjects compared to heathy controls, and correlated directly with worst Oxford MEST pathology score, a lower glomerular filtration rate (GFR), and hypertension [32].

4.3. Membranous Nephropathy

Membranous nephropathy (MN) is the second most commonly diagnosed GN, and the most common cause for nephrotic syndrome in adults (20–50%) [33]. Disease progression varies greatly with ~1/3 of patients undergoing spontaneous remission, ~1/3 developing progressive renal insufficiency, and ~1/3 maintaining normal GFR despite persistent proteinuria. MN is characterized by presence of anti-podocyte antibodies in the subepithelial space of glomerular capillary loops and granular deposits of IgG4 and C3. M-type phospholipase A2 receptor (PLA$_2$R) has been found as the main target podocyte antigen for autoantibodies in 70–80% of patients with primary MN, while antibodies against thrombospondin type 1 domain-containing 7A (THSD7A) are detected in a minority of patients [34]. Although antibodies from IgG4 subclass are poor classical complement pathway activators, deposition of C3 and breakdown of C4b products are detectable in almost all patients with a primary form of MN [27]. Mannose binding lectin and MBL-associated serine protease expression (MASP-1, MASP-2) are detected in PLA$_2$R positive patients' glomeruli, suggesting that complement activation proceeds through this pathway [35]. Hypogalactosylated IgG (including IgG4) binds MBL and activates the complement providing a possible explanation to the IgG4 conundrum [36]. Animal studies also indicate a role for MAC insertion into podocytes; blocking their formation prevents disease [37]. Sublytic activation alters podocyte cytoskeletal structure crucial for slit diaphragm integrity and function, leading to proteinuria [38,39].

4.4. Post Infectious Glomerulonephritis

Post infectious GN is a common cause of nephritic syndrome that develops after self-limited bacterial infections (most commonly from *streptococcal* or *staphylococcal* species). It occurs mainly in childhood, but can also be seen in adults. It is characterized by hypercellularity within the capillary loops (caused by neutrophils infiltration and endothelial proliferation) and strong C3 staining, usually in addition to IgG. Post infectious GN occurs due to passive glomerular trapping of circulating immune complexes composed of nephritogenic bacterial antigens and IgG, complement activation, and attraction of neutrophils responsible for glomerular injury [28]. However, levels of C1q and C4 deposition are lacking or low in most of the cases [40,41], suggesting contributions from lectin and alternative pathway. This is eventually triggered from specific pathogens' components; for example, streptococcal pyrogenic exotoxin B is a possible alternative pathway activation [42]. Autoantibodies with C3 nephritic factor (C3nef), activity that binds to and stabilizes C3 convertases, has also been reported in post-infectious GN and may be associated with an enhanced cleavage of C3 [28]. In some patients underlying genetic defects in the regulation of the alternative pathway, including mutations in complement regulators (fH or CFHR5) and presence of C3Nef, lead to persistent glomerular deposition of complement factors within the glomeruli and inflammatory infiltrates that resemble features of a persistent proliferative glomerulonephritis [43]. Interestingly, in few cases, post infectious GN evolved into C3 glomerulopathy (C3G) [44]: recent reports document repeat biopsies demonstrating transformation of post infectious GN to C3G, including identical appearing early lesions of C3G and initiation of C3G by streptococcal infection. Sethi et al. [43] described that most of the cases with biopsy-proven persistent post-infectious GN had underlying genetic mutations and/or auto-antibodies affecting regulation of the alternative complement pathway. These findings indicate that glomerular injuries initiated by infection may transfer to C3G by imbalanced alternative complement pathway activation: C3G is initiated by heterogeneous insults, leading to a final common pathway of alternative complement dysregulation.

4.5. Immune Complex-Mediated Membranoproliferative Glomerulonephritis (MPGN)

Membranoproliferative glomerulonephritis (MPGN) is a histopathological pattern of glomerular injury characterized by mesangial hypercellularity, capillary wall changes (i.e., "tram-tracking"), and endocapillary proliferation found in 7–10% of biopsy-diagnosed glomerulonephritis [45]. MPGN classification was based on electron micrograph ultrastructural findings but advances in our understanding of underlying pathomechanisms produced a rethinking of MPGN and a classification schema based on immunofluorescence findings; MPGN is caused by immune complex deposition, C3 dysregulation, or thrombotic microangiopathy (TMA) [45]. Immune complex-mediated MPGN is caused by immune complex deposition in the subendothelial space activating complement classical pathways and causing glomerular injury. When not linked to a systemic disease, it is termed 'idiopathic' but secondary forms more commonly occur in association with infections (e.g., hepatitis B, C, or tuberculosis), autoimmune diseases (e.g., Sjogren's Syndrome or systemic lupus erythematosus SLE), or monoclonal gammopathy. Clinical evidence of classical complement activation in immune complex-mediated MPGN includes preferential consumption of plasma C4 (although C3 is often low as well) and detection of C1q and terminal C5b-9 complex in glomeruli. This phase is followed by an influx of leukocytes, promoted by formation of the C3a and C5a anaphylatoxins, leading to capillary damage and proteinuria [46]. Activation of classical pathway through immunoglobulins is the most prominent pathogenic process, but heterozygous mutations in alternative pathway complement regulators and the presence of circulating C3nef factor are also identified in some patients with immune complex-mediated MPGN, suggesting additional contributions from the alternative pathway [47]. These findings raise the possibility that in individuals with genetic or acquired complement alternative pathway dysregulation, immune complex deposition initially triggers injury through the classical pathway but chronic kidney injury is sustained through the enhanced alternative pathway [46]. The complement also features prominently in the two other dominant etiologies of MPGN: C3 glomerulopathies and TMA from atypical Hemolytic Uremic Syndrome (aHUS), and these are discussed in detail later in this paper.

4.6. Anti-GBM Glomerulonephritis

Anti-glomerular basement membrane (GBM) is a rare life-threatening autoimmune disease, caused by IgG autoantibodies against alpha 3 NC1 domain of collagen IV of the GBM. Antibody binding to the GBM leads to injury characterized by strong complement activation, leukocyte infiltration, and proteinuria; leading to crescent formation, scarring, and, frequently, end-stage renal disease (ESRD). Evidence of complement pathogenic role comes from detection of complement components MBL, C1q, factor B (fB), properdin, C3d/C4d, and C5b-9 in GBM, and circulating MAC levels that correlate with kidney injury severity [48]. Local complement activation produces C3a- and C5a-mediated inflammation, as well as MAC-dependent sublytic activation of glomerular cells, which together enhance inflammation and extracellular matrix formation [49]. Pathways of complement activation in anti-GBM disease have been studied in murine models by injection of heterologous antibodies against GBM, where C3 and C4 deficiency prevented full manifestation of renal disease [46,50,51]. This evidence supports involvement of, at least, both classical and alternative pathways in anti-GBM disease.

4.7. ANCA Induced Renal Vasculitis

Antineutrophil cytoplasmic antibody (ANCA) associated vasculitides commonly target the kidney, with abundant complement component deposition in vessels and glomeruli without immunoglobulin (pauci-immune). Current research supports that vascular injury is due to cytokine-primed neutrophils displaying surface ANCA-binding antigens (myeloperoxidase and proteinase-3) that undergo degranulation while simultaneously activating alternative complement pathways which potentiates neutrophil recruitment via C5a [8]. C5a generation functions as an amplification loop for ANCA-mediated neutrophil activation, eventually culminating in the severe necrotizing inflammation of the vessel walls. Studies in animal models have also shown complement contributes to pathogenesis, and agents blocking C5 cleavage/C5a signaling or C5 and fB deficiency themselves are protective; conversely, preventing MAC formation is ineffective, supporting the importance of C5a in ANCA-mediated pathogenesis [52,53]. A recent trial of patients with ANCA vasculitis compared the use of rituximab/cyclophosphamide in addition to either placebo and high-dose steroids, avacopan (C5aR antagonist) plus reduced dose steroids, or avacopan and no steroids. Regimens with low or absent steroids were non-inferior to traditional regimens; this illustrates complement's essential role in ANCA vasculitis and suggests C5aR antagonism as a feasible alternative in patients where steroids are contraindicated [54].

4.8. Lupus Nephritis

Systemic lupus erythematosus (SLE) is an autoimmune disorder characterized by antibodies to self-antigens (e.g., anti-nuclear) leading to the formation of immune complexes that deposit in target organs. Lupus nephritis (LN) is one severe complication of SLE. Up to 50% of patients with SLE have clinically evident kidney disease at presentation, and up to 75% develop it during the course of the disease [55]. The hallmark of renal pathology is simultaneous glomerular deposition of IgG, IgM, IgA, C4, and C3, referring to the poker hand ranking, the "full house pattern" [55]. Complement deposition is not merely a biomarker of LN, as it mediates direct glomerular injury: Immune complex-mediated classical pathway plays a key pathogenic role through both intra capillary generation of neutrophil and macrophage chemotactic factors (class II–IV) and formation of MAC (class V) [56]. Circulating C3 and C4 levels are reduced in more than 90% of patients with diffuse proliferative LN and their decline often reflects a worsening in disease activity [57]. Extensive data from animal models also indicate a significant role for alternative pathway activation: Deletion of regulators (i.e., fH) or activators (i.e., fB and fD) worsen or ameliorate, respectively, experimental LN [58–60]. In humans, plasma Bb levels (but not C3) are associated with LN outcome and strongly correlated with MAC levels. In addition, Bb co-localized with MAC in the glomeruli with LN, overall supporting the concept that activation of MAC in LN reflects alternative pathway activation [57]. Experimental LN can be prevented by blockade of all complement pathways through the administration of CR2-*Crry* fusion protein [61]. Data also show that the disease severity can be ameliorated by C5aR blockade [62] or anti-C5 mAb [63], which suggests the potential clinical relevance of complement pathway intervention. A phase 1 human trial with eculizumab (anti-C5) suggested preliminary efficacy, but the treatment period was too short to draw definitive conclusions [64]. The complement system seems to have a paradoxical role in SLE: genetically determined complement deficiencies or development of anti-complement antibodies involving components of the classical pathway (anti-C1q or C1-INH) [65], are strong risk factors. Susceptibility is likely due to a defective clearance of nuclear antigens released by injured and apoptotic cells since experimental studies have shown that such deficiencies lead to autoantibody production and glomerular injury [66].

5. Disease with Complement Activation in the Absence of Detectable Serum Antibodies

5.1. Atypical Hemolytic Uremic Syndrome

Hemolytic uremic syndrome (HUS) is defined by the triad of mechanical hemolytic anemia, thrombocytopenia and acute kidney injury. Renal pathology shows typically diffuse fibrin thrombi, endothelial swelling and capillary lumens narrowed/collapsed (acute features), or reduplication of GMB, mesangiolysis, and vessels recanalization (chronic phase). Typical forms of HUS are related to infection by Shiga toxin (Stx) producing *Escherichia coli* (STEC), while aHUS) is a condition due to defects in alternative complement activation. It has been associated with a predisposing genotype, usually an inherited heterozygous mutation [67,68], rather than an acquired mutation or loss of complement proteins (e.g., fI, fH, MCP).

The first identified mutant gene encodes for fH [28], the most important alternative pathway regulator in plasma and on cell surfaces. Subsequently, over 100 mutations were identified and most commonly lead to normal levels of a protein that is unable to bind and regulate complement components on endothelial cells [69].

Most complement genes mutations associated with aHUS result in an altered cell surface regulation: MCP mutation and fI mutation prevent effective degradation of C3 convertase. Although rarer, factors C3/C3b or fB gain of function mutations have been described [28]. Formation of blocking antibodies direct against fH is also another possible pathogenic mechanism [46,68]. 3–5% of patients with aHUS also carry heterozygous mutation of thrombomodulin (THBD), a molecule that normally enhances fI function [70]. As discussed below, complement targeting therapies have been extremely effective in treating this condition.

5.2. C3 Nephropathy

C3 nephropathy (C3N) is a rare nephritic disease, with a poor long-term outcome. The membranoproliferative pattern is the most common (not unique) histological presentation of C3 nephropathy and is further divided in the two entities of: Dense deposit disease (DDD), with typical ultrastructural evidence of intramembranous highly electron-dense osmophilic deposits with or without IgG and C3 on immunofluorescence, and C3 glomerulonephritis (C3GN) diagnosed with C3 positive on IF while all others immunoglobulins are negative [71,72]. Low serum C3 and glomerular deposits of C3 are emblematic of alternative pathway dysregulation.

A major subset of C3 glomerulopathies arises from C3Nef autoantibodies (present in 40% of C3GN and 80% of DDD) stabilizing C3 convertases against complement regulatory proteins (CRegs), or from other antibodies (former anti-fB, anti-fH) targeting directly CRegs [47]. C3 glomerulopathy can be due to genetic missense or non-sense mutations, affecting genes that encode for complement components or regulators [46,73]. The most important seems to involve fH, fI, and CFHR proteins with loss of function [74]; C3 mutation with gain of function and resistance to fH is uncommon [75] and when C5 genes are affected a less severe form of GN occurs [76]. fH/fI deficiency/resistance play a critical role in developing the disease because the GBM does not express CRegs and therefore relies on circulating ones (i.e., fH/fI) to prevent excessive local fluid phase AP activation.

Several cases of familiar C3 glomerulopathy have also been described when mutation of CFHR gene cluster occurs; recently an autosomal dominant inheritance among some Cypriote families has been described. In this nephropathy, CFHR5 has reduced affinity for surface-bound complement [77], the glomeruli present with C3GN features but C3 levels in the serum tend to be normal suggesting that improper complement activation occurs in the glomerulus rather than plasma [46,78–81].

6. Other Glomerular Diseases

Focal Segmental Glomerulosclerosis

Focal segmental glomerulosclerosis (FSGS), is one of the leading causes of nephrotic syndrome in adults. Patients with non-nephrotic proteinuria have good prognosis and about 15% progress to ESRD over the course of 10 years, whereas 50% of patients with nephrotic-range proteinuria progress to ESRD over 5–10 years [82]. In patients with massive proteinuria (10–14 g/d), the course is malignant, resulting in ESRD by 2–3 years on average [82]. It is characterized by focal and segmental obliteration of glomerular capillary tufts, with an increase in matrix. The sources of podocyte damage are varied and not altogether known, but include circulating factors, genetic abnormalities, viral infection, and medications that produce common deleterious effects on podocytes. C3 and IgM glomerular deposition is typical, suggesting complement activation contributes to FSGS pathogenesis [83]. Sclerotic lesions are significantly higher in patients with C3 deposition combined with IgM; they have worse renal dysfunction and limited response to therapy [84]. Murine models of FSGS clarified that glomerular IgM deposits activate complement, suggesting that glomerular injury simultaneously increases classical pathway activation by natural IgM, which binds to injury associated epitopes, while also decreasing glomerular alternative complement regulating abilities [85]. Consistent with a pathogenic role for IgM, B cell absence in murine FSGS models prevents IgM deposition and albuminuria [85]. In humans, mutations in fH and C3 have been described in literature cases of biopsy documented FSGS [86] and FSGS patient urine and plasma are enriched with complement fragments C3a, C3b, Ba, Bb, C4a, sC5b-9 compared to samples from patients with other renal diseases [87].

7. Complement Inhibitory Drugs in Kidney Diseases

Identification of complement component contributions to renal pathogenesis recently spurred pharmaceutical industry efforts to therapeutically target complement

Many available agents target terminal complement molecules and more proximal roles, such as opsonization, remains preserved. Even so, since these agents are immunosuppressants, they convey increased infection risk. More importantly, relevant to kidney diseases, many upstream elements (e.g., C3a, C5a, and C3b) contribute to pathogenesis and are not effectively targeted by available compounds. Currently, Food and Drug Administration (FDA) approved complement inhibitors include the monoclonal anti-C5 antibody Eculizumab, and Cynrize an inhibitor of fragment C1 (C1-INH) [88–90].

7.1. Eculizumab

Eculizumab is a humanized murine monoclonal antibody to complement C5 that acts on the terminal complement cascade preventing the formation of C5a, C5b, and C5b-9. The drug use has been approved by European Medicines Agency's (EMA) and FDA for treatment of paroxysmal nocturnal hemoglobinuria (PNH) and aHUS [91]. The major side effect is predisposition to infections, especially from gram-negative bacteria; as such, all patients are advised to be immunized for *meningococcus* before receiving eculizumab. Eculizumab approval for aHUS treatment was given based on results from two prospective trials: one involving 17 aHUS patients with thrombocytopenia and the other with 20 aHUS patients requiring persistent plasma exchange (PE) [92]. Whole patients from these cohorts no longer required PE and 88% reached normal hematological values after median of 63 weeks of Eculizumab treatment. This medication has dramatically improved renal morbidity, with consistent decreases in ESRD risk, but its clinical use is still limited by uncertainty over patient selection, timing, and duration of treatment. An ongoing multi center single-arm trial is now testing the safety Eculizumab discontinuation in patients with aHUS (NCT02574403). Eculizumab has also been successfully used to prevent or treat recurrence of aHUS after kidney transplant [93–95], but appears ineffective in preventing delayed graft function (NCT01919346) [96] in sensitized kidney transplant recipients (NCT00670774, NCT01095887, NCT01327573) [97,98].

Eculizumab has successfully treated patients with DDD and C3GN highlighting its potential with these rare diseases. Treatment of six patients (three C3GN and three DDD) resulted in complete to partial remission in four patients at one year of follow-up [99]. This positive effect was limited to patients with crescentic rapidly progressive C3 glomerulopathy as opposed to a more insidious C3GN suggesting that it is specific to disease pathogenesis. Moreover, advantages are not seen so far in C3GN recurrence after kidney transplantation [100]. Eculizumab use in patients with glomerular diseases other than aHUS or C3GN/DDD is limited to case reports and of uncertain efficacy. The price of eculizumab is a factor that limits its use. Competitors have in clinical development both similar agents targeting C5 (e.g., Ravulizumab), as well as agents that affect complement component C5a (i.e., Avacoban).

7.2. C1 Inhibitor

Despite the potential advantages of terminal complement inhibition, these approaches may not be sufficient in conditions stemming from more proximal complement activation. Classical complement pathway activation occurs when C1q binds the Fc portion of antigen bound immunoglobulin. Preventing this process is C1-esterase inhibitor and its absence or mutated function produces the condition hereditary angioedema. *Cinryze*, a human serum derived C1 inhibitor (C1-INH) is FDA approved for treatment of hereditary angioedema. C1-INH does not have approved indications for kidney disease, but a phase I/II study was conducted on highly sensitized renal transplant recipients randomized to C1INH or placebo. Antibody mediated rejection was prevented in all 10 patients receiving C1INH group and 9/10 only receiving placebo. Efficacy and safety of C1INH for treatment of acute antibody mediated rejection in kidney transplantation is being evaluated in a randomized double-blind study of donor-sensitized kidney transplants recipients (NCT02052141, NCT02547220) [101]. Results may broaden its use to patients with antibody mediated rejection.

8. Conclusions

The complement system is a complex network of proteins that augment immune system function and, in many cases, contribute to kidney disease pathogenesis. Increasing research suggests that selective interventions to stop cascade activation can halt or even reverse renal disease. Ongoing research, both translational and in animal models, will help delineate which pathway(s), and at what level, intervention could be effective. Although infrequently a primary insult, common mutations affecting complement regulation synergize with other pathological features perpetuating inflammation and, ultimately, nephron loss. The advent of selective complement-targeting therapeutics offers the opportunity for new treatment strategies for renal disease, an area in desperate need of new options.

Author Contributions: S.A. and J.L. searched the literature and wrote the manuscript. G.Z. and P.C. contributed to the literature search and literature analysis. P.C. revised the manuscript. All authors read and approved the final manuscript.

Funding: Paolo Cravedi is funded by the NIH NIDDK grant R01DK119431-01.

Conflicts of Interest: The authors declare no conflict of interest.

References

1. Walport, M.J. Complement–First of Two Parts. *N. Engl. J. Med.* **2001**, *344*, 1058–1066. [CrossRef] [PubMed]
2. Walport, M.J. Complement: Second of two parts: Complement at the interface between innate and adaptive immunity. *N. Engl. J. Med.* **2001**, *344*, 1140–1144. [CrossRef] [PubMed]
3. Mizuno, M.; Suzuki, Y.; Ito, Y. Complement regulation and kidney diseases: Recent knowledge of the double-edged roles of complement activation in nephrology. *Clin. Exp. Nephrol.* **2018**, *22*, 3–14. [CrossRef] [PubMed]
4. Hourcade, D.E.; Spitzer, D.; Mitchell, L.M.; Atkinson, J.P. Properdin Can Initiate Complement Activation by Binding Specific Target Surfaces and Providing a Platform for De Novo. *J. Immunol. Ref.* **2007**, *179*, 2600–2608.
5. Holmskov, U.; Thiel, S.; Jensenius, J.C. Collectin and Ficolins: Humoral Lectins of the Innate Immune Defense. *Annu. Rev. Immunol.* **2003**, *21*, 547–578. [CrossRef]
6. Endo, Y.; Matsushita, M.; Fujita, T. The role of ficolins in the lectin pathway of innate immunity. *Int. J. Biochem. Cell Biol.* **2011**, *43*, 705–712. [CrossRef]
7. Forneris, F.; Ricklin, D.; Wu, J.; Tzekou, A.; Wallace, R.S.; Lambris, J.D.; Gros, P. Structures of C3b in Complex with Factors B and D Give Insight into Complement Convertase Formation. *Science* **2010**, *330*, 1816–1820. [CrossRef]
8. Mathern, D.R.; Heeger, P.S. Molecules Great and Small: The Complement System. *Clin. J. Am. Soc. Nephrol.* **2015**, *10*, 1636–1650. [CrossRef]
9. Ricklin, D.; Hajishengallis, G.; Yang, K.; Lambris, J.D. Complement-a key system for immune surveillance and homeostasis. *Nat. Immunol.* **2010**, *11*, 785. [CrossRef]

10. Guo, R.-F.; Ward, P.A. Role of C5a in inflamatory response. *Annu. Rev. Immunol.* **2005**, *23*, 821–852. [CrossRef]
11. Kwan, W.H.; van der Touw, W.; Paz-Artal, E.; Li, M.O.; Heeger, P.S. Signaling through C5a receptor and C3a receptor diminishes function of murine natural regulatory T cells. *J. Exp. Med.* **2013**, *210*, 257–268. [CrossRef] [PubMed]
12. Van Der Touw, W.; Cravedi, P.; Kwan, W.-H.; Paz-Artal, E.; Merad, M.; Heeger, P.S. Receptors for C3a and C5a modulate stability of alloantigen-reactive induced regulatory T cells. *J. Immunol.* **2013**, *190*, 5921–5925. [CrossRef] [PubMed]
13. Klos, A.; Tenner, A.J.; Johswich, K.-O.; Ager, R.R.; Reis, E.S.; Köhl, J. The Role of the Anaphylatoxins in Health and Disease. *Mol. Immunol.* **2009**, *46*, 2753–2766. [CrossRef] [PubMed]
14. Jane-wit, D.; Manes, T.D.; Yi, T.; Qin, L.; Clark, P.; Kirkiles-Smith, N.C.; Abrahimi, P.; Devalliere, J.; Moeckel, G.; Kulkarni, S.; et al. Alloantibody and Complement Promote T Cell-Mediated Cardiac Allograft Vasculopathy through Non-Canonical NF-κB Signaling in Endothelial Cells. *Circulation* **2013**, *128*, 2504–2516. [CrossRef]
15. Adler, S.; Baker, P.J.; Johnson, R.J.; Ochi, R.F.; Pritzl, P.; Couser, W.G. Complement Membrane Attack Complex. Stimulates Production of Reactive Oxygen Metabolites by Cultured Rat Mesangial Cells. *J. Clin. Investig.* **1996**, *77*, 762–767. [CrossRef]
16. Peake, P.W.; O'Grady, S.; Pussell, B.A.; Charlesworth, J.A. C3a is made by proximal tubular HK-2 cells and activates them via the C3a receptor. *Kidney Int.* **1999**, *56*, 1729–1736. [CrossRef]
17. Lalli, P.N.; Strainic, M.G.; Yang, M.; Lin, F.; Medof, M.E.; Heeger, P.S. Locally produced C5a binds to T cell-expressed C5aR to enhance effector T-cell expansion by limiting antigen-induced apoptosis. *Blood* **2008**, *11*, 1759–1766. [CrossRef]
18. Strainic, M.G.; Liu, J.; Huang, D.; An, F.; Lalli, P.N.; Muqim, N.; Shapiro, V.S.; Dubyak, G.R.; Heeger, P.S.; Medof, M.E. Locally Produced Complement Fragments C5a and C3a Provide Both Costimulatory and Survival Signals to Naive CD4 + T. Cells. *Immunity* **2008**, *28*, 425–435. [CrossRef]
19. Heeger, P.S.; Lalli, P.N.; Lin, F.; Valujskikh, A.; Liu, J.; Muqim, N; Xu, Y.; Medof, M.E. Decay-accelerating factor modulates induction of T cell immunity. *J. Exp. Med.* **2005**, *201*, 1523–1530. [CrossRef]
20. Hanko, J.B.; Mullan, R.N.; O'rourke, D.M.; Mcnamee, P.T.; Maxwell, A.P.; Courtney, A.E. The changing pattern of adult primary glomerular disease. *Nephrol. Dial. Transpl.* **2009**, *24*, 3050–3054. [CrossRef]
21. Nair, R.; Walker, P.D. Is IgA nephropathy the commonest primary glomerulopathy among young adults in the USA? *Kidney Int.* **2006**, *69*, 1455–1458. [CrossRef] [PubMed]
22. Wada Id, Y.; Matsumoto, K.; Suzuki, T.; Saito, T.; Kanazawa, N.; Tachibanaid, S.; Iseri, K.; Sugiyama, M.; Iyoda, M.; Shibata, T. Clinical significance of serum and mesangial galactose-deficient IgA1 in patients with IgA nephropathy. *PLoS ONE* **2018**, *13*, e0206865. [CrossRef] [PubMed]
23. Mestecky, J.; Raska, M.; Julian, B.A.; Gharavi, A.G.; Renfrow, M.B.; Moldoveanu, Z.; Novak, L.; Matousovic, K.; Novak, J. IgA Nephropathy: Molecular Mechanisms of the Disease. *Annu. Rev. Pathol: Mech. Dis.* **2012**, *8*, 217–240. [CrossRef] [PubMed]
24. Lafayette, R.A.; Kelepouris, E.; Lafayette, R. Immunoglobulin A Nephropathy: Advances in Understanding of Pathogenesis and Treatment. *Rev. Artic. Am. J. Nephrol* **2018**, *47*, 43–52. [CrossRef] [PubMed]
25. Oortwijn, B.D.; Eijgenraam, J.W.; Rastaldi, M.P.; Roos, A.; Daha, M.R.; van Kooten, C. The Role of Secretory IgA and Complement in IgA Nephropathy. *Semin. Nephrol.* **2008**, *28*, 58–65. [CrossRef] [PubMed]
26. Roos, A.; Rastaldi, M.P.; Calvaresi, N.; Oortwijn, B.D.; Schlagwein, N.; Van Gijlswijk-Janssen, D.J.; Stahl, G.L.; Matsushita, M.; Fujita, T.; Van Kooten, C.; et al. Glomerular Activation of the Lectin Pathway of Complement in IgA Nephropathy Is Associated with More Severe Renal Disease. *J. Am. Soc. Nephrol.* **2006**, *17*, 1724–1734. [CrossRef] [PubMed]
27. Thurman, J.M. Complement in Kidney Disease: Core Curriculum. *Am. J. Kidney Dis.* **2015**, *65*, 156–168. [CrossRef]
28. Couser, W.G. Pathogenesis and treatment of glomerulonephritis-an update. *J. Bras. Nefrol.* **2016**, *38*, 107–122. [CrossRef]
29. Gharavi, A.G.; Kiryluk, K.; Choi, M.; Li, Y.; Hou, P.; Xie, J.; Sanna-Cherchi, S.; Men, C.J.; Julian, B.A.; Wyatt, R.J.; et al. Genome-wide association study identifies susceptibility loci for IgA nephropathy. *Nat. Genet.* **2011**, *43*, 321–329. [CrossRef]
30. Xie, J.; Kiryluk, K.; Li, Y.; Mladkova, N.; Zhu, L.; Hou, P.; Ren, H.; Wang, W.; Zhang, H.; Chen, N.; et al. Fine Mapping Implicates a Deletion of CFHR1 and CFHR3 in Protection from IgA Nephropathy in Han Chinese. *J. Am. Soc. Nephrol.* **2016**, *27*, 3187–3194. [CrossRef]

31. Medjeral-Thomas, N.R.; Lomax-Browne, H.J.; Beckwith, H.; Willicombe, M.; McLean, A.G.; Brookes, P.; Pusey, C.D.; Falchi, M.; Cook, H.T.; Pickering, M.C. Circulating complement factor H–related proteins 1 and 5 correlate with disease activity in IgA nephropathy. *Kidney Int.* **2017**, *92*, 942–952. [CrossRef]
32. Zhu, L.; Guo, W.Y.; Shi, S.F.; Liu, L.J.; Lv, J.C.; Medjeral-Thomas, N.R.; Lomax-Browne, H.J.; Pickering, M.C.; Zhang, H. Circulating complement factor H–related protein 5 levels contribute to development and progression of IgA nephropathy. *Kidney Int.* **2018**, *94*, 150–158. [CrossRef] [PubMed]
33. Akiyama, S.I.; Imai, E.; Maruyama, S. Immunology of membranous nephropathy. *F1000 Res.* **2019**, *8*. [CrossRef] [PubMed]
34. Wang, Z.; Wen, L.; Dou, Y.; Zhao, Z. Human anti-thrombospondin type 1 domain-containing 7A antibodies induce membranous nephropathy through activation of lectin complement pathway. *Biosci. Rep.* **2018**, *38*. [CrossRef] [PubMed]
35. Yang, Y.; Wang, C.; Jin, L.; He, F.; Li, C.; Gao, Q.; Chen, G.; He, Z.; Song, M.; Zhou, Z.; et al. IgG4 anti-phospholipase A2 receptor might activate lectin and alternative complement pathway meanwhile in idiopathic membranous nephropathy: An inspiration from a cross-sectional study. *Immunol. Res.* **2016**, *64*, 919–930. [CrossRef] [PubMed]
36. Ma, H.; Sandor, D.G.; Beck, L.H., Jr. The role of complement in membranous nephropathy. *Semin. Nephrol.* **2013**, *33*, 531–542. [CrossRef]
37. Baker, P.J.; Ochi, R.F.; Schulze, M.; Johnson, R.J.; Campbell, C.; Couser, W.G. Depletion of C6 Prevents Development of Proteinuria in Experimental Membranous Nephropathy in Rats. *Am. J. Pathol.* **1989**, *135*, 185–194.
38. Saran, A.M.; Yuan, H.; Takeuchi, E.; McLaughlin, M.; Salant, D.J. Complement mediates nephrin redistribution and actin dissociation in experimental membranous nephropathy. *Kidney Int.* **2003**, *64*, 2072–2078. [CrossRef]
39. Yuan, H.; Takeuchi, E.; Taylor, G.A.; Mclaughlin, M.; Brown, D.; Salant, D.J. Nephrin Dissociates from Actin, and Its Expression Is Reduced in Early Experimental Membranous Nephropathy. *J. Am. Soc. Nephrol.* **2002**, *13*, 946–956.
40. Morel-Maroger, L.; Leathem, A.; Richet, G. Glomerular abnormalities in nonsystemic diseases. Relationship between findings by light microscopy and immunofluorescence in 433 renal biopsy specimens. *Am. J. Med.* **1972**, *53*, 170–184. [CrossRef]
41. Verroust, P.J.; Wilson, C.B.; Cooper, N.R.; Edgington, T.S.; Dixon, F.J. Glomerular Complement Components in Human Glomerulonephritis. *J. Clin. Investig.* **1974**, *53*, 77–84. [CrossRef] [PubMed]
42. Hisano, S.; Matsushita, M.; Fujita, T.; Takeshita, M.; Iwasaki, H. Activation of the lectin complement pathway in post-streptococcal acute glomerulonephritis. *Pathol. Int.* **2007**, *57*, 351–357. [CrossRef] [PubMed]
43. Sethi, S.; Fervenza, F.C.; Zhang, Y.; Zand, L.; Meyer, N.C.; Borsa, N.; Nasr, S.H.; Smith, R.J.H. Atypical post-infectious glomerulonephritis is associated with abnormalities in the alternative pathway of complement. *Kidney Int.* **2013**, *83*, 293–299. [CrossRef] [PubMed]
44. Ito, N.; Ohashi, R.; Nagata, M. C3 glomerulopathy and current dilemmas. *Clin. Exp. Nephrol.* **2017**, *21*, 541–551. [CrossRef]
45. Masani, N.; Jhaveri, K.D.; Fishbane, S. Update on membranoproliferative GN. *Clin. J. Am. Soc. Nephrol.* **2014**, *9*, 600–608. [CrossRef]
46. Noris, M.; Remuzzi, G. Glomerular Diseases Dependent on Complement Activation, Including Atypical Hemolytic Uremic Syndrome, Membranoproliferative Glomerulonephritis, and C3 Glomerulopathy: Core Curriculum 2015. *Am. J. Kidney Dis.* **2015**, *66*, 359–375. [CrossRef]
47. Servais, A.; Ne Noël, L.-H.; Roumenina, L.T.; Le Quintrec, M.; Ngo, S.; -Agnès Dragon-Durey, M.; Macher, M.-A.; Zuber, J.; Karras, A.; Provot, F.; et al. Acquired and genetic complement abnormalities play a critical role in dense deposit disease and other C3 glomerulopathies. *Kidney Int.* **2012**, *82*, 454–464. [CrossRef]
48. Ma, R.; Cui, Z.; Hu, S.-Y.; Jia, X.-Y.; Yang, R. The Alternative Pathway of Complement Activation May Be Involved in the Renal Damage of Human Anti-Glomerular Basement Membrane Disease. *PLoS ONE* **2014**, *9*, 91250. [CrossRef]
49. Minto, A.W.; Kalluri, R.; Togawa, M.; Bergijk, E.C.; Killen, P.D.; Salant, D.J. Augmented expression of glomerular basement membrane specific type IV collagen isoforms (alpha3-alpha5) in experimental membranous nephropathy. *Proc. Assoc. Am. Physicians* **1998**, *110*, 207–217.

50. Sheerin, N.S.; Springall, T.; Carroll, M.C.; Hartley, B.; Sacks, S.H. Protection against anti-glomerular basement membrane (GBM)-mediated nephritis in C3-and C4-deficient mice. *Clin. Exp. Immunol.* **1997**, *110*, 403–409. [CrossRef]
51. Fischer, E.G.; Lager, D.J. Anti-glomerular basement membrane glomerulonephritis: A morphologic study of 80 cases. *Am. J. Clin. Pathol.* **2006**, *125*, 445–450. [CrossRef] [PubMed]
52. Xiao, H.; Dairaghi, D.J.; Powers, J.P.; Ertl, L.S.; Baumgart, T.; Wang, Y.; Seitz, L.C.; Penfold, M.E.; Gan, L.; Hu, P.; et al. C5a Receptor (CD88) Blockade Protects against MPO-ANCA GN Necrotizing and crescentic GN (NCGN) and vasculitis are associated with ANCA. *J. Am. Soc. Nephrol.* **2014**, *25*, 225–231. [CrossRef] [PubMed]
53. Xiao, H.; Schreiber, A.; Heeringa, P.; Falk, R.J.; Jennette, J.C. Alternative complement pathway in the pathogenesis of disease mediated by anti-neutrophil cytoplasmic autoantibodies. *Am. J. Pathol.* **2007**, *170*, 52–64. [CrossRef] [PubMed]
54. Jayne, D.R.W.; Bruchfeld, A.N.; Harper, L.; Schaier, M.; Venning, M.C.; Hamilton, P.; Burst, V.; Grundmann, F.; Jadoul, M.; Szombati, I.; et al. Randomized trial of C5a receptor inhibitor avacopan in ANCA-associated vasculitis. *J. Am. Soc. Nephrol.* **2017**, *28*, 2756–2767. [CrossRef] [PubMed]
55. Markowitz, G.S.; D'Agati, V.D. Classification of lupus nephritis. *Curr. Opin. Nephrol. Hypertens.* **2009**, *18*, 220–225. [CrossRef] [PubMed]
56. Couser, W.G. Basic and Translational Concepts of Immune-Mediated Glomerular Diseases. *J. Am. Soc. Nephrol.* **2012**, *23*, 381–399. [CrossRef] [PubMed]
57. Song, D.; Guo, W.Y.; Wang, F.M.; Li, Y.Z.; Song, Y.; Yu, F.; Zhao, M.H. Complement Alternative Pathway's Activation in Patients with Lupus Nephritis. *Am. J. Med. Sci.* **2017**, *353*, 247–257. [CrossRef]
58. Pickering, M.C.; Botto, M. Are anti-C1q antibodies different from other SLE autoantibodies? *Nat. Publ. Gr.* **2010**, *6*, 490–493. [CrossRef]
59. Bao, L.; Haas, M.; Quigg, R.J. Complement Factor H Deficiency Accelerates Development of Lupus Nephritis. *J. Am. Soc. Nephrol.* **2011**, *22*, 285–295. [CrossRef]
60. Bao, L.; Quigg, R.J. Complement in Lupus Nephritis: The Good, the Bad, and the Unknown. *Semin. Nephrol.* **2007**, *27*, 69–80. [CrossRef]
61. Tomlinson, S.; Atkinson, C.; Qiao, F.; Song, H.; Gilkeson, G.S. Mice lpr MRL/ Manifestations of Autoimmune Disease in Protects against Renal Disease and Other Low-Dose Targeted Complement Inhibition. *J. Immunol. Ref.* **2019**, *180*, 1231–1238.
62. Bao, L.; Osawe, I.; Puri, T.; Lambris, J.D.; Haas, M.; Quigg, R.J. C5a promotes development of experimental lupus nephritis which can be blocked with a specific receptor antagonist. *Eur. J. Immunol.* **2005**, *35*, 2496–2506. [CrossRef] [PubMed]
63. Wang, Y.; Hu, Q.; MADRIt, J.A.; Rollins, S.A.; Chodera, A.; Matis, L.A.; Talmage, D.W. Amelioration of lupus-like autoimmune disease in NZB/W F1 mice after treatment with a blocking monoclonal antibody specific for complement component C5. *Proc. Natl. Acad. Sci. USA* **1996**, *93*, 8563–8568. [CrossRef] [PubMed]
64. Murdaca, G.; Colombo, B.M.; Puppo, F. Emerging biological drugs: A new therapeutic approach for Systemic Lupus Erythematosus. An update upon efficacy and adverse events. *Autoimmun. Rev.* **2011**, *11*, 56–60. [CrossRef] [PubMed]
65. Mészáros, T.; Füst, G.; Farkas, H.; Jakab, L.; Temesszentandrási, G.; Nagy, G.; Kiss, E.; Gergely, P.; Zeher, M.; Griger, Z.; et al. C1-inhibitor autoantibodies in SLE. *Lupus* **2010**, *19*, 634–638.
66. Al-Mayouf, S.M.; Abanomi, H.; Eldali, A. Impact of C1q deficiency on the severity and outcome of childhood systemic lupus erythematosus. *Int. J. Rheum. Dis.* **2011**, *14*, 81–85. [CrossRef]
67. Heurich, M.; Martínez-Barricarte, R.; Francis, N.J.; Roberts, D.L.; Rodríguez De Córdoba, S.; Morgan, B.P.; Harris, C.L. Common polymorphisms in C3, factor B, and factor H collaborate to determine systemic complement activity and disease risk. *Proc. Natl. Acad. Sci. USA* **2011**, *108*, 8761–8766. [CrossRef]
68. Noris, M.; Caprioli, J.; Bresin, E.; Mossali, C.; Pianetti, G.; Gamba, S.; Daina, E.; Fenili, C.; Castelletti, F.; Sorosina, A.; et al. Relative Role of Genetic Complement Abnormalities in Sporadic and Familial aHUS and Their Impact on Clinical Phenotype. *Clin. J. Am. Soc. Nephrol.* **2010**, *5*, 1844–1859. [CrossRef]
69. Manuelian, T.; Hellwage, J.; Meri, S.; Caprioli, J.; Noris, M.; Heinen, S.; Jozsi, M.; Neumann, H.P.H.; Remuzzi, G.; Zipfel, P.F. Mutations in factor H reduce binding affinity to C3b and heparin and surface attachment to endothelial cells in hemolytic uremic syndrome. *J. Clin. Invest.* **2003**, *111*, 1181–1190. [CrossRef]

70. Caprioli, J.; Noris, M.; Brioschi, S.; Pianetti, G.; Castelletti, F.; Bettinaglio, P.; Mele, C.; Bresin, E.; Cassis, L.; Gamba, S.; et al. Genetics of HUS: The impact of MCP, CFH, and IF mutations on clinical presentation, response to treatment, and outcome. *Blood* **2006**, *108*, 1267–1279. [CrossRef]
71. Sethi, S.; Haas, M.; Markowitz, G.S.; D'agati, V.D.; Rennke, H.G.; Jennette, J.C.; Bajema, I.M.; Alpers, C.E.; Chang, A.; Cornell, L.D.; et al. Mayo Clinic/Renal Pathology Society Consensus Report on Pathologic Classification, Diagnosis, and Reporting of GN. *J. Am. Soc. Nephrol.* **2016**, *27*, 1278–1287. [CrossRef] [PubMed]
72. Sethi, S.; Fervenza, F.C. Pathology of Renal Diseases Associated with Dysfunction of the Alternative Pathway of Complement: C3 Glomerulopathy and Atypical Hemolytic Uremic Syndrome (aHUS). *Semin. Thromb. Hemost.* **2014**, *40*, 416–421. [PubMed]
73. Łukawska, E.; Polcyn-Adamczak, M.; Niemir, Z.I. The role of the alternative pathway of complement activation in glomerular diseases. *Clin. Exp. Med.* **2018**, *18*, 297–318. [CrossRef] [PubMed]
74. Barbour, T.D.; Pickering, M.C.; Cook, H.T. Recent insights into C3 glomerulopathy. *Nephrol. Dial. Transpl.* **2013**, *28*, 1685–1693. [CrossRef] [PubMed]
75. Schramm, E.C.; Roumenina, L.T.; Rybkine, T.; Chauvet, S.; Vieira-Martins, P.; Hue, C.; Maga, T.; Valoti, E.; Wilson, V.; Jokiranta, S.; et al. Mapping interactions between complement C3 and regulators using mutations in atypical hemolytic uremic syndrome. *Blood* **2015**, *125*, 2359–2369. [CrossRef]
76. Pickering, M.C.; Warren, J.; Rose, K.L.; Carlucci, F.; Wang, Y.; Walport, M.J.; Cook, H.T.; Botto, M. Prevention of C5 activation ameliorates spontaneous and experimental glomerulonephritis in factor H-deficient mice. *Proc. Natl. Acad. Sci. USA* **2006**, *103*, 9649–9654. [CrossRef]
77. Gale, D.P.; De Jorge, E.G.; Cook, H.T.; Martinez-Barricarte, R.; Hadjisavvas, A.; McLean, A.G.; Pusey, C.D.; Pierides, A.; Kyriacou, K.; Athanasiou, Y.; et al. Identification of a mutation in complement factor H-related protein 5 in patients of Cypriot origin with glomerulonephritis. *Lancet* **2010**, *376*, 794–801. [CrossRef]
78. Xiao, X.; Ghossein, C.; Tortajadam, A.; Zhang, Y.; Meyer, N.; Jones, M.; Borsa, N.G.; Nester, C.M.; Thomas, C.P.; de Córdoba, S.R.; et al. Familial C3 glomerulonephritis caused by a novel CFHR5-CFHR2 fusion gene. *Mol. Immunol.* **2016**, *77*, 89–96. [CrossRef]
79. Chen, Q.; Wiesener, M.; Eberhardt, H.U.; Hartmann, A.; Uzonyi, B.; Kirschfink, M.; Amann, K.; Buettner, M.; Goodship, T.; Hugo, C.; et al. Complement factor H-related hybrid protein deregulates complement in dense deposit disease. *J. Clin. Investig.* **2014**, *124*, 145–155. [CrossRef]
80. Kościelska-Kasprzak, K.; Bartoszek, D.; Myszka, M.; Zabińska, M.; Klinger, M. The Complement Cascade and Renal Disease. *Arch. Immunol. Ther. Exp.* **2014**, *62*, 47–57. [CrossRef]
81. Kim, M.-K.; Maeng, Y.-I.; Lee, S.-J.; Lee, I.H.; Bae, J.; Kang, Y.-N.; Park, B.-T.; Park, K.-K. Pathogenesis and significance of glomerular C4d deposition in lupus nephritis: Activation of classical and lectin pathways. *Int. J. Clin. Exp. Pathol.* **2013**, *6*, 2157–2167. [PubMed]
82. Korbet, S.M. Treatment of Primary FSGS in Adults. *J. Am. Soc. Nephrol.* **2012**, *23*, 1769–1776. [CrossRef] [PubMed]
83. D'Agati, V.D.; Fogo, A.B.; Bruijn, J.A.; Jennette, J.C. Pathologic Classification of Focal Segmental Glomerulosclerosis: A Working Proposal. *Am. J. Kidney Dis.* **2004**, *43*, 368–382. [CrossRef] [PubMed]
84. Zhang, Y.; Gu, Q.; Huang, J.; Qu, Z.; Wang, X.; Meng, L.; Wang, F.; Liu, G.; Cui, Z.; Zhao, M. Article Clinical Significance of IgM and C3 Glomerular Deposition in Primary Focal Segmental Glomerulosclerosis. *Clin. J. Am. Soc. Nephrol.* **2016**, *11*, 1582–1589. [CrossRef]
85. Strassheim, D.; Renner, B.; Panzer, S.; Fuquay, R.; Kulik, L.; Ljubanovic, D.; Holers, V.M.; Thurman, J.M. IgM Contributes to Glomerular Injury in FSGS. *J. Am. Soc. Nephrol.* **2013**, *24*, 393–406. [CrossRef]
86. Sethi, S.; Fervenza, F.C.; Zhang, Y.; Smith, R.J. Secondary Focal and Segmental Glomerulosclerosis Associated with Single-Nucleotide Polymorphisms in the Genes Encoding Complement Factor H and C3 HHS Public Access. *Am. J. Kidney Dis.* **2012**, *60*, 316–321. [CrossRef]
87. Thurman, J.M.; Wong, M.; Renner, B.; Frazer-Abel, A.; Giclas, P.C.; Joy, M.S.; Jalal, D.; Radeva, M.K.; Gassman, J.; Gipson, D.S.; et al. Complement Activation in Patients with Focal Segmental Glomerulosclerosis. *PLoS ONE* **2015**, *10*, e0136558. [CrossRef]
88. Tomlinson, S.; Thurman, J.M. Tissue-targeted complement therapeutics. *Mol. Immunol.* **2018**, *102*, 120–128. [CrossRef]
89. Horiuchi, T.; Tsukamoto, H. Complement-targeted therapy: Development of C5-and C5a-targeted inhibition. *Inflamm. Regen.* **2016**, *36*, 11. [CrossRef]

90. Cicardi, M.; Aberer, W.; Banerji, A.; Bas, M.; Bernstein, J.A.; Bork, K.; Caballero, T.; Farkas, H.; Grumach, A.; Kaplan, A.P.; et al. Classification, diagnosis, and approach to treatment for angioedema: Consensus report from the Hereditary Angioedema International Working Group. *Allergy* **2014**, *69*, 602–616. [CrossRef]
91. Rother, R.P.; Rollins, S.A.; Mojcik, C.F.; Brodsky, R.A.; Bell, L. Discovery and development of the complement inhibitor eculizumab for the treatment of paroxysmal nocturnal hemoglobinuria. *Nat. Biotechnol.* **2007**, *25*, 1256–1264. [CrossRef] [PubMed]
92. Legendre, C.M.; Licht, C.; Muus, P.; Greenbaum, L.A.; Babu, S.; Bedrosian, C.; Bingham, C.; Cohen, D.J.; Delmas, Y.; Douglas, K.; et al. Terminal complement inhibitor eculizumab in atypical hemolytic-uremic syndrome. *N. Engl. J. Med.* **2013**, *368*, 2169–2181. [CrossRef] [PubMed]
93. Chatelet, V.; Frémeaux, V.; Frémeaux-Bacchi, F.; Lobbedez, T.; Ficheux, M.; Hurault De Ligny, B. Safety and Long-Term Efficacy of Eculizumab in a Renal Transplant Patient with Recurrent Atypical Hemolytic-Uremic Syndrome. *Am. J. Transpl.* **2009**, *9*, 2644–2645. [PubMed]
94. Wong, E.K.S.; Goodship, T.H.J.; Kavanagh, D. Complement therapy in atypical haemolytic uraemic syndrome (aHUS). *Mol. Immunol.* **2013**, *56*, 199–212. [CrossRef]
95. Kaabak, M.; Babenko, N.; Shapiro, R.; Zokoyev, A. A prospective randomized, controlled trial of eculizumab to prevent ischemia-reperfusion injury in pediatric kidney transplantation. *Pediatr. Transpl.* **2018**, *22*. [CrossRef]
96. Marks, W.H.; Mamode, N.; Montgomery, R.A.; Stegall, M.D.; Ratner, L.E.; Cornell, L.D.; Rowshani, A.T.; Colvin, R.B.; Dain, B.; Boice, J.A.; et al. Safety and efficacy of eculizumab in the prevention of antibody-mediated rejection in living-donor kidney transplant recipients requiring desensitization therapy: A randomized trial. *Am. J. Transpl.* **2019**, 1–13. [CrossRef]
97. Glotz, D.; Russ, G.; Rostaing, L.; Legendre, C.; Tufveson, G.; Chadban, S.; Grinyó, J.; Mamode, N.; Rigotti, P.; Couzi, L.; et al. Safety and efficacy of eculizumab for the prevention of antibody-mediated rejection after deceased-donor kidney transplantation in patients with preformed donor-specific antibodies. *Am. J. Transpl.* **2019**, *19*, 2865–2875. [CrossRef]
98. Bomback, A.S.; Smith, R.J.; Barile, G.R.; Zhang, Y.; Heher, E.C.; Herlitz, L.; Stokes, B.M.; Markowitz, G.S.; D'agati, V.D.; Canetta, P.A.; et al. Article Eculizumab for Dense Deposit Disease and C3 Glomerulonephritis. *Clin. J. Am. Soc. Nephrol.* **2012**, *7*, 748–756. [CrossRef]
99. Radhakrishnan, S.; Lunn, A.; Kirschfink, M.; Thorner, P.; Hebert, D.; Langlois, V.; Pluthero, F.; Licht, C. Eculizumab and refractory membranoproliferative glomerulonephritis. *N. Engl. J. Med.* **2012**, *366*, 1165–1166. [CrossRef]
100. Mccaughan, J.A.; O'rourke, D.M.; Courtney, A.E. Recurrent Dense Deposit Disease After Renal Transplantation: An Emerging Role for Complementary Therapies. *Am. J. Transpl.* **2012**, *12*, 1046–1051. [CrossRef]
101. Thurman, J.M.; Le Quintrec, M. Targeting the complement cascade: Novel treatments coming down the pike. *Kidney Int.* **2016**, *90*, 746–752. [CrossRef] [PubMed]

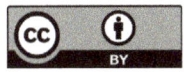

© 2019 by the authors. Licensee MDPI, Basel, Switzerland. This article is an open access article distributed under the terms and conditions of the Creative Commons Attribution (CC BY) license (http://creativecommons.org/licenses/by/4.0/).

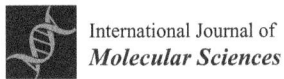

Review

A Narrative Review on C3 Glomerulopathy: A Rare Renal Disease

Francesco Paolo Schena [1,2,*], Pasquale Esposito [3] and Michele Rossini [1]

1. Department of Emergency and Organ Transplantation, Renal Unit, University of Bari, 70124 Bari, Italy; michelerossini@libero.it
2. Schena Foundation, European Center for the Study of Renal Diseases, 70010 Valenzano, Italy
3. Department of Internal Medicine, Division of Nephrology, Dialysis and Transplantation, University of Genoa and IRCCS Ospedale Policlinico San Martino, 16132 Genova, Italy; p.esposito@smatteo.pv.it
* Correspondence: paolo.schena@uniba.it

Received: 5 December 2019; Accepted: 10 January 2020; Published: 14 January 2020

Abstract: In April 2012, a group of nephrologists organized a consensus conference in Cambridge (UK) on type II membranoproliferative glomerulonephritis and decided to use a new terminology, "C3 glomerulopathy" (C3 GP). Further knowledge on the complement system and on kidney biopsy contributed toward distinguishing this disease into three subgroups: dense deposit disease (DDD), C3 glomerulonephritis (C3 GN), and the CFHR5 nephropathy. The persistent presence of microhematuria with or without light or heavy proteinuria after an infection episode suggests the potential onset of C3 GP. These nephritides are characterized by abnormal activation of the complement alternative pathway, abnormal deposition of C3 in the glomeruli, and progression of renal damage to end-stage kidney disease. The diagnosis is based on studying the complement system, relative genetics, and kidney biopsies. The treatment gap derives from the absence of a robust understanding of their natural outcome. Therefore, a specific treatment for the different types of C3 GP has not been established. Recommendations have been obtained from case series and observational studies because no randomized clinical trials have been conducted. Current treatment is based on corticosteroids and antiproliferative drugs (cyclophosphamide, mycophenolate mofetil), monoclonal antibodies (rituximab) or complement inhibitors (eculizumab). In some cases, it is suggested to include sessions of plasma exchange.

Keywords: C3 glomerulopathy; Dense deposits disease; C3 glomerulonephritis; CFHR5 nephropathy

1. Introduction

Membranoproliferative or mesangiocapillary glomerulonephritis (MPGN) has been traditionally classified based on the light and electron microscopy (EM) findings; here, there are three categories: type I, characterized by the presence of immune deposits in the subendothelial space and mesangium of glomeruli; type II, characterized by C3 deposits within the mesangium and in the basement membranes highly osmiophilic on electron microscopy (dense deposits disease; DDD); and type III, which is a variant of type I [1].

In August 2012, a group of experts in renal pathology, nephrology, complementology, and complement therapeutics organized a consensus conference on the C3 glomerulopathy (C3 GP), meeting in Cambridge, UK [2]. Subsequently, new information on the complement system has increased our understanding of the MPGN, which has been divided into two groups: (i) MPGN caused by immune complexes (IC-MPGN) that can be caused by polyclonal or monoclonal IgG and (ii) complement-mediated glomerulonephritis (Figure 1).

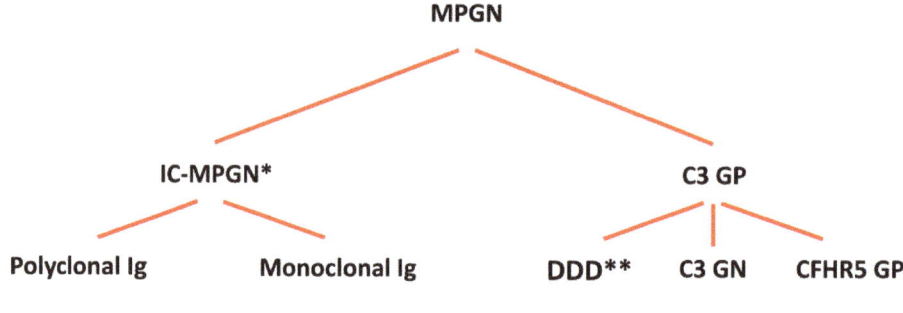

Figure 1. Classification of the membranoproliferative glomerulonephritis (MPGN). Abbreviations: IC-MPGN (immune complex MPGN); Ig (immunoglobulin); C3 GP (C3 glomerulopathy); DDD (dense deposits disease); C3 GN (C3 glomerulonephrits); CFHR5 GP (complement factor H-related protein 5 glomerulopathy).

The term C3 GP includes a group of nephritides based on the abnormal control of the alternative pathway of the complement system that causes a dominant accumulation of C3 fragments in glomeruli, as evidenced by an intense staining of C3 with absence or low presence of immunoglobulins and components of the classical complement pathway in the immunofluorescence pattern of a kidney biopsy [3]. This form of nephritis can be detected in individuals with defects in the complement activation that is induced by circulating factors or the presence of rare gene variants in complement components of the alternative pathway.

In a recent classification proposed by Cook and Pickering [4], C3 GP was shown to be principally composed of three major subgroups (Figure 1): (i) *DDD* is characterized by intramembranous glomerular deposits of dense osmophilic material; (ii) *C3 glomerulonephritis* (C3 GN) is based on the presence of less dense deposits of C3 in the mesangial, subendothelial, and subepithelial areas of glomeruli; it also appears with the presence of circulating auto-antibodies against C3bBb, factor B (FB), and factor H (FH); (iii) *complement factor H-related 5 glomerulopathy* (CFHR5 GP) is caused by genetic variants of CFHR5. Differences in these three nephritides are based on the interpretation of data obtained by light microscopy, immunofluorescence/immunohistochemistry and EM, laboratory complement findings, and clinical data. However, in some cases, there is an overlap of clinical data and laboratory findings, suggesting the possibility of a disease continuum based on the dysregulation of the complement alternative pathway; this would be caused by acquired factors (autoantibodies) or genetic variants of some complement components of the alternative pathway.

2. Pathogenesis

The complement system is the first cornerstone of innate immunity, and in the presence of various infections, it induces the lysis of agents through the generation of the membrane attack complex (MAC) [5]. Moreover, the system modulates adaptive immunity.

The complement system can be activated through three different pathways, as illustrated in Figure 2.

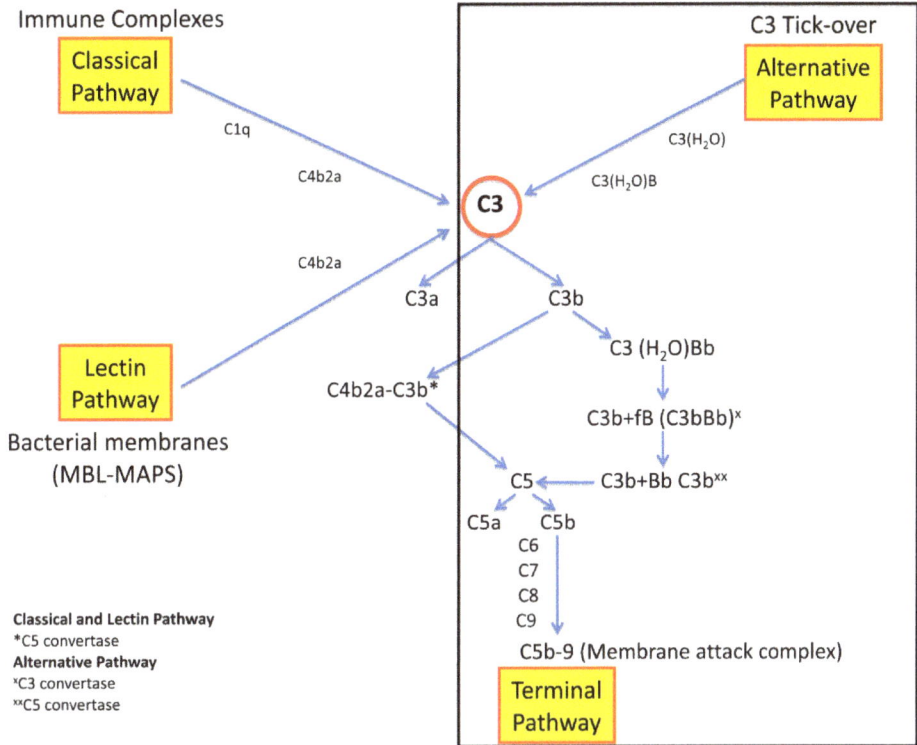

Figure 2. Complement system pathways.

The *classical pathway* is activated by circulating immune complexes, whereas the *lectin pathway* is activated by bacteria or their membrane fragments. Both pathways cleave C3 into C3a and C3b. C3a is an anaphylatoxin with a proinflammatory effect, whereas C3b binds a fragment of factor B (Bb), thus forming the C3 convertase (C3bBb). Additional production of C3b promotes the formation of the complex C3bBbC3b (C5 convertase), which cleaves C5 into C5a and C5b and combines with C6, C7, C8, and C9, thus forming the membrane attack complex (C5b-9) that induces the lysis of cellular membranes and the glomerular basement membrane (GBM).

The *alternative pathway* is continuously activated by the C3 tick-over at a low rate with the constant generation of C3b, which here is rapidly degraded. In this physiological process, C3 is hydrolyzed to $C3(H_2O)$ and combines with fB the complex $C3(H_2O)B$. Then, this complex cleaves C3, generating C3b, which combines with Bb and forms the C3 convertase of the alternative pathway (C3bBb). In the presence of further C3b, the formed C5 convertase (C3bBbC3b) activates C5 with the sequential induction of the *terminal complement pathway* (C5b-9).

The three pathways of the complement system are modulated by proteins that regulate the system in the blood (fluid phase) and on the surface of cells (surface phase). In the fluid phase, the C1-inhibitor (C1-INH) downregulates the classical and lectin pathways; the C4 binding protein (C4bp) downregulates the classical pathway; clusterin and vimentin regulate C5b-9. The regulators of the complement in the surface phase system are the membrane cofactor protein (MCP, named CD46), CD59 that is a regulator of MAC formation, the decay accelerating factor (DAF, named CD55), and the complement receptor 1 (CR1).

The alternative pathway is regulated by properdin, FB, FI, FH, and FH-related proteins. Properdin enhances the formation of C3 convertase and stabilizes it; thus, properdin prevents the action of FH.

FH is the principal regulator of the alternative pathway both in the fluid phase and on the cellular surface; it inhibits the binding of C3b with FB, enhances C3 convertase dissociation, and the activity of FI, which cleaves C3b into inactivated C3b (iC3b). A dysregulated control of C3 convertase (C3bBb) can be caused by the abnormal activity of FH, as illustrated in Figure 3. The regulatory activity of this factor can be inhibited by the presence of genetic FH deficiency or autoantibodies against FH, which have been found in patients with C3 GP [6–9].

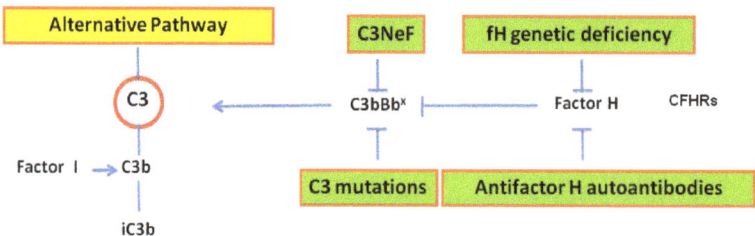

Figure 3. Schematic dysregulation of the C3 activation in C3 GP.

The activity of FH is regulated by the group of CFHRs that activate the alternative pathway by binding C3b and the activity of C3bBb convertase. CFHRs also compete with FH when attempting to bind to C3b deposited on the cellular surfaces. Therefore, the competition between FH and CFHRs influences the degree of C3b by inhibiting (predominant FH binding) or allowing (predominant FHR binding) to this process. The CFHR system is composed of five proteins that are coded by genes (CFHR1 to CFHR5) located near the CFH gene. CFHR genes may have rearrangements because the deletion or duplication of the first two consensus repeats with the presence of altered activity of CFHR proteins. Abnormal rearrangements include intragenic duplication in CFHR1 and CFHR5 and the presence of hybrid CFHR2-CFHR5 and CFHR3-CFHR1 genes. A deletion of the CFHR1 gene is associated with the abnormal activity of FH and reduced control of the activation of the alternative complement pathway in the circulation system.

CFHR5 interacting with CFHR1 and CFHR2 may generate abnormal CFHR proteins that impact the function of C3 and/or C5 convertases in the fluid phase or on the glomeruli, causing C3 GP. More than 20 different mutations have been identified in the CFH-CFHR gene family of patients affected by C3 GP, as reported by Xiao et al. [10] and Merinero et al. [11]. A recent review on the process of CFH deregulation that is responsible for the C3 activation has been published by Barbour et al. [12].

An excessive activation of the alternative pathway may be caused by the presence of autoantibodies against the C3 convertase of the alternative pathway (C3NeF) and C3 convertase of the classical pathway (C4NeF) (Figure 3). In 1969, NeF was detected for the first time in a case of MPGN with persistent hypocomplementemia [13]. The serum of this patient was able to break down into C3 when it was incubated with normal human serum. The activity of NeF was attributed to the stabilization of the alternative complement pathway convertase (C3bBb), and it was named C3NeF [13,14]. Then, further studies [15–18] described various types of NeF stabilizing different convertases, thus preventing their cleavage and causing continuous activation of the complement system. Marinozzi et al. [19] detected a C3NeF that stabilizes the C5 convertase of the alternative pathway (C5NeF). C4NeF was first detected in a case of patients with postinfection glomerulonephritis and who had persistent low levels of C3 and C5 [20], and it was also discovered in a case of MPGN. C3NeF and C4NeF may coexist in the same patient [21], but plasma C3, consumption, and disease severity do not always correlate with the presence and activity of C3NeF in individuals with MPGN [22]. Other autoantibodies related to complement components, such as FB, FH, and C3b have been detected in a smaller percentage of patients [23]. A recent review regarding the use of diagnostic tools to detect and characterize NeFs was published by Donadelli et al. [24].

In conclusion, various autoantibodies enhance the activity of the alternative pathway in different ways. C3NeF binds and stabilizes the C3 convertase in the presence of properdin. C4NeF binds and stabilizes C3 convertase (C4bC2a) of the classical pathway, thus causing more production of C3b and C3bBb. Autoantibodies against factor H eliminate the regulatory function of this factor [25], whereas autoantibodies against factor B stabilize the enhancing function of factor B [26,27]. The presence of one of these autoantibodies is responsible for the development of C3 GP caused by an abnormal control of alternative complement pathway activation with reduced C3 degradation and increased C3 fragment deposition in the GBM.

3. Epidemiology

C3 GP is a rare disease, so its frequency can only be approximately calculated. Cohort studies and an analysis of data from C3 GP registry have estimated an annual incidence of biopsy-proven DDD and C3 GN of one to two cases per million, with both sexes being affected equally [28]. The prevalence has been calculated as less than five cases per 1,000,000 in the United States and ~0.2–1.0 cases per 1,000,000 among the European population [25,29].

Instead, for CFHR5 GP, which was first observed in patients from Cyprus, data of incidences are lacking, while the prevalence value has been estimated at 140 cases per 1,000,000 Cypriot individuals [30].

4. Clinical Manifestations

Because of the low frequency of C3 GP, patient cohort studies are important and can provide valuable information regarding clinical presentation, pathological and laboratory features, and their correlation with disease outcomes.

Table 1 shows the clinical and laboratory data of patients affected by C3 GP in different cohorts, as described by many investigators [23,25,29,31–36]. C3 GP involves mainly children and young people and may develop after an infectious episode (i.e., streptococcal infection) of the upper respiratory tract. However, the presence of rare variants linked to C3 and other components of the alternative pathway predisposes an individual to C3 GP susceptibility.

The onset of the disease is characterized by micro- or macroscopic hematuria, light or heavy proteinuria, and a progressive reduction of renal function. Microhematuria is present in 90% of individuals, and episodes of gross hematuria may occur in 20% of patients in concomitance with upper respiratory tract infections. At the beginning of the disease and mainly in adults, light proteinuria may be present, which then becomes heavy over the course of the disease. The impairment of renal function is more frequent in adults and elderly subjects.

These clinical manifestations are common in all subtypes of C3 GP based on the aberrant control of the alternative complement pathway and sequential deposition of C3 in glomeruli. Therefore, renal biopsy remains the main approach for diagnosis.

In **DDD**, the onset is characterized by nephrotic syndrome in 50% of the patients and acute nephritic syndrome in the other 50%. Hypertension may be present at the onset of the disease or detected during the course of the disease. These clinical manifestations are preceded by an acute episode of upper respiratory tract infection.

In a few cases, DDD shows at the fundus oculi drusen bodies that are electron-dense deposits of complement factors between the Bruch's membrane and the retinal epithelium. This abnormality may be present at all ages and comes with a modest risk of progressive visual loss.

In some cases, patients with DDD may show acquired partial lipodistrophy that is characterized by the absence of subcutaneous fat in the face, but can also be present in the arms and upper portions of the trunk. However, partial lipodistrophy is more frequent in MPGN.

Table 1. Clinical and laboratory characteristics of patients affected by C3 GP enrolled in cohort studies.

Author-Year (Ref. No.)	Study Population				Clinical Findings				Histology				Complement Findings §		
	Country	C3 GP Class	N	Age at Diagnosis (Years)	Male Sex (%)	Median SCr at Diagnosis (mg/dL)	Median UP at Diagnosis (g/24 h)	Main Clinical Presentation	Main Histological Patterns (%)	Low C3 (%)	Low C4 (%)	C3Nef No. (%)	Complement Gene Variant Identified No. (%)	Other Complement Antibodies No. (%)
Athanasiou, 2011 [31]	Cyprus	CFHR5 GP	91	Range 12–88	47	N/A	N/A	H 90 Pu 38	MES	0	0	N/A	91/91 (100)	N/A
Servais, 2012 [32]	France	C3 GN	56	30	58.6	1.3	3.6	H 64 NS 27	MPGN (71), MES (29)	40	0	25 (45)	10 (18)	N/A
		DDD	29	12	43	1.6	5.6	H 76 NS 30		59	4	25 (86)	5 (17)	N/A
Mejeral-Thomas, 2014 [25]	UK/Ireland	C3 GN	59	26	54	1.4	3	H 87 NS 44	MPGN (52), MES (24), Crescentic (5)	48	36	N/A	N/A	N/A
		DDD	21	12	43	0.9	3	H 86 NS 43	MPGN (62), MES (14), Crescentic (19)	79	15	N/A	N/A	N/A
Rabasco, 2015 [33]	Spain	C3 GN	60	27	57	1.4	3.8	NS 52 H 49	MPGN (75), MES (15)	63	N/A	11/23 (48)	3/23 (13)	0
Iatropoulos, 2016 [34]	Italy	C3 GN	52	14.6	42	N/A	N/A	H 86 NS 29	N/A	69	N/A	23/52 (44)	10/52 (20)	N/A
		DDD	21	15.9	38	N/A	N/A	H 90 NS29		86	N/A	16/21 (78)	3/21 (14)	N/A
Caliskan, 2017 [35]	Turkey	C3 GN (no subclass)	66	36	54	1.6	3.8	H 89 NS 48	MPGN (75), MES (24)	41	4	N/A	N/A	N/A
Bomback, 2018 [29]	USA	C3 GN	87	28.3	63.2	2	3.7	H 59 NS 33	MPGN (68.8), MES (17.5)	65	14	13/42 (31)	12/42 (28)	3/42 (7)
		DDD	24	40	67	2.1	4.4	H 82 NS 17	MPGN (45.8), MES (29.3)	64	14	1/9 (11)	3/9 (33)	1/9 (11)
Le Quintrec, 2018 [36]	France	C3 GN (no subclass)	26	17.5	48	1	4.1	NS 73	MPGN (62)	88	N/A	16/24 (67)	5/22 (23)	2/22 (9)
Ravindran, 2018 [23]	USA *	C3 GN	102	41.5	59	1.6	2.5	H 87 Pu 38	MPGN (52), MES (34), Crescentic (7)	42	12	27/60 (46)	21/61 (39)	8/60 (13)
		DDD	12	31.5	25	1.4	6.5	H 92 Pu 75	MPGN (45), MES (27), Crescentic (16)	58	8	3/10 (30)	2/9 (22)	1/8 (12)

Abbreviations: C3G = C3 glomerulopathy; CeGN = C3 glomerulonephritis; DDD = dense deposition disease; CFHR5N = CFHR5 nephropathy; SCr = serum creatinine; UP = urinary protein; H = hematuria, Pu = proteinuria; NS = nephrotic syndrome; MPGN = Membrano-Proliferative Glomerulonephritis; MES = Mesangial expansion; C3Nef = C3 Nephritic factors; N/A = data not available from the study. Notes: * including 36 patients with Monoclonal immunoglobulin; § complement findings were often evaluated only in a part of the studied patients.

The outcome of DDD patients is poor, given that 50% of individuals progress to end-stage kidney disease (ESKD) within 10 years of diagnosis.

In **C3 GN**, the onset of the disease is characterized by microhematuria associated with hypertension in one-third of patients and nephritic syndrome in another third. The percentage of patients with ESKD is similar to that of patients with DDD. The disease involves mainly children and young adults. Microhematuria is present in 90% of individuals, and episodes of gross hematuria may occur in 20% of patients, along with upper respiratory tract infections. At the beginning of the disease light proteinuria that becomes heavy during the course of the disease is present but mainly in adults. The impairment of renal function is more frequent in adults.

CFHR5 glomerulopathy (CHFR5 GP) has been described in family studies; here, the abnormal activity of the complement factor H-related (CFHR) proteins or deregulation of CFH caused by CFH gene polymorphisms segregates in some members of the family [33,37,38]. Individuals with these genomic abnormalities show persistent microscopic hematuria that may be associated with proteinuria. The development of chronic renal failure progressing to ESKD is more frequent in men with proteinuria. In other patients, the usual presentation may be macroscopic hematuria in the concomitance of upper respiratory tract infection, as in IgA nephropathy, which mainly occurs in children.

However, familial cases of C3 GP have been observed in the presence of CFHR3-1 protein abnormalities [39] or the internal duplication of CFHR1 [40] or CFHR5, specifically in members of a Cypriot family [41].

5. Renal Biopsy

A renal biopsy is essential to identify C3 GP because it is the correct approach for distinguishing the different subtypes of MPGN.

5.1. Immunofluorescence Microscopy

The diagnosis of C3 GP is based on an immunofluorescence (IF) technique, which reveals C3 dominant staining, with C3 being the only positive immunoreactant or with others (IgG, IgA, IgM, C1q) but C3 at least 2 + stronger [42].

In DDD, C3 deposits are arranged in a ribbon-like ("garland") pattern in the glomerular basement membranes with sometimes ring-shaped mesangial deposits (Figure 4a). Broad linear tubular basement membranes (~60%) (Figure 4b) and Bowman capsule deposits (~30%) can also be present in DDD.

In C3 GN, prominent granular C3 deposits are seen in the mesangium and/or glomerular basement membranes (Figure 4c,d).

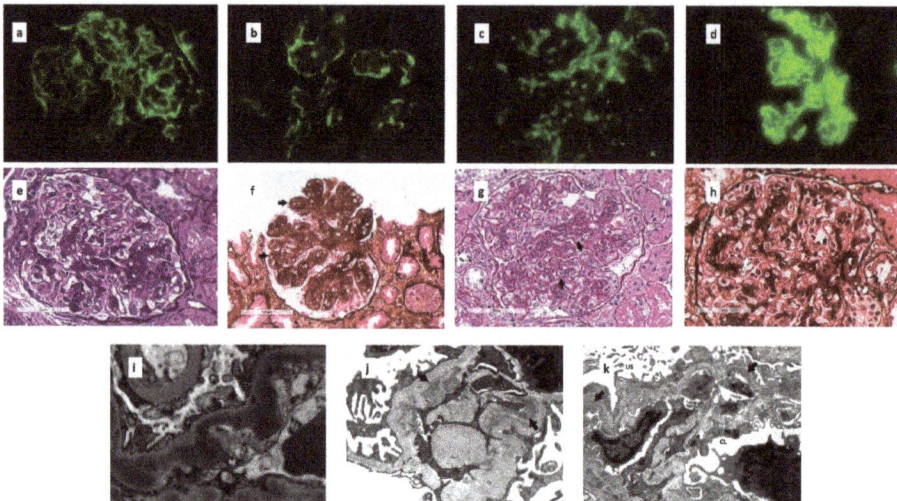

Figure 4. (**a**) Ribbon like pattern of C3 deposition along glomerular basement membrane in a patient with DDD (×400). (**b**) Linear C3 deposition along tubular basement membrane in DDD (×400). (**c**) Granular mesangial C3 deposits in a patient with a mesangial proliferative C3 GN (×400). (**d**) Coarsely granular mesangial and glomerular capillary wall C3 deposits in a patient with membranoproliferative pattern of C3 GN (×400). (**e**) Glomerulus with segmental mesangial proliferation in a patient with C3 GN (PAS). (**f**) Glomerulus with global membranoproliferative pattern of injury in a patient with C3 GN. Several aspects of glomerular basement membrane double contours (black arrows) are present (Jones silver stain). (**g**) Glomerulus with thickened strongly PAS positive glomerular basement membranes with several double contours (black arrows) (PAS) in a patient with DDD. (**h**) Silver negative glomerular basement membrane in a patient with DDD (white arrows). Glomerular basement membranes appear eosinophilic and refractile (Jones silver stain). (**i**) Highly osmiophilic electron dense deposits permeating lamina densa in a patient with DDD (TEM, ×8900). (**j**) Mesangial electron dense deposits (black arrows) in a patient with mesangial proliferative C3 GN (TEM, ×11000). (**k**) Subendothelial electron dense deposits (black arrows) with newly formed lamina densa (i.e., double contours) and cellular interposition (white arrow) in a patient with membranoproliferative patter of C3 GN (US: urinary space, CL: capillary lumen) (TEM, ×8900).

The absence of C4d in the kidney biopsy from proliferative GN has been found to be helpful, as noted by Sethi et al. [43], in distinguishing C3 GP from Ig complex-mediated and postinfection glomerulonephritis. Although helpful, this feature has been questioned by other studies [44].

C3 GP has now been included among the possible manifestations of monoclonal gammopathy of renal significance (MGRS) because 30–50% of patients >50 years of age with C3 GP have a detectable monoclonal Ig [45]. For this reason, careful examination of a renal biopsy and searching for a monoclonal Ig or light chain is mandatory. Failing to detect a monoclonal protein using an immunofluorescence technique from fresh frozen tissue should prompt reprocessing to formalin-fixed-paraffin-embedded tissue after pronase digestion. Actually, 10–20% of patients with a serum monoclonal component and finding of C3 GP on immunofluorescence have a proliferative GN with masked monoclonal deposits [45].

It is important to distinguish C3 deposition in C3 GN from other forms of glomerulonephritis, such as postinfection glomerulonephritis, in which immunoglobulin deposition occurs in the first phase of the disease and then disappears. In this case, persistence of heavy proteinuria and/or double contours on light microscopy (LM) may suggest the occurrence of C3 GP.

5.2. Light Microscopy

LM can vary greatly, presenting with different morphologic patterns. Mesangial proliferative glomerulonephritis (Figure 4e) and membranoproliferative glomerulonephritis (Figure 4f) are the most common patterns found, respectively, 33.3% and 50.8% of a cohort of 114 patients with C3 GP from the Mayo Clinic [23]. The membrane proliferative pattern in light microscopy is not different from that seen in idiopathic forms with Ig deposits. It is characterized by the thickening of glomerular basement membranes with double contours and cellular interposition. The features of exudative glomerulonephritis with endocapillary hypercellularity with or without polymorphonucleates are observed in 10–20% of cases. Extracellular proliferation with a crescent formation can also be present. In chronic phases of injury focal, segmental and/or global glomerulosclerosis and a fibrous crescent can be found. Fibrinoid necrosis is uncommon.

In DDD, glomerular basement membranes appear eosinophilic and refractile and stain brightly with periodic acid-Schiff (PAS) and poorly with a Jones silver stain (Figure 4g,h).

5.3. Electron Microscopy

EM studies have refined the G3 GP classification into further categories (DDD and C3 GN) based on the appearance of deposits.

In DDD (formerly MPGN type II), EM shows highly osmiophilic dense deposits in the lamina densa of the glomerular basement membranes, resulting in an electron-dense appearance (Figure 4i). These deposits can also be found in the mesangium, Bowman capsule, tubular basement membranes, and small vessel walls.

In C3 GN, the "usual" electron-dense deposits are found in various locations: the mesangial (Figure 4j), subendothelial (Figure 4k), and intramembranous areas. Subepithelial humps can be found both in DDD and C3 GN.

6. Diagnosis

A single algorithm cannot define the diagnostic approach to C3 GP, which is based on the interpretation of individual cases through the integration of the information provided by the renal biopsy together with clinical, serological, and genetic assessments.

Because the clinical presentation of C3 GP in its different forms may vary from asymptomatic hematuria to nephrotic syndrome and acute kidney injury, a diagnosis of C3 GP should be taken into consideration virtually in all patients presenting features of glomerulonephritis (proteinuria, hematuria, renal failure, or active urine sediment).

The clinical and laboratory work-up for the diagnosis of C3 GP is illustrated in Figure 5. After collecting the medical history and providing an accurate examination of the physical status, the patient usually undergoes general laboratory evaluation, looking at immunity (measurement of the serum levels of immunoglobulins and detection of serum cryoglobulins) and the complement system (hemolytic assay of the classical and alternative pathway). In the presence of the specific activation of the alternative complement pathway (i.e., reduced C3 and normal C4 serum levels) C3 GP is highly suspected although not yet determined. The diagnosis of C3 GP is exclusively made based on renal histological findings. In particular, as previously shown, LM is not specific enough for C3 GP, but IF and EM are necessary to make a diagnosis of C3 GP and to distinguish between C3 GN and DDD.

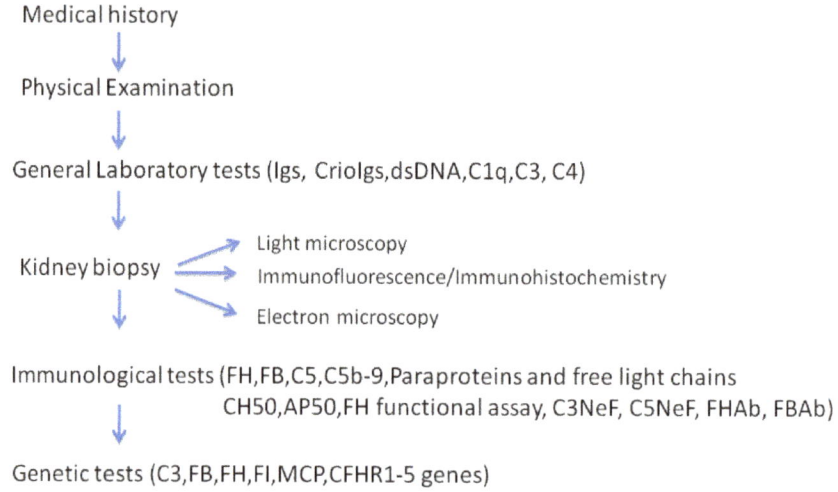

Figure 5. Clinical and Laboratory Work-up for diagnosis of C3 glomerulopathy.

C3-dominant glomerulonephritis is defined as C3 deposition in renal tissue of at least two orders of magnitude greater than that for any other immunoreactant (including Ig, C4, C1q, etc.). However, even when a C3 prevailing deposition is found, only a suspected diagnosis of C3 GP may be formulated, while the definitive diagnosis might require an ultra-structural analysis by EM.

Once the histological diagnosis of C3 GP has been realized, additional laboratory tests should be done to evaluate the serum levels of other components of the complement system, such as FH, FB, C5, and other complement regulatory proteins. Then, the work-up proceeds to a differential diagnosis and excludes secondary forms of glomerulonephritis. Investigations of the medical history should include a possible familial story of glomerulonephritis, unclear renal insufficiency, prior episodes of hematuria and/or proteinuria, and secondary causes, such as infections, autoimmune diseases, and paraproteinemia. Particular attention should be paid to recent infective episodes that may represent a trigger for complement activation. Moreover, all patients (especially if the age is more than 50 years) should be screened for the presence of paraproteins by serum electrophoresis-immunofixation and serum-free light chain measurement. Indeed, it has been shown that monoclonal gammopathy may be common in patients with a histological diagnosis of C3 GP [46]. If paraproteins are present, the patient should be referred to hematology consultation because in these cases, a clone-guided treatment might improve renal outcomes.

If secondary forms of complement activation are unlikely or excluded, all patients with C3 GP should undergo a comprehensive evaluation of the complement system, which includes measurements of the complement hemolytic activity, screening for circulating autoantibodies and genetic studies, which can help in defining the diagnosis and choosing the therapeutic approach [47].

The evaluation of the overall complement activity may be performed by evaluating the total complement hemolytic activity (CH50), the complement alternative pathway activity (AP50), or the complement FH functional activity [48]. Although functional tests may be considered the gold standard for studying the complement activity, they may actually have a significant rate of false-negative results, and their use still needs to be validated.

Moving to the specific details, serological studies of the complement AP should include the quantification of individual complement components, here bearing in mind that the results of these studies may change over the course of the disease. The most important complement components to evaluate are C3 and C4. Low C3 is found in a substantial number of patients with C3 GN (40–75%) and DDD (60%), while serum C4 levels are usually normal [23]. Moreover, serum FB, FH, FI, properdin, and membrane cofactor proteins (MCP or CD46) should also be tested, considering that a deficiency of these factors, often accompanied by low C3 levels, can be associated with altered AP activation [49]. However, complement activation may also be detected by measuring the decay products of complement activation; when elevated, they may reflect an increased turnover of C3 (C3a, C3d), C5 (C5a), and FB (Bb) [50]. Finally, considering that the activation of all complement pathways leads to the generation of the membrane attack complex (C5b-9), soluble levels of C5b-9 should be evaluated as an additional marker of complement activation [49]. Interestingly, it should be noted that small differences in complement biomarkers between C3 GN and DDD exist. For example, in C3 GN, the plasma properdin reduction and soluble C5b-9 elevation tend to be higher than in DDD. Thus, a complement component evaluation may also provide an indication of the disease in the differential diagnosis between C3GN and DDD.

Serological studies in patients with C3 GP should also include screening for autoantibodies, which may constitute the acquired causes of C3 GP. C3NeF and C5NeF are the most frequently identified autoantibodies (Figure 5). Various diagnostic tools can be used to detect NeFs [51]. Three of these tools are functional and hemolytic assays. The first method consists of the measurement of C3 fragments in the serum's patient by two-dimensional immunoelectrophoresis, immunofixation electrophoresis, or Western blotting. The second test is based on a hemolytic assay that measures the lysis of sheep or rabbits erythrocytes after incubation with the serum or plasma of the patient. Finally, the presence of NeFs can be detected through the quantification of C3a and C5a anaphylotoxins. NeFs can be measured by binding assays that detect C3NeF by various ELISA techniques. Actually, they encompass a heterogeneous group of IgG and IgM autoantibodies that stabilize the alternative pathway of C3 and C5 convertase (C3bBb and C3bBbC3b, respectively), prolonging their survival and promoting massive C3 or C5 consumption [51]. C3NeF is found in 80% of patients affected by DDD and in 50% of patients affected by C3 GN. Detecting C3NeF can be done in many different ways, including ELISA, C3 convertase surface assay, and electrophoresis [52]. In addition, C4 nephritic factor (C4NeF), which stabilizes the C3 convertase of the classical and lectin pathways, has been identified in a small subset of patients with C3 GP, even if its role remains unclear [53]. Antifactor H antibodies are another group of auto-antibodies described in patients affected by C3 GP; they may be detected using an enzyme-linked immunosorbent assay and have been related to the presence of monoclonal gammopathy [54]. Finally, anti-FB antibodies have rarely been described, but their detection remains confined to research laboratories [26].

Because genetic factors have been reported in cohorts of patients with C3 GP, genetic testing should be considered in these patients [32] (Figure 5). In particular, genetic screening should include the evaluation of the C3, FB, FH, MCP, CFHR1-5, and FI genes to detect single nucleotide changes, small insertions and deletions, or more complex rearrangements, such as copy number variations [34]. However, the interpretation of a genetic analysis in C3 GP is often difficult for several reasons. First, genetic defects have been identified only in a small number of patients with C3 GP. Second, the actual pathogenetic and functional meaning of many mutations is still not defined. Finally, most genetic variants have a low penetrance, and combined variants may coexist, which also involves other genes, such as thrombomodulin (THBD) and diacylglycerol kinase-epsilon (DGKE) [55]. Thus, it is necessary to cautiously analyze the detected gene alterations to determine if they are specifically disease associated.

A different situation is found in the familial forms of C3 GP, where disease-specific gene mutations have been characterized. This is the case of patients affected by CFHR5 GP and who are of Cypriot origin, in which an internal duplication in the CFHR5 gene has been described as causative [37]. Interestingly, other forms of familial C3 GP have been related to rearrangements of the CFHR2-CFHR5 hybrid gene and abnormalities in CFHR1 and CFHR5 [39,40], suggesting that the CFHR1-5 gene family should be carefully assessed in all C3 GP cases. A detailed description of the methods to quantify the CFHR proteins in the serum and detect circulating autoantibodies has recently been published by Sanchez-Corral et al. [56].

In any case, although the precise value of genetic testing remains to be defined in a general clinical setting for C3 GP, a genetic cause of the disease should be taken into consideration, and genetic screening should be offered to all the family members of affected patients who carry a potentially causative mutation.

7. Differential Diagnosis

A differential diagnosis should be done in the presence of diagnosed C3 GP on either a native or transplanted kidney. In this case, it is necessary to investigate the concomitant presence of low plasma levels of C4, occurrence of C4NeF (C4bC2a), and paraproteins (i.e., monocolonal gammopathy) because in this case, the patient is affected by MPGN type 1.

C3 GP must be differentiated from other types of glomerulonephritides that have excessive activation of the C system in the presence of circulating immune complexes, causing postinfection glomerulonephritis or secondary glomerulonephritides (lupus nephritis, essential cryoglobulinemia, and others) [1]. Because the clinical presentation in these cases is similar, it is suggested that an accurate study of the complement system and genetic tests in specialized laboratories be carried out. However, a kidney biopsy is diriment in these patients because it shows a prevalent deposition of immunoglobulins, which is the characteristic pattern of these nephritides. In addition, postinfection glomerulonephritis should be differentiated from C3 GP when there is no spontaneous resolution of the disease within one to two months.

G3 GP can be diagnosed in the presence of false-negative staining for immunoglobulins by immunofluorescence on the frozen renal tissue sections of patients with essential cryoglobulinemia. In these cases, it is suggested to investigate the presence of C4 in a kidney biopsy to discover the potential occurrence of the low serum levels of circulating immune complexes or cryoglobulins.

In many cases, the prognosis of C3 GP is severe when it comes to the progression of renal damage to ESKD [28,32]. It is less severe in CFHR5 GP.

8. Recurrence or De Novo C3 GP after Kidney Transplatation

Patients with C3 GP are at high risk to develop the disease after kidney transplantation. Therefore, post-transplant monitoring and available optional therapies are necessary for improving the outcome of the patients. The recurrence is at high rate for both DDD and C3 GN. The recurrence of CHFR5 GP has been observed in the kidney allograft of patients, allowing for a family with CFHR gene abnormalities [57]. C3 GP occurs in over 50% of patients with native C3 GP [58]. The timing and clinical presentation may be different with DDD recurrence in later post-transplant time. The appearance of hematuria, proteinuria and reduction of eGFR is a strong indicator of C3 GP recurrence. However, LM, IF, and EM studies are necessary for a correct diagnosis. A recent report [59] suggests that aggressive renal lesions in native kidney and hybrid CFHR3 1 gene-related C3 GN contribute to more recurrence of the disease in the post-transplant time.

The approach to therapy has not been established because different treatments have been used in these patients. Recent data from Bomback et al. [60] in a prospective open-label, uncontrolled trial and by other investigators [61–63] suggest the administration of eculizumab which induces reduction of proteinuria and stabilization of the renal function. However, the heterogeneous treatment response suggests the opportunity to design a larger multicenter study in C3 GP patients after kidney transplantation. For this reason in 2017, a group of researchers across Europe and North and South America initiated the post-TrANsplant GlOmerular (TANGO) disease study, an observational multicenter cohort study with the aim to enroll patients who arrived to ESKD for different forms of glomerulonephritis, mainly C3 GP [64].

If eculizumab represents a successful therapy in atypical hemolytic uremic syndrome (AHUS) [65], the response rate is heterogeneous in patients with C3 GP [66]. The different response is due to the correct blockage of the terminal complement pathway in AHUS, whereas this therapy is questionable in patients with C3 GP because the disease is characterized by abnormal activation of the alternative complement pathway, abnormal cleavage of C3 and continuous deposition of C3 split products in glomeruli. This provides different response rate between the two diseases.

Some considerations should be done on the use of anti-CD 20 (rituximab) that has been used in a small number of cases with different response to the treatment. This drug is correctly indicated in patients with kidney graft who develop MPGN with monoclonal IgG deposits caused by dysregulated B cells or plasma cells alone without hematologic malignancy [67]. However, sporadic use of rituximab in association with immunosuppressive drugs has shown failure in the treatment of many cases [62,68,69].

Recurrence or *de novo* C3 GP may receive other therapies that are under trough evaluation as (i) compostatin that is a C3 inhibitory peptide; (ii) CP40 is a compostatin analog [70]; (iii) monoclonal antibodies against C3b [71], FB [72] and properdin [73]. Moreover, soluble complement receptor 1(CR1)) may prevent the dysregulated alternative pathway caused by abnormal production of C3 convertase.

All these drugs can block the dysregulated alternative complement pathway induced by autoantibodies or genetic mutations.

9. Therapy

The current gap in the treatment of C3 GP derives from the absence of a robust understanding of its natural outcomes. Therefore, a specific treatment for different types of C3 GP has not been established. Recommendations have been obtained from case series and observational studies [12] because there are no randomized clinical trials for treatments. Current treatment is based on the inhibition of factors that activate the complement pathways, which is done by administering the available drugs as corticosteroids and antiproliferative drugs (cyclophoshamide, mycophenolate mofetil), monoclonal antibodies (rituximab), or complement inhibitors (eculizumab).

Children and adults with C3 GP in presence of mild or moderate proteinuria should receive supportive therapy with angiotensin-converting enzyme inhibitors or angiotensin receptor blockers. Patients with nephrotic syndrome and a decline in renal function should receive oral CYC or MMF plus a low dose of daily or alternate-day corticosteroids [33]. If despite this treatment nephrotic syndrome persists or the renal function impairs, tacrolimus or RTX can be considered although the percentage of its beneficial effect is very low [35,70].

Treatment with chemotherapeutic agents, immune-suppressive drugs, and complement inhibitors confer infection risks. Indeed, Koopman et al. [71] suggest vaccination prophylaxis against Streptococcus pneumonia, Neisseria meningitis, and Hemophilus influenzae.

In patients with C3 GN with abnormal deposition of C3 because of persistent activation of the alternative complement pathway, it is suggested that treatment with eculizumab (monoclonal anti-C5 antibody) may be administered. A prospective clinical trial in which six patients with native or post-transplant recurrent DDD or C3 GN received eculizumab therapy was the first clinical study to evaluate the benefit of this monoclonal antibody [60]. Other case reports described by Barbour et al. [12] have shown complete or partial remission of the clinical findings (significant reduction of serum creatinine and/or proteinuria). Recently, Le Quintrec et al. [36] evaluated a cohort of 26 patients (13 children/adolescents) with C3 GP who were treated with eculizumab. At the initiation of eculizumab, 40% of the patients had chronic kidney disease, while about 30% had a rapidly progressive disease. After eculizumab treatment, six (23%) patients achieved a complete clinical response, defined as a >50% decrease in serum creatinine and proteinuria, while six (23%) and 14 (54%) had partial or no response, respectively. Interestingly, at the time of diagnosis, patients who had a complete clinical response, when compared with others, presented a more severe disease associated with more extracapillary proliferation on kidney biopsy, suggesting that different response profiles to eculizumab treatment among C3 GP patients could be recognized.

In individuals with monoclonal gammopathy that causes C3 GP (proteinuria and decline of renal function), a retrospective study of 50 patients with various types of monoclonal gammopathy [72] demonstrated that chemotherapy reduced proteinuria and improved renal function in 74% of patients, mainly in patients who had a reduction of gammopathy. Moreover, the hazard of ESRD was 83%

lower in patients with reduced gammopathy. The same improvement was observed in other patients who received chemotherapy [23] in the presence of gammopathy because of lymphoproliferative disorders [73,74]. Many patients have shown an improvement in the clinical course, which is characterized by a reduction of proteinuria and improvement of renal function. However, the role of eculizumab remains to be defined. C3 GP remains the ideal disease in which anticomplement drugs (compostatin, monoclonal antibodies against C3, FB, properdin) can be tested [75–78].

Plasma exchange removes autoantibodies such as NeFs and mutated proteins, but it must be associated with immunosuppressive therapy for blocking antibody production. This approach has been used successfully in patients with CFH mutations [79–81]. The Consensus Report on C3 GP [2] concluded that an international pathology registry is necessary to define the different spectra of this disease and to divide patients into appropriate subgroups. Thus, the combination of well-defined clinical studies associated with a robust complement study would be ideal before enrolling patients in clinical trials. The final aim will be to treat homogenous cohorts before enrolling patients in clinical trials.

10. Conclusions

C3 GPs are orphan diseases of which the understanding of the pathophysiology of the complement system has improved laboratory and clinical diagnosis. However, a multidisciplinary approach that involves nephrologists, renal pathologists, and geneticists is helpful for a correct diagnosis and for choosing optimum therapeutic plans. More comprehensive genetic and biomarker studies are needed to refine our diagnostic approach. We should continue to improve the clinicopathological phenotype for designing correct multicenter trials that will give more information on the clinical course of the disease and the effect of new drugs. Treatment with a combination of immune-suppressive drugs or anticomplement agents can induce complete or partial remission in 50% of patients. Remission is more frequent in C3 GN than in DDD, whereas spontaneous remission is very rare. These diseases lead to ESKD in 50% of patients; some of them have persistent heavy proteinuria that is nonresponsive to therapy, ranging from ACEi-ARB to immunosuppressive drugs. Older age reduced renal function, and nephrotic syndrome at presentation are unfavorable prognostic factors. The recurrence of these diseases in patients after kidney transplantation is very frequent; therefore, post-transplant monitoring and available treatment options should be taken into consideration. Newer therapies such as monoclonal antibodies and recombinant proteins may be promising strategies in the near future.

Author Contributions: The authors contributed equally to the conception of the work and to the acquisition, analysis and interpretation of data from the literature. All authors have read and agreed to the published version of the manuscript.

Funding: This research was funded by the Schena Foundation.

Conflicts of Interest: The authors declare no conflict of interest. The sponsor had no role in the design, execution, interpretation or writing of the study.

References

1. Schena, F.P.; Alpers, G.E. Membranoproliferative glomerulonephritis and cryoglobulinemic glomerulonephritis. In *Comprehensive Clinical Nephrology*, 5th ed.; Elsevier: Sanders, PA, USA, 2015; pp. 253–260.
2. Pickering, M.C.; D'Agati, V.D.; Nester, C.M.; Smith, R.J.; Haas, M.; Appel, G.B.; Alpers, C.E.; Bajema, I.M.; Bedrosian, C.; Braun, M.; et al. C3 glomerulopathy: Consensus report. *Kidney Int.* **2013**, *84*, 1079–1089. [CrossRef]
3. Fakhouri, F.; Frémeaux-Bacc, V.; Noël, L.H.; Cook, H.T.; Pickering, M.C. C3 glomerulopathy: A new classification. *Nat. Rev. Nephrol.* **2010**, *6*, 494–499. [CrossRef]
4. Cook, H.T.; Pickering, M.C. Clusters Not Classifications: Making Sense of Complement-Mediated Kidney Injury. *J. Am. Soc. Nephrol.* **2019**, *29*, 9–12. [CrossRef]

5. Ricklin, D.; Mastellos, D.C.; Reis, E.S.; Lambris, J.D. The renaissance of complement therapeutics. *Nat. Rev. Nephrol.* **2018**, *14*, 26–47. [CrossRef]
6. Jokiranta, T.S.; Solomon, A.; Pangburn, M.K.; Zipfel, P.F.; Meri, S. Nephritogenic lambda light chain dimer: A unique human miniautoantibody against complement factor H. *J Immunol.* **1999**, *163*, 4590–4596.
7. Goodship, T.H.; Pappworth, I.Y.; Toth, T.; Denton, M.; Houlberg, K.; McCormick, F.; Warland, D.; Moore, I.; Hunze, E.M.; Staniforth, S.J.; et al. Factor H autoantibodies in membranoproliferative glomerulonephritis. *Mol. Immunol.* **2012**, *52*, 200–206. [CrossRef]
8. Nozal, P.; Strobel, S.; Ibernon, M.; López, D.; Sánchez-Corral, P.; Rodríguez de Córdoba, S.; Józsi, M.; López-Trascasa, M. Anti-factor H antibody affecting factor H cofactor activity in a patient with dense deposit disease. *Clin. Kidney J.* **2012**, *5*, 133–136. [CrossRef] [PubMed]
9. Blanc, C.; Togarsimalemath, S.K.; Chauvet, S.; Le Quintrec, M.; Moulin, B.; Buchler, M.; Jokiranta, T.S.; Roumenina, L.T.; Fremeaux-Bacchi, V.; Dragon-Durey, M.A. Anti-factor H autoantibodies in C3 glomerulopathies and in atypical hemolytic uremic syndrome: One target, two diseases. *J. Immunol.* **2015**, *194*, 5129–5138. [CrossRef] [PubMed]
10. Xiao, X.; Pickering, M.C.; Smith, R.J. C3 glomerulopathy: The genetic and clinical findings in dense deposit disease and C3 glomerulonephritis. *Semin. Thromb. Hemost.* **2014**, *40*, 465–471. [CrossRef] [PubMed]
11. Merinero, H.M.; García, S.P.; García-Fernández, J.; Arjona, E.; Tortajada, A.; Rodríguez de Córdoba, S. Complete functional characterization of disease-associated genetic variants in the complement factor H gene. *Kidney Int.* **2018**, *93*, 470–481. [CrossRef]
12. Barbour, T.D.; Ruseva, M.M.; Pickering, M.C. Update on C3 glomerulopathy. *Nephrol. Dial. Transplant.* **2016**, *31*, 717–725. [CrossRef] [PubMed]
13. Spitzer, R.E.; Vallota, E.H.; Forristal, J.; Sudora, E.; Stitzel, A.; Davis, N.C.; West, C.D. Serum C'3 lytic system in patients with glomerulonephritis. *Science* **1969**, *164*, 436–437. [CrossRef] [PubMed]
14. Arroyave, C.M.; Vallota, E.H.; Müller-Eberhard, H.J. Lysis of human erythrocytes due to activation of the alternate complement pathway by nephritic factor (C3NeF). *J. Immunol.* **1974**, *113*, 764–768. [PubMed]
15. Daha, M.R.; Fearon, D.T.; Austen, K.F. Formation in the presence of C3 nephritic factor (C3NeF) of an alternative pathway C3 convertase containing uncleaved B. *Immunology* **1976**, *31*, 789–796. [PubMed]
16. Daha, M.R.; Austen, K.F.; Fearon, D.T. The incorporation of C3 nephritic factor (C3NeF) into a stabilized C3 convertase, C3bBb (C3NeF), and its release after decay of convertase function. *J. Immunol.* **1977**, *119*, 812–817.
17. Williams, D.G.; Bartlett, A.; Duffus, P. Identification of nephritic factor as an immunoglobulin. *Clin. Exp. Immunol.* **1978**, *33*, 425–429.
18. Józsi, M.; Reuter, S.; Nozal, P.; López-Trascasa, M.; Sánchez-Corral, P.; Prohászka, Z.; Uzonyi, B. Autoantibodies to complement components in C3 glomerulopathy and atypical hemolytic uremic syndrome. *Immunol. Lett.* **2014**, *160*, 163–171. [CrossRef]
19. Marinozzi, M.C.; Chauvet, S.; Le Quintrec, M.; Mignotet, M.; Petitprez, F.; Legendre, C.; Cailliez, M.; Deschenes, G.; Fischbach, M.; Karras, A.; et al. C5 nephritic factors drive the biological phenotype of C3 glomerulopathies. *Kidney Int.* **2017**, *92*, 1232–1241. [CrossRef]
20. Halbwachs, L.; Leveillé, M.; Lesavre, P.; Wattel, S.; Leibowitch, J. Nephritic factor of the classical pathway of complement: Immunoglobulin G autoantibody directed against the classical pathway C3 convetase enzyme. *J. Clin. Investig.* **1980**, *65*, 1249–1256. [CrossRef]
21. Tanuma, Y.; Ohi, H.; Hatano, M. Two types of C3 nephritic factor: Properdin-dependent C3NeF and properdin-independent C3NeF. *Clin. Immunol. Immunopathol.* **1990**, *56*, 226–238. [CrossRef]
22. Schena, F.P.; Pertosa, G.; Stanziale, P.; Vox, E.; Pecoraro, C.; Andreucci, V.E. Biological significance of the C3 nephritic factor in membranoproliferative glomerulonephritis. *Clin. Nephrol.* **1982**, *18*, 240–246. [PubMed]
23. Ravindran, A.; Fervenza, F.C.; Smith, R.J.H.; De Vriese, A.S.; Sethi, S. C3 Glomerulopathy: Ten Years' Experience at Mayo Clinic. *Mayo Clin. Proc.* **2018**, *93*, 991–1008. [CrossRef] [PubMed]
24. Donadelli, R.; Pulieri, P.; Piras, R.; Iatropoulos, P.; Valoti, E.; Benigni, A.; Remuzzi, G.; Noris, M. Unraveling the Molecular Mechanisms Underlying Complement Dysregulation by Nephritic Factors in C3G and IC-MPGN. *Front. Immunol.* **2018**, *9*, 2329. [CrossRef] [PubMed]
25. Medjeral-Thomas, N.R.; O'Shaughnessy, M.M.; O'Regan, J.A.; Traynor, C.; Flanagan, M.; Wong, L.; Teoh, C.W.; Awan, A.; Waldron, M.; Cairns, T.; et al. C3 glomerulopathy: Clinicopathologic features and predictors of outcome. *Clin. J. Am. Soc. Nephrol.* **2014**, *9*, 46–53. [CrossRef]

26. Strobel, S.; Zimmering, M.; Papp, K.; Prechl, J.; Józsi, M. Anti-factor B autoantibody in dense deposit disease. *Mol. Immunol.* **2010**, *47*, 1476–1483. [CrossRef]
27. Chen, Q.; Müller, D.; Rudolph, B.; Hartmann, A.; Kuwertz-Bröking, E.; Wu, K.; Kirschfink, M.; Skerka, C.; Zipfel, P.F. Combined C3b and factor B autoantibodies and MPGN type II. *N Engl. J. Med.* **2011**, *365*, 2340–2342. [CrossRef]
28. Smith, R.J.H.; Alexander, J.; Barlow, P.N.; Botto, M.; Cassavant, T.L.; Cook, H.T.; deCórdoba, S.R.; Hageman, G.S.; Jokiranta, T.S.; Kimberling, W.J.; et al. Dense Deposit Disease Focus Group. New approaches to the treatment of dense deposit disease. *J. Am. Soc. Nephrol.* **2007**, *18*, 2447–2456. [CrossRef]
29. Bomback, A.S.; Santoriello, D.; Avasare, R.S.; Regunathan-Shenk, R.; Canetta, P.A.; Ahn, W.; Radhakrishnan, J.; Marasa, M.; Rosenstiel, P.E.; Herlitz, L.C.; et al. C3 glomerulonephritis and dense deposit disease share a similar disease course in a large United States cohort of patients with C3 glomerulopathy. *Kidney Int.* **2018**, *93*, 977–985. [CrossRef]
30. Smith, R.J.H.; Appel, G.B.; Blom, A.M.; Cook, H.T.; D'Agati, V.D.; Fakhouri, F.; Fremeaux-Bacchi, V.; Józsi, M.; Kavanagh, D.; Lambris, J.D.; et al. C3 glomerulopathy—Understanding a rare complement-driven renal disease. *Nat. Rev. Nephrol.* **2019**, *15*, 129–143. [CrossRef]
31. Athanasiou, Y.; Voskarides, K.; Gale, D.P.; Damianou, L.; Patsias, C.; Zavros, M.; Maxwell, P.H.; Cook, H.T.; Demosthenous, P.; Hadjisavvas, A.; et al. Familial C3 glomerulopathy associated with CFHR5 mutations: Clinical characteristics of 91 patients in 16 pedigrees. *Clin. J. Am. Soc. Nephrol.* **2011**, *6*, 1436–1446. [CrossRef]
32. Servais, A.; Noël, L.H.; Roumenina, L.T.; Le Quintrec, M.; Ngo, S.; Dragon-Durey, M.A.; Macher, M.A.; Zuber, J.; Karras, A.; Provot, F.; et al. Acquired and genetic complement abnormalities play a critical role in dense deposit disease and other C3 glomerulopathies. *Kidney Int.* **2012**, *82*, 454–464. [CrossRef] [PubMed]
33. Rabasco, C.; Cavero, T.; Román, E.; Rojas-Rivera, J.; Olea, T.; Espinosa, M.; Cabello, V.; Fernández-Juarez, G.; González, F.; Ávila, A.; et al. Spanish Group for the Study of Glomerular Diseases (GLOSEN). Effectiveness of mycophenolate mofetil in C3 glomerulonephritis. *Kidney Int.* **2015**, *88*, 1153–1160. [CrossRef] [PubMed]
34. Iatropoulos, P.; Noris, M.; Mele, C.; Piras, R.; Valoti, E.; Bresin, E.; Curreri, M.; Mondo, E.; Zito, A.; Gamba, S.; et al. Complement gene variants determine the risk of immunoglobulin-associated MPGN and C3 glomerulopathy and predict long-term renal outcome. *Mol. Immunol.* **2016**, *71*, 131–142. [CrossRef] [PubMed]
35. Caliskan, Y.; Torun, E.S.; Tiryaki, T.O.; Oruc, A.; Ozluk, Y.; Akgul, S.U.; Temurhan, S.; Oztop, N.; Kilicaslan, I.; Sever, M.S. Immunosuppressive Treatment in C3 Glomerulopathy: Is it Really Effective? *Am. J. Nephrol.* **2017**, *46*, 96–107. [CrossRef] [PubMed]
36. Le Quintrec, M.; Lapeyraque, A.L.; Lionet, A.; Sellier-Leclerc, A.L.; Delmas, Y.; Baudouin, V.; Daugas, E.; Decramer, S.; Tricot, L.; Cailliez, M.; et al. Patterns of Clinical Response to Eculizumab in Patients with C3 Glomerulopathy. *Am. J. Kidney Dis.* **2018**, *72*, 84–92. [CrossRef] [PubMed]
37. Gale, D.P.; Goicoechea de Jorge, E.G.; Cook, H.T.; Martinez-Barricate, R.; Hadjisavvas, A.; McLean, A.G. Identification of a mutation in complement factor H-related protein 5 in patients of Cypriot origin with glomerulonephritis. *Lancet* **2010**, *376*, 794–801. [CrossRef]
38. Martínez-Barricarte, R.; Heurich, M.; Valdes-Cañedo, F.; Vazquez-Martul, E.; Torreira, E.; Montes, T.; Tortajada, A.; Pinto, S.; Lopez-Trascasa, M.; Morgan, B.P.; et al. Human C3 mutation reveals a mechanism of dense deposit disease pathogenesis and provides insights into complement activation and regulation. *J. Clin. Investig.* **2010**, *120*, 3702–3712. [CrossRef]
39. Malik, T.H.; Lavin, P.J.; Goicoechea de Jorge, E.; Vernon, K.A.; Rose, K.L.; Patel, M.P.A. A hybrid CFHR3-1 gene causes familial C3 glomerulopathy. *J. Am. Soc. Nephrol.* **2012**, *23*, 1155–1160. [CrossRef]
40. Tortajada, A.; Ye'benes, H.; Abarrategui-Garrido, C.; Anter, J.; García-Fernández, J.M.; Martínez-Barricarte, R.; Alba-Domínguez, M.; Malik, T.H.; Bedoya, R.; Cabrera Pérez, R.; et al. C3 glomerulopathy associated CFHR1 mutation alters FHR oligomerization and complement regulation. *J. Clin. Investig.* **2013**, *123*, 2434–2446. [CrossRef]
41. Medjeral-Thomas, N.R.; Troldborg, A.; Constantinou, N.; Lomax-Browne, H.J.; Hansen, A.G.; Willicombe, M.; Pusey, C.D.; Cook, H.T.; Thiel, S.; Pickering, M.C. Progressive IgA Nephropathy is Associated with low circulating mannan-binding lectin-associated serine protease-3 (MASP-3) and increased glomerular factor H-related protein-5 (FHR5) Deposition. *Kidney Int. Rep.* **2017**, *3*, 426–438. [CrossRef]

42. Hou, J.; Markowitz, G.S.; Bomback, A.S.; Appel, G.B.; Herlitz, L.C.; Barry Stokes, M.; D'Agati, V.D. Toward a working definition of C3 glomerulopathy by immunofluorescence. *Kidney Int.* **2014**, *85*, 450–456. [CrossRef] [PubMed]

43. Sethi, S.; Nasr, S.H.; De Vriese, A.S.; Fervenza, F.C. C4d as a diagnostic tool in proliferative GN. *J. Am. Soc. Nephrol.* **2015**, *26*, 2852–2859. [CrossRef] [PubMed]

44. Singh, G.; Singh, S.K.; Nalwa, A.; Lavleen, S.; Pradeep, I.; Barwad, A.; Sinha, A.; Hari, P.; Bagga, A.; Bagchi, S.; et al. Glomerular C4d staining does not exclude a C3 Glomerulopathy. *Kidney Int. Rep.* **2019**, *4*, 698–709. [CrossRef] [PubMed]

45. Leung, N.; Bridoux, F.; Batuman, V.; Chaidos, A.; Cockwell, P.; D'Agati, V.D.; Dispenzieri, A.; Fervenza, F.C.; Fermand, J.P.; Gibbs, S.; et al. The evaluation of monoclonal gammopathy of renal significance: A consensus report of the International Kidney and Monoclonal Gammopathy Research Group. *Nat. Rev. Nephrol.* **2019**, *15*, 121–135. [CrossRef]

46. Zand, L.; Kattah, A.; Fervenza, F.C.; Smith, R.J.; Nasr, S.H.; Zhang, Y.; Vrana, J.A.; Leung, N.; Cornell, L.D.; Sethi, S. C3 glomerulonephritis associated with monoclonal gammopathy: A case series. *Am. J. Kidney Dis.* **2013**, *62*, 506–514. [CrossRef]

47. Angioi, A.; Fervenza, F.C.; Sethi, S.; Zhang, Y.; Smith, R.J.; Murray, D.; Van Praet, J.; Pani, A.; De Vriese, A.S. Diagnosis of complement alternative pathway disorders. *Kidney Int.* **2016**, *89*, 278–288. [CrossRef]

48. Grumach, A.S.; Kirschfink, M. Are complement deficiencies really rare? Overview on prevalence, clinical importance and modern diagnostic approach. *Mol. Immunol.* **2014**, *61*, 110–117. [CrossRef]

49. Zhang, Y.; Nester, C.M.; Martin, B.; Skjoedt, M.O.; Meyer, N.C.; Shao, D.; Borsa, N.; Palarasah, Y.; Smith, R.J. Defining the complement biomarker profile of C3 glomerulopathy. *Clin. J. Am. Soc. Nephrol.* **2014**, *9*, 1876–1882. [CrossRef]

50. Fervenza, F.C.; Sethi, S. Circulating complement levels and C3 glomerulopathy. *Clin. J. Am. Soc. Nephrol.* **2014**, *9*, 1829–1831. [CrossRef]

51. Corvillo, F.; Okrój, M.; Nozal, P.; Melgosa, M.; Sánchez-Corral, P.; López-Trascasa, M. Nephritic Factors: An Overview of Classification, Diagnostic Tools and Clinical Associations. *Front. Immunol.* **2019**, *10*, 886. [CrossRef]

52. Zhang, Y.; Meyer, N.C.; Wang, K.; Nishimura, C.; Frees, K.; Jones, M.; Katz, L.M.; Sethi, S.; Smith, R.J. Causes of alternative pathway dysregulation in dense deposit disease. *Clin. J. Am. Soc. Nephrol.* **2012**, *7*, 265–274. [CrossRef] [PubMed]

53. Ohi, H.; Yasugi, T. Occurrence of C3 nephritic factor and C4 nephritic factor in membranoproliferative glomerulonephritis (MPGN). *Clin. Exp. Immunol.* **1994**, *95*, 316–321. [CrossRef] [PubMed]

54. Watson, R.; Lindner, S.; Bordereau, P.; Hunze, E.M.; Tak, F.; Ngo, S.; Zipfel, P.F.; Skerka, C.; Dragon-Durey, M.A.; Marchbank, K.J. Standardisation of the factor H autoantibody assay. *Immunobiology* **2014**, *219*, 9–16. [CrossRef] [PubMed]

55. Osborne, A.J.; Breno, M.; Borsa, N.G.; Bu, F.; Frémeaux-Bacchi, V.; Gale, D.P.; van den Heuvel, L.P.; Kavanagh, D.; Noris, M.; Pinto, S.; et al. Statistical Validation of Rare Complement Variants Provides Insights into the Molecular Basis of Atypical Hemolytic Uremic Syndrome and C3 Glomerulopathy. *J. Immunol.* **2018**, *200*, 2464–2478. [CrossRef] [PubMed]

56. Sánchez-Corral, P.; Pouw, R.B.; López-Trascasa, M.; Józsi, M. Self-Damage Caused by Dysregulation of the Complement Alternative Pathway: Relevance of the Factor H Protein Family. *Front. Immunol.* **2018**, *12*, 1607. [CrossRef]

57. Vernon, K.A.; Gale, D.P.; de Jorge, E.G.; McLean, A.G.; Galliford, J.; Pierides, A.; Maxwell, P.H.; Taube, D.; Pickering, M.C.; Cook, H.T. Recurrence of complement factor H-related protein 5 nephropathy in a renal transplant. *Am. J. Transplant.* **2011**, *11*, 152–155. [CrossRef]

58. Cochat, P.; Fargue, S.; Mestrallet, G.; Jungraithmayr, T.; Koch-Nogueira, P.; Ranchin, B.; Zimmerhackl, L.B. Disease recurrence in paediatric renal transplantation. *Pediatr. Nephrol.* **2009**, *11*, 2097–2108. [CrossRef]

59. Wong, L.; Moran, S.; Lavin, P.J.; Dorman, A.M.; Conlon, P.J. Kidney transplant outcomes in familial C3 glomerulopathy. *Clin. Kidney J.* **2016**, *3*, 403–407. [CrossRef]

60. Bomback, A.S.; Smith, R.J.; Barile, G.R.; Zhang, Y.; Heher, E.C.; Herlitz, L.; Stokes, M.B.; Markowitz, G.S.; D'Agati, V.D.; Canetta, P.A.; et al. Eculizumab for dense deposit disease and C3 glomerulonephritis. *Clin. J. Am. Soc. Nephrol.* **2012**, *7*, 748–756. [CrossRef]

61. Abbas, F.; El Kossi, M.; Kim, J.J.; Shaheen, I.S.; Sharma, A.; Halawa, A. Complement-mediated renal diseases after kidney transplantation—Current diagnostic and therapeutic options in de novo and recurrent diseases. *World J. Transplant.* **2018**, *8*, 203–219. [CrossRef]
62. Sánchez-Moreno, A.; De la Cerda, F.; Cabrera, R.; Fijo, J.; López-Trascasa, M.; Bedoya, R.; Rodríguez de Córdoba, S.; Ybot-González, P. Eculizumab in dense-deposit disease after renal transplantation. *Pediatr. Nephrol.* **2014**, *29*, 2055–2059. [CrossRef] [PubMed]
63. Lim, W.H.; Shingde, M.; Wong, G. Recurrent and de novo Glomerulonephritis after Kidney Transplantation. *Front. Immunol.* **2019**, *10*, 1944. [CrossRef] [PubMed]
64. Uffing, A.; Pérez-Sáez, M.J.; La Manna, G.; Comai, G.; Fischman, C.; Farouk, S.; Manfro, R.C.; Bauer, A.C.; Lichtenfels, B.; Mansur, J.B.; et al. A large, international study on post-transplant glomerular diseases: The TANGO project. *BMC Nephrol.* **2018**, *19*, 229. [CrossRef] [PubMed]
65. Legendre, C.M.; Licht, C.; Muus, P.; Greenbaum, L.A.; Babu, S.; Bedrosian, C.; Bingham, C.; Cohen, D.J.; Delmas, Y.; Douglas, K.; et al. Terminal complement inhibitor eculizumab in atypical hemolytic-uremic syndrome. *N. Engl. J. Med.* **2013**, *368*, 2169–2181. [CrossRef]
66. Welte, T.; Arnold, F.; Kappes, J.; Seidl, M.; Häffner, K.; Bergmann, C.; Walz, G.; Neumann-Haefelin, F. Treating C3 glomerulopathy with eculizumab. *BMC Nephrol.* **2018**, *19*, 7. [CrossRef]
67. Von Visger, J.; Cassol, C.; Nori, U.; Franco-Ahumada, G.; Nadasdy, T.; Satoskar, A.A. Complete biopsy-proven resolution of deposits in recurrent proliferative glomerulonephritis with monoclonal IgG deposits (PGNMIGD) following rituximab treatment in renal allograft. *BMC Nephrol.* **2019**, *20*, 53. [CrossRef]
68. McCaughan, J.A.; O'Rourke, D.M.; Courtney, A.E. Recurrent dense deposit disease after renal transplantation: An emerging role for complementary therapies. *Am. J. Transplant.* **2012**, *12*, 1046–1051. [CrossRef]
69. Zand, L.; Lorenz, E.C.; Cosio, F.G.; Fervenza, F.C.; Nasr, S.H.; Gandhi, M.J.; Smith, R.J.; Sethi, S. Clinical findings, pathology, and outcomes of C3GN after kidney transplantation. *J. Am. Soc. Nephrol.* **2014**, *25*, 1110–1117. [CrossRef]
70. Rudnicki, M. Rituximab for Treatment of Membranoproliferative Glomerulonephritis and C3 Glomerulopathies. *BioMed Res. Int.* **2017**, *2017*, 2180508. [CrossRef]
71. Koopman, J.J.E.; Teng, Y.K.O.; Boon, C.J.F.; van den Heuvel, L.P.; Rabelink, T.J.; van Kooten, C.; de Vries, A.P.J. Diagnosis and treatment of C3 glomerulopathy in a center of expertise. *Neth. J. Med.* **2019**, *77*, 10–18.
72. Chauvet, S.; Roumenina, L.T.; Aucouturier, P.; Marinozzi, M.C.; Dragon-Durey, M.A.; Karras, A.; Delmas, Y.; Le Quintrec, M.; Guerrot, D.; Jourde-Chiche, N.; et al. Both Monoclonal and Polyclonal Immunoglobulin Contingents Mediate Complement Activation in Monoclonal Gammopathy Associated-C3 Glomerulopathy. *Front. Immunol.* **2018**, *9*, 2260. [CrossRef] [PubMed]
73. Chauvet, S.; Frémeaux-Bacchi, V.; Petitprez, F.; Karras, A.; Daniel, L.; Burtey, S.; Choukroun, G.; Delmas, Y.; Guerrot, D.; François, A.; et al. Treatment of B-cell disorder improves renal outcome of patients with monoclonal gammopathy-associated C3 glomerulopathy. *Blood* **2017**, *129*, 1437–1447. [CrossRef] [PubMed]
74. Sethi, S.; Sukov, W.R.; Zhang, Y.; Fervenza, F.C.; Lager, D.J.; Miller, D.V.; Cornell, L.D.; Krishnan, S.G.; Smith, R.J. Dense deposit disease associated with monoclonal gammopathy of undetermined significance. *Am. J. Kidney Dis.* **2010**, *56*, 977–982. [CrossRef] [PubMed]
75. Zhang, Y.; Shao, D.; Ricklin, D.; Hilkin, B.M.; Nester, C.M.; Lambris, J.D.; Smith, R.J. Compstatin analog Cp40 inhibits complement dysregulation in vitro in C3 glomerulopathy. *Immunobiology* **2015**, *220*, 993–998. [CrossRef] [PubMed]
76. Paixão-Cavalcante, D.; Torreira, E.; Lindorfer, M.A.; Rodriguez de Cordoba, S.; Morgan, B.P.; Taylor, R.P.; Llorca, O.; Harris, C.L. A humanized antibody that regulates the alternative pathway convertase: Potential for therapy of renal disease associated with nephritic factors. *J. Immunol.* **2014**, *192*, 4844–4851. [CrossRef] [PubMed]
77. Subías, M.; Tortajada, A.; Gastoldi, S.; Galbusera, M.; López-Perrote, A.; Lopez, L.J.; González-Fernández, F.A.; Villegas-Martínez, A.; Dominguez, M.; Llorca, O.; et al. A novel antibody against human factor B that blocks formation of the C3bB proconvertase and inhibits complement activation in disease models. *J. Immunol.* **2014**, *193*, 5567–5575. [CrossRef]
78. Pauly, D.; Nagel, B.M.; Reinders, J.; Killian, T.; Wulf, M.; Ackerman, S.; Ehrenstein, B.; Zipfel, P.F.; Skerka, C.; Weber, B.H. A novel antibody against human properdin inhibits the alternative complement system and specifically detects properdin from blood samples. *PLoS ONE* **2014**, *9*, e96371. [CrossRef]

79. Krmar, R.T.; Holtbäck, U.; Linné, T.; Berg, U.B.; Celsi, G.; Söderberg, M.P.; Wernerson, A.; Szakos, A.; Larsson, S.; Skattum, L.; et al. Acute renal failure in dense deposit disease: Complete recovery after combination therapy with immunosuppressant and plasma exchange. *Clin. Nephrol.* **2011**, *75*, 4–10.
80. Häffner, K.; Michelfelder, S.; Pohl, M. Successful therapy of C3Nef-positive C3 glomerulopathy with plasma therapy and immunosuppression. *Pediatr. Nephrol.* **2015**, *30*, 1951–1959. [CrossRef]
81. Kurtz, K.A.; Schlueter, A.J. Management of membranoproliferative glomerulonephritis type II with plasmapheresis. *J. Clin. Apher.* **2002**, *17*, 135–137. [CrossRef]

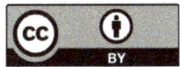

© 2020 by the authors. Licensee MDPI, Basel, Switzerland. This article is an open access article distributed under the terms and conditions of the Creative Commons Attribution (CC BY) license (http://creativecommons.org/licenses/by/4.0/).

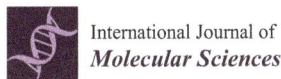

Review

Nephrocalcinosis: A Review of Monogenic Causes and Insights They Provide into This Heterogeneous Condition

Fay J. Dickson [1] and John A. Sayer [2,3,4,*]

1. Hull University Teaching Hospitals, Anlaby Road, Hull HU3 2JZ, UK; fayhill@gmail.com
2. Translational and Clinical Research Institute, Faculty of Medical Sciences, Newcastle University, Central Parkway, Newcastle upon Tyne NE1 3BZ, UK
3. The Newcastle upon Tyne NHS Hospitals Foundation Trust, Newcastle upon Tyne NE7 7DN, UK
4. NIHR Newcastle Biomedical Research Centre, Newcastle upon Tyne NE4 5PL, UK
* Correspondence: john.sayer@ncl.ac.uk; Tel.: +44-191-2418608

Received: 2 December 2019; Accepted: 2 January 2020; Published: 6 January 2020

Abstract: The abnormal deposition of calcium within renal parenchyma, termed nephrocalcinosis, frequently occurs as a result of impaired renal calcium handling. It is closely associated with renal stone formation (nephrolithiasis) as elevated urinary calcium levels (hypercalciuria) are a key common pathological feature underlying these clinical presentations. Although monogenic causes of nephrocalcinosis and nephrolithiasis are rare, they account for a significant disease burden with many patients developing chronic or end-stage renal disease. Identifying underlying genetic mutations in hereditary cases of nephrocalcinosis has provided valuable insights into renal tubulopathies that include hypercalciuria within their varied phenotypes. Genotypes affecting other enzyme pathways, including vitamin D metabolism and hepatic glyoxylate metabolism, are also associated with nephrocalcinosis. As the availability of genetic testing becomes widespread, we cannot be imprecise in our approach to nephrocalcinosis. Monogenic causes of nephrocalcinosis account for a broad range of phenotypes. In cases such as Dent disease, supportive therapies are limited, and early renal replacement therapies are necessitated. In cases such as renal tubular acidosis, a good renal prognosis can be expected providing effective treatment is implemented. It is imperative we adopt a precision-medicine approach to ensure patients and their families receive prompt diagnosis, effective, tailored treatment and accurate prognostic information.

Keywords: nephrocalcinosis; nephrolithiasis; hypercalciuria; monogenic; precision medicine

---

1. Introduction

Nephrocalcinosis can broadly be defined as the deposition of calcium, either as calcium phosphate or calcium oxalate, within the interstitium of the kidney [1]. Whilst Oliver Wrong's original classification sub-divided nephrocalcinosis into being either molecular, microscopic or macroscopic, in clinical practice the term commonly refers to macroscopic nephrocalcinosis that can be detected radiologically [2]. Rarely, asymmetric presentation of nephrocalcinosis localised to the renal cortex may represent calcium release from tissue breakdown, for example in renal transplant rejection or renal infarction [3]. However, in the majority of cases, nephrocalcinosis affects the renal medulla and can be detected as bilateral, symmetrical increased echogenicity within the renal pyramids on ultrasound imaging [4]. This non-invasive imaging modality is utilised either as a screening tool, or as a method of assessing disease progression/response to treatment, as medullary nephrocalcinosis can be reliably graded (Grade I–III) according to the extent of increased echogenicity affecting the medullary pyramids [5].

Whilst the exact pathogenesis of nephrocalcinosis remains under investigation, it is acknowledged medullary nephrocalcinosis is a consequence of hypercalciuria. Increased urinary calcium load arises either through increased calcium absorption (extra-renal causes) or impaired calcium reabsorption within the renal tubule [2]. The majority of calcium reabsorption (~65%) occurs in the proximal tubule, whilst ~25% is reabsorbed in the thick ascending limb of the loop of Henle [6] and ~5% is reabsorbed from the cortical collecting duct [2]. Identification of monogenic causes of nephrocalcinosis affecting these areas has provided valuable insights into the pathogenesis of this heterogeneous condition. Interestingly, although a further ~7–10% of calcium is reabsorbed within the distal convoluted tubule, no monogenic causes of nephrocalcinosis have been identified which affect this section of the renal tubule [2].

Hypercalciuria, in addition to being part of the underlying pathological process for nephrocalcinosis, also predisposes patients to renal stone formation (nephrolithiasis). Nephrocalcinosis and nephrolithiasis will therefore commonly co-exist within the phenotypes of these rare monogenic conditions, and nephrolithiasis onset at a young age may prompt investigations for nephrocalcinosis and uncover an inherited condition [7].

Nephrocalcinosis in itself is a rare disorder, and consequently monogenic forms affect even smaller numbers of the population. For those individuals affected by nephrocalcinosis, however, a tailored, individualised approach to their initial diagnostic work-up is imperative. Presentation at a young age, a family history of an affected individual or carrier, or a history of consanguinity in the family is often suggestive of an inherited tubulopathy. Several factors, including recessive inheritance patterns and varied phenotype presentation, dictate that a family history is often not present, and suspicion of a monogenic cause should not be dismissed simply due to absence of the above factors.

The morbidity associated with nephrolithiasis and nephrocalcinosis is widely accepted [8]. Whilst an overall approach may focus upon slowing progression of associated chronic kidney disease (CKD), specific treatment strategies, such as dietary modifications or use of thiazide diuretics, will vary depending upon the underlying disease process. Widespread adoption of precision medicine within this field is likely to have significant advantages for both current and future patients. Several monogenic causes of nephrocalcinosis are associated with rapid progression of CKD, often requiring initiation of renal replacement therapies before adulthood. Early diagnosis of a monogenic cause is vital for providing accurate prognostic information for the patient and their family, including the opportunity to screen other family members or offer pre-implantation genetic diagnosis (PGD) testing for subsequent pregnancies. Perhaps most significantly, a prompt diagnosis may also avoid the individual being exposed to unnecessary or harmful treatments. For example, a patient with *OCRL* mutations (Dent disease 2) was reported to receive immunosuppressive therapies including corticosteroids and cyclophosphamide, based on a misdiagnosis of nephrotic syndrome, before their inherited tubulopathy was correctly identified [9]. Commonly used medications may easily inadvertently worsen the condition of patients with other inherited tubulopathies: loop diuretic use can potentiate hypercalciuria and worsen nephrolithiasis/nephrocalcinosis burden, whereas use of potassium-sparing diuretics should be avoided in patients with distal renal tubular acidosis [10]. Furthermore, in cases where a proactive approach to personalised genetic medicine has been taken, next generation sequencing has identified *CLCN5* mutations (Dent disease 1) in patients for whom only low-molecular weight proteinuria was present at diagnosis, i.e., before the full phenotype had emerged [11]. Finally, given the current paucity of treatment options for nephrocalcinosis, it is potentially from the study of these rare monogenic causes that key future therapeutic targets may emerge which could revolutionise our management of the condition (Table A1).

2. Monogenic Causes of Nephrocalcinosis

2.1. CLCN5 Mutations

The proximal tubule represents the site of greatest calcium reabsorption within the renal tubule, and it is mutations in the ClC-5 chloride transporter in this region, encoded by *CLCN5*, that give rise to Dent disease type 1 [12]. This condition demonstrates an X-linked recessive pattern of inheritance; affected males usually display a triad of low molecular weight (LMW) proteinuria, hypercalciuria and nephrocalcinosis, although the triad may be incomplete at initial presentation [11]. Female carriers are usually asymptomatic, but may occasionally have LMW proteinuria, hypercalciuria or nephrolithiasis [12].

Dent disease 1 (*CLCN5* mutations) accounts for 60% of Dent disease cases. *OCRL* mutations, which may result in a spectrum of phenotypes ranging from Dent disease 2 to the more severe Lowe oculocerebrorenal syndrome, account for a further 15% of cases, whilst the underlying genetic mutation remains unascertained in 25% of cases [12]. The varied phenotypes of Dent disease may also include a partial Fanconi syndrome as the initial clue indicating proximal tubular dysfunction [13], whilst nephrolithiasis or haematuria can also feature alongside the cardinal LMW proteinuria [11]. Although genetic conditions with a Fanconi syndrome, including Lowe oculocerebrorenal syndrome (*OCRL* mutations) and cystinosis (*CTNS* mutations) may also feature nephrocalcinosis [14,15], it remains more commonly associated with Dent disease 1 (*CLCN5* mutations) [16].

Patients with Dent disease carry a poor prognosis in terms of renal function: 30–80% of males develop end-stage renal disease (ESRD) by middle-age [12]. The development of CKD has been hypothesised to be linked to nephrocalcinosis, although this theory does not explain Dent disease patients without nephrocalcinosis who also develop progressive CKD, and it is probable more than one mechanism exists [16,17].

Treatment options for Dent disease are limited. Early diagnosis is crucial in order to prioritise preservation of renal function for as long as possible and offer accurate prognostic information [11]. Patients should undergo careful CKD monitoring with control of variables such as blood pressure. A strategy to try and reduce nephrocalcinosis development is to reduce urinary calcium excretion; thiazide diuretics may be used but in some patients their role is limited by unacceptable side effects including hypokalaemia, muscle cramps and dehydration [12]. The majority of patients will reach ESRD by the age of 40 [18]; renal transplantation offers the best outcomes as there is no recurrence in the renal allograft due to the donor kidney not carrying the causative mutation [12].

2.2. CYP24A1 Mutations

Nephrocalcinosis occurs as a result of impaired renal calcium handling; disorders of vitamin D metabolism can result in elevated calcium levels and represent a different pathway predisposing to nephrocalcinosis formation. The second stage of vitamin D activation takes place within the kidney, resulting in production of the active metabolite 1,25-dihydroxyvitamin D^3. Mutations in *CYP24A1*, which encodes 1,25-hydroxyvitamin-D_3-24-hydroxylase, result in an inability to catabolise this active vitamin D metabolite [19]. *CYP24A1* mutations were first detected following reports of a small cohort of babies developing adverse effects (including hypercalcemia and nephrocalcinosis) as a result of the public health intervention to routinely supplement formula milk with vitamin D [20]. Following further analysis, two distinct phenotypes resulting from *CYP24A1* mutations have been recognised, both of which frequently include nephrocalcinosis [19].

The first phenotype, idiopathic infantile hypercalcaemia (IIH) presents in childhood, and is classified as hypercalcaemia, infantile 1 (HCINF1). Affected infants often present with symptomatic hypercalcaemia, severe dehydration, vomiting and failure to thrive [21]. Nephrocalcinosis is often detectable on ultrasound imaging at diagnosis [21]. Management of these patients focusses upon removing exogenous sources of vitamin D (e.g., supplements), fluid resuscitation and future conservative measures (high fluid intake, dietary adjustments, avoidance of tanning beds) to prevent further nephrolithiasis/nephrocalcinosis formation.

A second, later-onset, phenotype has also been demonstrated in adults who present with nephrolithiasis, hypercalciuria or incidentally detected nephrocalcinosis [22]. This phenotype is usually less severe, and a history of vitamin D supplementation is not universally present. Treatment strategies focus upon low calcium and oxalate diet, avoidance of vitamin D supplementation and excessive sunlight exposure [19]. Use of azole antifungal agents (fluconazole, ketoconazole) have shown benefit as non-specific P450 enzyme inhibitors which inhibit 1α-hydroxylase (encoded by CYP27B1), thereby reducing production of the active form of vitamin D [19,23]. However, lifelong treatment with these agents may be undesirable owing to their side effect profile, including hepatotoxicity. Recently, rifampicin was demonstrated to reduce hypercalcaemia and effectively control 1,25-dihydroxyvitamin D^3 levels in patients with CYP24A1 mutations [24]. Rifampicin acts upon an alternative vitamin D catabolism pathway as a potent inducer of CYP3A4 [24]. This provides an alternative therapy that may be better tolerated as a lifelong treatment.

2.3. SLC34A1 Mutations

Autosomal recessive inheritance of mutations in the sodium-phosphate co-transporter NaPi2a, encoded by SLC34A1, cause idiopathic infantile hypercalcaemia (IIH), classified as hypercalcaemia, infantile 2 (HCINF2), in a subgroup of patients without CYP24A1 mutations [25]. In addition to the classic biochemical features associated with IIH of hypercalcaemia, hypercalciuria and high levels of 1,25-dihydroxyvitamin D_3, patients with SLC34A1 loss-of-function mutations exhibit hypophosphatemia [26]. This hypophosphatemia arises as a result of renal phosphate wasting within the proximal tubule, driving excessive production of 1,25-dihydroxyvitamin D_3 and subsequent hypercalcaemia and hypercalciuria.

Nephrocalcinosis is a common phenotypical feature in patients with SLC34A1 mutations [27]. In the acute presentation, where patients may have classical features of IIH such as failure to thrive, dehydration and vomiting, they should be fluid resuscitated and may receive loop diuretics (furosemide) to induce calciuresis [27]. Similar to patients with CYP24A1 mutations, an azole antifungal agent (ketoconazole or fluconazole) may be used to inhibit 1α-hydroxylase, thereby reducing the high calcium levels predisposing to nephrocalcinosis through reduction in levels of 1,25-dihydroxyvitamin D_3 [26]. The long-term management of these patients, however, should focus upon a low calcium diet and avoidance of vitamin D supplementation or heightened vitamin D exposure, in order to minimise the risk of nephrocalcinosis.

2.4. CLDN16 and CLDN19 Mutations

The thick ascending limb (TAL) of loop of Henle, where ~25% of calcium reabsorption [6] and ~60% of magnesium reabsorption usually takes place [28], is the site of two rare autosomal recessive channelopathies affecting calcium and magnesium absorption. Mutations in CLDN16 and CLDN19, which encode the tight junction proteins claudin-16 and claudin-19 respectively, give rise to the condition familial hypomagnesaemia with hypercalciuria and nephrocalcinosis (FHHNC) [29].

Patients are symptomatic from a young age, although initial presenting features may be non-specific such as polyuria/polydipsia, failure to thrive and vomiting. The biochemical profile of FHHNC phenotypes includes excessive loss of calcium and magnesium in the urine, with normal serum calcium levels and low serum magnesium levels [28]. Importantly, serum hypomagnesaemia is not universally present, and a fractional excretion value of magnesium (FeMg%) should be calculated using serum magnesium, serum creatinine and urinary magnesium levels to ensure diagnostic accuracy [30]. Nephrocalcinosis is a universal feature which develops early in the disease course of FHHNC, and hypercalciuria is one predisposing factor for this [30]. A further predisposing factor for nephrolithiasis and nephrocalcinosis in FHHNC is hypocitraturia, which removes the protective effect of urinary citrate against precipitation of calcium salts in the urine [30]. The renal prognosis for FHHNC is poor;

many patients progress to ESRD during adolescence [28]. Rapid progression of CKD in these patients may not be attributable solely to nephrocalcinosis, as their renal dysfunction is more severe/presents earlier than that observed in other tubulopathies predisposing to nephrocalcinosis such as primary distal renal tubular acidosis or Bartter syndrome [30]. *CLDN19* mutations are associated with severe ocular abnormalities as claudin-19 is also expressed in the retinal epithelium [28].

Treatment strategies for FHHNC patients focus initially on supportive measures aimed at reducing hypercalciuria and replacing magnesium; thiazide diuretics and oral magnesium supplements are used for this respectively, although their impact on total urine calcium and serum magnesium levels is not always significant [28,30]. Overall, these supportive treatments do not negate the progression of renal dysfunction, and renal replacement therapies are commonly necessitated before adulthood. Renal transplantation is the ideal option: the loss-of-function channelopathy is not present in the renal allograft so renal calcium and magnesium handling are normalised and there is no disease recurrence [31].

2.5. Bartter Syndromes

The Bartter syndromes describe five channelopathies affecting thick ascending limb (TAL) transporter proteins involved in sodium chloride (NaCl) re-absorption. Autosomal recessive inheritance of these gene mutations results in salt-losing tubulopathies characterised by excessive urinary sodium losses, with corresponding hypokalaemia, metabolic alkalosis and secondary hyperaldosteronism [32]. Nephrocalcinosis has been described in all Bartter syndromes but is most frequently associated with Bartter I, II and V [2]. The pathogenesis of nephrocalcinosis in Bartter syndromes is not fully understood, although it is most probably a consequence of hypercalciuria seen within the Bartter syndrome phenotypes [33]. Early identification of the Bartter syndrome genotype is clinically advantageous, especially given the fact nephrocalcinosis and other renal manifestations are not uniformly represented across the different Bartter syndrome phenotypes. Several clinical features, including age of onset, presence of transient hyperkalaemia, severity of hypokalaemia, sensorineural deafness and renal impairment may provide vital clues about the likely underlying genotype which can guide genetic testing.

Bartter syndromes I and II, caused by mutations in *SLC12A1* and *KCNJ1* respectively, usually present during the antenatal/postnatal period, and have been traditionally referred to as antenatal Bartter syndromes (aBS). Polyhydramnios, premature birth and low-birth weight are classic features of aBS, and nephrocalcinosis is frequently already detectable at this young age [34]. *KCNJ1* mutations, encoding the ROMK potassium channel, often display transient hyperkalaemia in the neonatal period prior to development of classic hypokalaemia [32]. Early treatment to correct electrolyte disturbance, rehydrate patients and minimise growth retardation is necessitated [35]. Cyclo-oxygenase inhibitors (e.g., indomethacin), which target the elevated prostaglandin levels seen within aBS, are an effective treatment and can lead to effective catch-up growth [33,35].

Our understanding of Bartter syndrome II has recently expanded to include a late-onset phenotype following case reports of two adults found to have *KCNJ1* mutations after incidental nephrocalcinosis detection. Both patients had nephrocalcinosis and mild renal impairment at diagnosis, and were treated with oral potassium supplementation, and either a potassium-sparing diuretic or angiotensin-converting enzyme inhibitor respectively [33,35].

Bartter syndrome III occurs as a result of mutations in *CLCNKB* which encode the chloride channel ClC-Kb. The syndrome often has a milder phenotype with later-onset of symptoms, although presentations within the neonatal period have been reported [32]. Patients with Bartter III often have a more severe hypokalaemic alkalosis which is the most likely clinical clue to their underlying genotype [32]. Hypercalciuria and nephrocalcinosis are less frequently associated with the Bartter III phenotype compared to Bartter I and II [32].

Mutations in *BSND*, which encode Barttin (a chaperone protein for ClC-Ka and ClC-Kb) account for Bartter syndrome IV. Sensorineural deafness is part of the Bartter IV phenotype [36]. An association between Bartter syndrome IV and renal impairment has been reported. Patients frequently develop CKD at a very young age, and may not respond to indomethacin, in contrast to those with other aBS genotypes [36].

Although the term Bartter syndrome V is sometimes used in the literature to describe gain-of-function mutations in *CASR* encoding the calcium-sensing receptor (CaSR), according to OMIM classification Bartter syndrome V instead refers to mutations in the *MAGED2* gene, causing an X-linked recessively inherited transient antenatal BS [37]. To avoid this nomenclature issue, CaSR mutations are described separately in the section below.

2.6. CASR Mutations

The calcium-sensing receptor (CaSR), expressed in the parathyroid gland and kidney, responds to changes in serum calcium levels, acting to inhibit parathyroid hormone (PTH) secretion and renal tubular calcium reabsorption [38]. A total of 112 mutations of the *CASR* gene have been reported, of which 48 are gain-of-function mutations, including those associated with autosomal dominant hypocalcaemia (ADH)/autosomal dominant hypocalcemic hypercalciuria (ADHH) [38].

Patients with ADH exhibit a biochemical phenotype which includes serum hypocalcemia, low-normal levels of PTH, hypercalciuria, and polyuria [39]. It is essential to distinguish these patients from those with hypoparathyroidism: ADH patients given vitamin D supplementation are likely to develop worsening hypercalciuria, nephrocalcinosis and renal impairment as 1,25-dihydroxyvitamin D upregulates transcription of the *CASR* gene [40]. Instead, a low-normal serum PTH (in contrast to a very low or undetectable level) and low urinary calcium levels in a hypocalcemic patient should prompt clinicians to screen for *CASR* mutations [40]. Patients with ADH should receive treatment for their hypocalcemia only if it is symptomatic, and should aim for symptom control rather than normalised serum calcium levels [40]. Gain-of-function *CASR* mutations that inhibit activity of NKCC2 and ROMK channels in the thick ascending limb (TAL) of loop of Henle have been reported to produce a Bartter-like phenotype, which may include hypokalaemia and hyperreninemic hyperaldosteronism, in addition to hypocalcemia [41,42].

2.7. ADCY10 Mutations

Mutations in *ADCY10*, which encodes the soluble adenylyl cyclase gene, have been linked to familial idiopathic hypercalciuria, also known as Absorptive Hypercalciuria, 2 (HCA2) [43]. HCA2 displays autosomal dominant inheritance, with a phenotype including frequent calcium nephrolithiasis [44]. The underlying aetiology of the condition has not been fully delineated, but it is known increased intestinal calcium absorption is responsible for the hypercalciuria seen in these patients. Alongside the common clinical finding of calcium nephrolithiasis, increased renal calcium handling predisposes these patients to nephrocalcinosis formation [44].

2.8. Primary Distal Renal Tubular Acidosis

In distal renal tubular acidosis (dRTA), affected patients have a hyperchloremic normal anion-gap metabolic acidosis and alkaline urine (pH > 5.3) [10]. This characteristic biochemical profile arises as a consequence of type A intercalated cells in the collecting duct failing to acidify the urine [45].

Under normal physiological conditions, H^+ and HCO_3^- are produced within the type A intercalated cells. Mutations in either the vacuolar H^+-ATPase pump, which excretes H^+ into the urine, or the chloride bicarbonate counter transporter anion exchanger (AE1), which reabsorbs HCO_3^- into the circulation, account for 85% of known causes of primary dRTA [10]. Mutations in the B1 and A4 subunit of the vacuolar H^+-ATPase pump, encoded by *ATP6V1B1* and *ATP6V0A4* respectively, demonstrate autosomal recessive transmission and produce a phenotype frequently associated with sensorineural hearing loss as well as the commonly recognised biochemical abnormalities [45]. Mutations in *SLC4A1*, which encodes AE1, can occur with either autosomal dominant or autosomal recessive transmission: autosomal recessive cases are associated with earlier age of symptom onset and a more severe phenotype [10]. Red blood cell abnormalities may also form part of the phenotype for patients with *SLC4A1* mutations [45]. More recently, mutations in Forkhead box protein I1 (encoded by *FOXI1*) and WD repeat-containing protein 72 (encoded by *WDR72*) have been recognised as alternative underlying genetic mutations in a small number of families with autosomal recessive inheritance of dRTA [46,47]. At present the underlying genetic defect remains unknown in approximately 15% of cases of primary dRTA [10].

Nephrocalcinosis is an extremely common feature within the phenotype of primary dRTA patients [48]. Calcium phosphate precipitates at higher pH; the alkaline urine of dRTA patients acts as a predisposing factor for nephrolithiasis and nephrocalcinosis formation [45]. In addition, chronic metabolic acidosis leads to excessive bone demineralisation often resulting in hypercalciuria: this also increases the likelihood of nephrocalcinosis developing if patients do not receive early diagnosis and treatment [48].

Treatment strategies for dRTA focus primarily on correcting the underlying metabolic acidosis; patients are maintained on oral potassium citrate which must be taken at regular intervals given its short half-life. This treatment may soon become less cumbersome for patients, as a controlled-release preparation of potassium bicarbonate and potassium citrate designed to be taken twice daily is undergoing phase three trials [10]. Primary distal renal tubular acidosis carries a good prognosis providing prompt diagnosis and treatment initiation are achieved. In patients on treatment with a corrected metabolic acidosis, it has been noted nephrocalcinosis does not progress and their renal function usually remains preserved [10]. However, potassium citrate treatment cannot reverse nephrocalcinosis if already present. Long-term follow-up of dRTA patients should include annual ultrasound screening to monitor for nephrocalcinosis and nephrolithiasis, as well as monitoring of their renal function [45].

2.9. Primary Hyperoxaluria

Primary hyperoxaluria describes a group of inborn errors of metabolism where defective liver enzymes involved in glyoxylate metabolism result in excess production of oxalate [49]. The predominant route of oxalate excretion is via the kidneys, with enteric excretion also playing a role when renal function is impaired [50]. In primary hyperoxaluria, excessive oxalate levels supersaturate renal excretion mechanisms, leading initially to calcium oxalate deposition within the kidney, and subsequently systemic oxalosis (deposition of oxalate within other systems) affecting the skeleton, heart, liver and other organs [49].

Currently there are three known types of primary hyperoxaluria which all display autosomal recessive inheritance. Reports of phenotypically similar cases with no proven monogenic cause increase the likelihood of further pathogenic mutations being discovered over time [49]. Recurrent calcium-oxalate nephrolithiasis and nephrocalcinosis are a central feature of primary hyperoxaluria phenotypes. Treatment options and renal prognosis vary considerably between the three genotypes however, making early genetic diagnosis imperative.

Primary hyperoxaluria type 1 (PH1) is the commonest form of primary hyperoxaluria and displays the most severe phenotype, with 50% of patients developing ESRD before the age of 25 [51]. Mutations in *AGXT*, which encode the hepatic alanine-glyoxylate aminotransferase (AGT) enzyme, result in an inability to break down glyoxylate into glycine. Instead, glyoxylate is converted to oxalate, leading to pathological hyperoxaluria [49]. Pyridoxine (vitamin B6) is a co-factor for AGT, and therefore offers a therapeutic target unique to PH1. An estimated 10–40% of PH1 patients respond to pyridoxine supplementation, which can delay progression to ESRF and allow consideration of isolated renal transplantation rather than simultaneous liver/kidney transplantation providing the patient is fully pyridoxine sensitive [51,52]. Early initiation of conservative measures such as high fluid intake and use of potassium citrate may reduce the incidence of nephrolithiasis and delay progression to ESRD [51]. However, due to the risk of systemic oxalosis, renal replacement therapy (RRT) must be initiated once plasma oxalate levels > 30–45 µmol/L, often resulting in patients commencing dialysis at much higher GFR levels than for other renal conditions [52].

PH1 is far more prevalent in developing countries (likely related to higher consanguinity rates) meaning access to liver transplantation is limited [51]. Even in countries where transplantation is more accessible, it carries significant risks for the patient [52]. The evolution of our treatment of this condition therefore hinges upon identifying therapeutic targets which do not necessitate organ transplantation to replace the defective enzyme. Trials utilising the oxalate-metabolising bacterium *Oxabacter formigenes* to increase gut excretion of oxalate and reduce urinary oxalate excretion reached phase II/III trials but did not significantly reduce urinary oxalate excretion [50]. Animal studies have shown oxalate decarboxylase enzymes can effectively reduce urinary oxalate levels, providing an alternative potential future therapy for reduction of calcium-oxalate nephrocalcinosis in primary hyperoxaluria [53,54].

Primary hyperoxaluria type 2 (PH2) occurs as a result of mutations in *GRHPR* which encodes the glyoxylate reductase/hydroxypyruvate reductase enzyme. PH2 exhibits a less severe phenotype, with lower incidence of nephrolithiasis and nephrocalcinosis. It is rare for PH2 patients to progress to ESRD or develop systemic oxalosis [51].

Primary hyperoxaluria type 3 (PH3) account for only 10% of PH patients [49]. Mutations in *HOGA1*, which encodes the hepatic enzyme 4-hydroxy-2-oxoglutarate aldolase, underlie the condition. PH3 has a milder phenotype, with lower nephrolithiasis burden, and nephrocalcinosis and renal impairment being less common

2.10. GDNF Mutations

Medullary sponge kidney (MSK) is a congenital disorder resulting in ectatic collecting ducts within one or both kidneys. The clinical sequelae of nephrolithiasis, nephrocalcinosis, recurrent urinary tract infections and urinary acidification defects are often not apparent until adulthood [55]. The underlying pathogenesis of MSK is yet to be fully elicited. Whilst once considered a sporadic disorder, evidence of MSK cases showing likely autosomal dominant inheritance have emerged, intensifying the search for underlying genetic causes [56]. Identification of mutations in *GDNF*, which encodes glial cell-derived neurotrophic factor, have now been identified in some MSK patients and may account for the underlying pathophysiological process in a subset of MSK patients [57].

3. Other Genetic Conditions That May Feature Nephrocalcinosis within Their Clinical Phenotype

Hypercalciuria acts as a predisposing factor for medullary nephrocalcinosis formation; any condition associated with excess urinary calcium excretion may lead to cases of nephrocalcinosis. Hypercalciuria and nephrocalcinosis have been described in association with the inherited conditions Wilson's disease, Williams-Beuren syndrome and cystic fibrosis.

Wilson's disease, a rare autosomal recessive condition characterised by *ATP7B* mutations leading to defective copper excretion, can feature a renal Fanconi syndrome [58,59]. In Wilson's disease patients exhibiting hypercalciuria, nephrolithiasis and nephrocalcinosis have been described [59].

Williams-Beuren syndrome is a developmental disorder occurring as a result of a microdeletion on the q arm of chromosome 7. The classical phenotype includes a distinctive facial appearance, intellectual disability and cardiovascular problems. However, patients with this syndrome have been found to be at increased risk of hypercalcaemia; the combination of resulting dehydration and hypercalciuria have led to cases of nephrocalcinosis being described [60].

Cystic fibrosis, caused by mutations in the *CFTR* gene, has been associated with hypercalciuria and microscopic nephrocalcinosis. However, the patients described did not demonstrate any signs of renal dysfunction associated with their microscopic nephrocalcinosis [61].

Amelogenesis Imperfecta describes a group of inherited enamel defects; there have been case reports of nephrocalcinosis detection in some of these patients in association with a distal renal tubular acidosis. However, in contrast to Wilson's disease, Williams-Beuren syndrome and cystic fibrosis, these patients have not demonstrated hypercalciuria, indicating different underlying pathophysiology [62].

4. Conclusions

Monogenic causes of nephrocalcinosis account for a rare set of conditions with a low population frequency. However, the clinical course for affected patients is very different depending on their underlying genotype. Accurate, prompt diagnosis allows early initiation of conservative measures, which in some cases can halt nephrocalcinosis or delay progression of renal impairment. Establishing the underlying genetic mutation also allows accurate prognostic information to be given and can help facilitate screening of other family members. As our understanding of these rare inherited conditions increases, it is hoped further treatment targets that address underlying enzymatic/protein defects will emerge. However, at present for the majority of cases treatment strategies focus upon supportive treatments to correct biochemical parameters, and careful monitoring of disease progression.

Funding: This research received no external funding.

Conflicts of Interest: The authors declare no conflict of interest.

Appendix A

Table A1. Monogenic causes of nephrocalcinosis.

Gene	Encoded Protein	Site of Action	Clinical Condition	Inheritance	Phenotype
CLCN5	ClC-5 chloride transporter	Renal proximal tubule	Dent disease 1	X-linked recessive	Low molecular-weight (LMW) proteinuria, hypercalciuria, nephrocalcinosis/nephrolithiasis, progression to ESRD [1] by middle-age
OCRL	Inositol polyphosphate 5-phosphatase OCRL-1	Renal proximal tubule	Dent disease 2; Lowe oculocerebrorenal syndrome	X-linked recessive	Low molecular-weight (LMW) proteinuria, hypercalciuria, nephrocalcinosis/nephrolithiasis (less frequently than in Dent disease 1) Mild intellectual disability, cataracts Lowe oculocerebrorenal syndrome: more severe phenotype including ocular abnormalities, intellectual disability, amino aciduria, renal dysfunction, vitamin-D resistant rickets
CYP24A1	1,25-hydroxyvitamin-D_3-24-hydroxylase	Kidney	Hypercalcemia, Infantile, 1: HCINF1 [2]	AR [3]	Hypercalcemia, hypercalciuria, high 1,25-dihydroxyvitamin D_3 (a) Early presentation with vomiting, dehydration, failure to thrive, nephrocalcinosis (b) Adult presentation with nephrocalcinosis, nephrolithiasis
SLC34A1	Sodium-phosphate co-transporter NaPi2a	Renal proximal tubule	Hypercalcemia, Infantile 2: HCINF2 [4]	AR	Hypercalcemia, hypercalciuria, high 1,25-dihydroxyvitamin D_3, hypophosphatemia, vomiting, dehydration, failure to thrive, nephrocalcinosis
CLDN16	Tight junction protein claudin-16	Thick ascending limb (TAL)	FHHNC [5]	AR	Hypomagnesaemia, high urinary Mg^{2+}/Ca^{2+}, polyuria/polydipsia, failure to thrive, nephrocalcinosis, progression to ESRD in adolescence
CLDN19	Tight junction protein claudin-19	Thick ascending limb (TAL)	FHHNC with severe ocular involvement	AR	Hypomagnesaemia, high urinary Mg^{2+}/Ca^{2+}, polyuria/polydipsia, failure to thrive, nephrocalcinosis, progression to ESRD in adolescence severe ocular abnormalities
SLC12A1	Sodium-potassium-chloride cotransporter NKCC2	Thick ascending limb (TAL)	Bartter syndrome Type 1, Antenatal (BARTS1)	AR	Antenatal/neonatal presentation with polyhydramnios, premature birth and low-birth weight, nephrocalcinosis, hypokalaemia, metabolic alkalosis, secondary hypoaldosteronism

Table A1. Cont.

Gene	Encoded Protein	Site of Action	Clinical Condition	Inheritance	Phenotype
KCNJ1	ROMK potassium channel	Thick ascending limb (TAL)	Bartter syndrome Type 2, Antenatal (BARTS2)	AR	Often antenatal/neonatal presentation with polyhydramnios, premature birth and low-birth weight, nephrocalcinosis, hypokalaemia, metabolic alkalosis, secondary hypoaldosteronismFew reports of later-onset (adult) presentation with nephrocalcinosis and CKD [6]
CLCNKB	Chloride channel ClC-Kb	Thick ascending limb (TAL)	Bartter syndrome, Type 3 (BARTS3)	AR	Severe hypokalaemic metabolic alkalosis, secondary hypoaldosteronism Usually later symptom-onset but few cases of neonatal onset
BSND	Barttin, chaperone protein for ClC-Ka and ClC-Kb	Thick ascending limb (TAL)	Bartter syndrome, Type 4: BSND [7]	AR	Severe hypokalaemic metabolic alkalosis, secondary hypoaldosteronism, sensorineural deafness, development of CKD in childhood
CASR	Gain-of-function mutation in Calcium-sensing receptor (CaSR)	Thick ascending limb (TAL), parathyroid gland	Hypocalcemia, autosomal dominant 1 (HYPOC1)	AD [8]	Serum hypocalcaemia, low serum PTH, hypercalciuria, nephrocalcinosis
ADCY10	Soluble Adenylate cyclase 10	Increased intestinal calcium reabsorption	Familial idiopathic hypercalciuria	AD	Hypercalciuria, calcium nephrolithiasis, nephrocalcinosis
ATP6V1B1	B1 subunit vacuolar H+-ATPase pump	Collecting duct	distal RTA [9] with deafness	AR	Hyperchloremic normal anion-gap metabolic acidosis, alkaline urine sensorineural deafness, nephrocalcinosis Good renal prognosis once on treatment
ATP6V0A4	A4 subunit vacuolar H+-ATPase pump	Collecting duct	distal RTA	AR	Hyperchloremic normal anion-gap metabolic acidosis, alkaline urine, sensorineural deafness, nephrocalcinosis Good renal prognosis once on treatment
SLC4A1	AE1	Collecting duct	distal RTA	AD or AR	Hyperchloremic normal anion-gap metabolic acidosis, alkaline urine nephrocalcinosis, red blood cell abnormalities Good renal prognosis once on treatment
FOXI1	Forkhead box protein I1	Collecting duct	distal RTA	AR	Hyperchloremic normal anion-gap metabolic acidosis, alkaline urine, nephrocalcinosis. Good renal prognosis once on treatment
WDR72	WD repeat-containing protein 72	Collecting duct	distal RTA	AR	Hyperchloremic normal anion-gap metabolic acidosis, alkaline urine nephrocalcinosis. Good renal prognosis once on treatment

Table A1. Cont.

Gene	Encoded Protein	Site of Action	Clinical Condition	Inheritance	Phenotype
AGXT	Alanine-glyoxylate aminotransferase	Hepatic peroxisomes	Hyperoxaluria, primary, type 1	AR	Early onset recurrent calcium oxalate nephrolithiasis, nephrocalcinosis Frequent progression to ESRD Systemic oxalosis affecting multiple organs including kidney, bones, heart, liver
GRHPR	Glyoxylate reductase/hydroxypyruvate reductase	Liver, leucocytes, kidney	Hyperoxaluria, primary, type 2	AR	Recurrent nephrolithiasis, nephrocalcinosis Milder phenotype than PH1, only some patients progress to ESRD
HOGA1	4-hydroxy-2-oxoglutarate aldolase	Liver	Hyperoxaluria, primary, type 3	AR	Nephrolithiasis ± rarely nephrocalcinosis, renal impairment rare
GDNF	Glial cell-derived neurotrophic factor	Kidney	Medullary sponge kidney	Sporadic or AD	Nephrolithiasis, nephrocalcinosis, recurrent urinary tract infection, urinary acidification defects

[1] ESRD = End stage renal disease, [2] HCINF1 = Hypercalcemia, idiopathic, of infancy type 1, [3] AR = Autosomal Recessive, [4] HCINF2 = Hypercalcaemia, idiopathic, of infancy type 2, [5] FHHNC = Familial hypomagnesaemia with hypercalciuria and nephrocalcinosis, [6] CKD = Chronic kidney disease, [7] BSND = Bartter Syndrome, Neonatal, with Sensorineural Deafness, [8] AD = Autosomal Dominant, [9] Distal RTA = distal renal tubular acidosis.

References

1. Shavit, L.; Jaeger, P.; Unwin, R.J. What is nephrocalcinosis? *Kidney Int.* **2019**, *88*, 35–43. [CrossRef]
2. Oliveira, B.; Kleta, R.; Bockenhauer, D.; Walsh, S.B. Genetic, pathophysiological, and clinical aspects of nephrocalcinosis. *Am. J. Physiol.* **2016**, *311*, F1243–F1252. [CrossRef] [PubMed]
3. Barratt, J.; Harris, K.; Topham, P. *Oxford Desk Reference Nephrology*; Oxford University Press: New York, NY, USA, 2008; pp. 278–279.
4. Glazer, G.M.; Callen, P.W.; Filly, R.A. Medullary nephrocalcinosis: Sonographic evaluation. *Am. J. Roentgenol.* **1982**, *138*, 55–57. [CrossRef] [PubMed]
5. Dick, P.T.; Shuckett, B.M.; Tang, B.; Daneman, A.; Kooh, S.W. Observer reliability in grading nephrocalcinosis on ultrasound examinations in children. *Pediatr. Radiol.* **1999**, *29*, 68–72. [CrossRef] [PubMed]
6. Moor, M.B.; Bonny, O. Ways of calcium reabsorption in the kidney. *Am. J. Physiol.* **2016**, *310*, F1337–F1350. [CrossRef] [PubMed]
7. Daga, A.; Majmundar, A.J.; Braun, D.A.; Gee, H.Y.; Lawson, J.A.; Shril, S.; Jobst-Schwan, T.; Vivante, A.; Schapiro, D.; Tan, W.; et al. Whole exome sequencing frequently detects a monogenic cause in early onset nephrolithiasis and nephrocalcinosis. *Kidney Int.* **2018**, *93*, 204–213. [CrossRef]
8. Weigert, A.; Hoppe, B. Nephrolithiasis and nephrocalcinosis in childhood- risk factor related current and future treatment options. *Front. Pediatr.* **2018**, *6*, 98. [CrossRef]
9. He, G.; Zhang, H.; Cao, S.; Xiao, H.; Yao, Y. Dent's disease complicated by nephrotic syndrome: A case report. *Intractable Rare Dis. Res.* **2016**, *5*, 297–300. [CrossRef]
10. Alexander, R.; Law, L.; Gil-Pena, H.; Greenbaum, L.; Santos, F. Hereditary distal tubular acidosis. In *GeneReviews, 2019*; Adam, M., Ardinger, H., Pagon, R., Wallace, S., Bean, L., Stephens, K., Amemiya, A., Eds.; University of Washington: Seattle, WA, USA, 2019. Available online: https://www.ncbi.nlm.nih.gov/pubmed/31600044/ (accessed on 24 November 2019).
11. Wen, M.; Shen, T.; Wang, Y.; Li, Y.; Shi, X.; Dang, X. Next-Generation Sequencing in Early Diagnosis of Dent Disease 1: Two Case Reports. *Front. Med.* **2018**, *5*, 347. [CrossRef]
12. Lieske, J.C.; Milliner, D.S.; Beara-Lasic, L.; Harris, P.; Cogal, A.; Abrash, E. Dent Disease. In *GeneReviews, 2017*; Adam, M., Ardinger, H., Pagon, R., Wallace, S., Bean, L., Stephens, K., Amemiya, A., Eds.; University of Washington: Seattle, WA, USA, 2019. Available online: https://www.ncbi.nlm.nih.gov/books/NBK99494/ (accessed on 20 November 2019).
13. Hodgin, J.B.; Corey, H.E.; Kaplan, B.S.; D'Agati, V.D. Dent disease presenting as partial Fanconi syndrome and hypercalciuria. *Kidney Int.* **2008**, *73*, 1320–1323. [CrossRef]
14. Bökenkamp, A.; Ludwig, M. The oculocerebrorenal syndrome of Lowe: An update. *Pediatr. Nephrol.* **2016**, *31*, 2201–2212. [CrossRef]
15. Elmonem, M.A.; Veys, K.R.; Soliman, N.A.; van Dyck, M.; van den Heuvel, L.P.; Levtchenko, E. Cystinosis: A review. *Orphanet J. Rare Dis.* **2016**, *11*, 47. [PubMed]
16. Anglani, F.; D'Angelo, A.; Bertizzolo, L.M.; Tosetto, E.; Ceol, M.; Cremasco, D.; Bonfante, L.; Addis, M.A.; Del Prete, D. Nephrolithiasis, kidney failure and bone disorders in Dent disease patients with and without CLCN5 mutations. *Springerplus* **2015**, *4*, 492. [CrossRef] [PubMed]
17. Anglani, F.; Gianesello, L.; Beara-Lasic, L.; Lieske, J. Dent disease: A window into calcium and phosphate transport. *J. Cell. Mol. Med.* **2019**, *23*, 7132–7142. [CrossRef] [PubMed]
18. Blanchard, A.; Curis, E.; Guyon-Roger, T.; Kahila, D.; Treard, C.; Baudouin, V.; Bérard, E.; Champion, G.; Cochat, P.; Dubourg, J.; et al. Observations of a large Dent disease cohort. *Kidney Int.* **2016**, *90*, 430–439. [CrossRef]
19. Hill, F.; Sayer, J.A. Clinical and biochemical features of patients with CYP24A1 mutations. In *A Critical Evaluation of Vitamin D*, 1st ed.; Gowder, S., Ed.; IntechOpen: London, UK, 2017; pp. 91–101. [CrossRef]
20. British Paediatric Association. Hypercalcemia in infants and vitamin D. *Br. Med. J.* **1956**, *2*, 149. [CrossRef]
21. Schlingmann, K.P.; Kaufmann, M.; Weber, S.; Irwin, A.; Goos, C.; John, U.; Misselwitz, J.; Klaus, G.; Kuwertz-Bröking, E.; Fehrenbach, H.; et al. Mutations in CYP24A1 and Idiopathic Infantile Hypercalcemia. *N. Engl. J. Med.* **2011**, *365*, 410–421. [CrossRef]
22. Dganit, D.; Pazit, B.; Liat, G.; Karen, T.; Zemach, E.; Holtzman, E.J. Loss-of-Function Mutations of CYP24A1, the Vitamin D 24-Hydroxylase Gene, Cause Long-standing Hypercalciuric Nephrolithiasis and Nephrocalcinosis. *J. Urol.* **2013**, *190*, 552–557.

23. Sayers, J.; Hynes, A.M.; Srivastava, S.; Dowen, F.; Quinton, R.; Datta, H.K.; Sayer, J.A. Successful treatment of hypercalcaemia associated with a CYP24A1 mutation with fluconazole. *Clin. Kidney J.* **2018**, *8*, 453–455. [CrossRef]
24. Hawkes, C.P.; Li, D.; Hakonarson, H.; Meyers, K.E.; Thummel, K.E.; Levine, M.A. CYP3A4 Induction by Rifampin: An Alternative Pathway for Vitamin D Inactivation in Patients With CYP24A1 Mutations. *J. Clin. Endocrinol. Metab.* **2017**, *102*, 1440–1446. [CrossRef]
25. Schlingmann, K.P.; Ruminska, J.; Kaufmann, M.; Dursun, I.; Patti, M.; Kranz, B.; Pronicka, E.; Ciara, E.; Akcay, T.; Bulus, D.; et al. Autosomal-Recessive Mutations in SLC34A1 Encoding Sodium-Phosphate Cotransporter 2A Cause Idiopathic Infantile Hypercalcemia. *J. Am. Soc. Nephrol.* **2016**, *27*, 604–614. [CrossRef] [PubMed]
26. De Paolis, E.; Scaglione, G.; De Bonis, M.; Minucci, A.; Capoluongo, E. CYP24A1 and SLC34A1 genetic defects associated with idiopathic infantile hypercalcemia: From genotype to phenotype. *Clin. Chem. Lab. Med.* **2019**, *57*, 1650. [CrossRef]
27. Kang, S.J.; Lee, R.; Kim, H.S. Infantile hypercalcemia with novel compound heterozygous mutation in SLC34A1 encoding renal sodium-phosphate cotransporter 2a: A case report. *Ann. Pediatr. Endocrinol. Metab.* **2019**, *24*, 64–67. [CrossRef]
28. Claverie-Martin, F. Familial hypomagnesaemia with hypercalciuria and nephrocalcinosis: Clinical and molecular characteristics. *Clin. Kidney J.* **2015**, *8*, 656–664. [CrossRef] [PubMed]
29. Viering, D.H.H.M.; de Baaij, J.H.F.; Walsh, S.B.; Kleta, R.; Bockenhauer, D. Genetic causes of hypomagnesemia, a clinical overview. *Pediatr. Nephrol.* **2017**, *32*, 1123–1135. [CrossRef] [PubMed]
30. Sikora, P.; Zaniew, M.; Haisch, L.; Pulcer, B.; Szczepańska, M.; Moczulska, A.; Rogowska-Kalisz, A.; Bieniaś, B.; Tkaczyk, M.; Ostalska-Nowicka, D.; et al. Retrospective cohort study of familial hypomagnesaemia with hypercalciuria and nephrocalcinosis due to CLDN16 mutations. *Nephrol. Dial. Transplant.* **2014**, *30*, 636–644. [CrossRef]
31. Vianna, J.G.P.; Simor, T.G.; Senna, P.; De Bortoli, M.R.; Costalonga, E.F.; Seguro, A.C.; Luchi, W.M. Atypical presentation of familial hypomagnesemia with hypercalciuria and nephrocalcinosis in a patient with a new claudin-16 gene mutation. *Clin. Nephrol. Case Stud.* **2019**, *7*, 27–34. [CrossRef]
32. Brochard, K.; Boyer, O.; Blanchard, A.; Loirat, C.; Niaudet, P.; Macher, M.A.; Deschenes, G.; Bensman, A.; Decramer, S.; Cochat, P.; et al. Phenotype-genotype correlation in antenatal and neonatal variants of Bartter syndrome. *Nephrol. Dial. Transplant.* **2008**, *24*, 1455–1464. [CrossRef]
33. Gollasch, B.; Anistan, Y.M.; Canaan-Kühl, S.; Gollasch, M. Late-onset Bartter syndrome type II. *Clin. Kidney J.* **2017**, *10*, 594–599. [CrossRef]
34. Walsh, P.R.; Tse, Y.; Ashton, E.; Iancu, D.; Jenkins, L.; Bienias, M.; Kleta, R.; van't Hoff, W.; Bockenhauer, D. Clinical and diagnostic features of Bartter and Gitelman syndromes. *Clin. Kidney J.* **2017**, *11*, 302–309. [CrossRef]
35. Huang, L.; Luiken, G.P.M.; van Riemsdijk, I.C.; Petrij, F.; Zandbergen, A.A.M.; Dees, A. Nephrocalcinosis as adult presentation of Bartter syndrome type II. *Neth. J. Med.* **2014**, *72*, 91–93. [PubMed]
36. Jeck, N.; Reinalter, S.C.; Henne, T.; Marg, W.; Mallmann, R.; Pasel, K.; Vollmer, M.; Klaus, G.; Leonhardt, A.; Seyberth, H.W.; et al. Hypokalemic Salt-Losing Tubulopathy With Chronic Renal Failure and Sensorineural Deafness. *Pediatrics* **2001**, *108*, e5. [CrossRef] [PubMed]
37. Online Mendelian Inheritance in Man, OMIM. OMIM Entry-#300971. Available online: https://www.omin.org/entry/300971#editHistory (accessed on 29 December 2019).
38. Pidasheva, S.; D'Souza-Li, L.; Canaff, L.; Cole, D.E.C.; Hendy, G.N. CASRdb: Calcium-sensing receptor locus-specific database for mutations causing familial (benign) hypocalciuric hypercalcemia, neonatal severe hyperparathyroidism, and autosomal dominant hypocalcemia. *Hum. Mutat.* **2004**, *24*, 107–111. [CrossRef] [PubMed]
39. Vargas-Poussou, R.; Huang, C.; Hulin, P.; Houillier, P.; Jeunemaître, X.; Paillard, M.; Planelles, G.; Déchaux, M.; Miller, R.T.; Antignac, C. Functional Characterization of a Calcium-Sensing Receptor Mutation in Severe Autosomal Dominant Hypocalcemia with a Bartter-Like Syndrome. *J. Am. Soc. Nephrol.* **2002**, *13*, 2259–2266. [CrossRef] [PubMed]
40. Pearce, S.H.S.; Williamson, C.; Kifor, O.; Bai, M.; Coulthard, M.G.; Davies, M.; Lewis-Barned, N.; McCredie, D.; Powell, H.; Kendall-Taylor, P.; et al. A Familial Syndrome of Hypocalcemia with Hypercalciuria Due to Mutations in the Calcium-Sensing Receptor. *N. Engl. J. Med.* **1996**, *335*, 1115–1122. [CrossRef]

41. Vezzoli, G.; Arcidiacono, T.; Paloschi, V.; Terranegra, A.; Biasion, R.; Weber, G.; Mora, S.; Syren, M.L.; Coviello, D.; Cusi, D.; et al. Autosomal dominant hypocalcemia with mild type 5 Bartter syndrome. *J. Nephrol.* **2006**, *19*, 525–528.
42. Hannan, F.M.; Thakker, R.V. Calcium-sensing receptor (CaSR) mutations and disorders of calcium, electrolyte and water metabolism. *Best Pract. Res. Clin. Endocrinol. Metab.* **2013**, *27*, 359–371. [CrossRef]
43. Online Mendelian Inheritance in Man, OMIM. OMIM Entry-#143870. Available online: https://www.omim.org/entry/143870#8 (accessed on 29 December 2019).
44. Reed, B.Y.; Heller, H.J.; Gitomer, W.L.; Pak, C.Y.C. Mapping a Gene Defect in Absorptive Hypercalciuria to Chromosome 1q23.3–q241. *J. Clin. Endocrinol. Metab.* **1999**, *84*, 3907–3913. [CrossRef]
45. Watanabe, T. Improving outcomes for patients with distal renal tubular acidosis: Recent advances and challenges ahead. *Pediatr Heal Med Ther.* **2018**, *9*, 181–190. [CrossRef]
46. Enerbäck, S.; Nilsson, D.; Edwards, N.; Heglind, M.; Alkanderi, S.; Ashton, E.; Deeb, A.; Kokash, F.E.; Bakhsh, A.R.; van't Hoff, W.; et al. Acidosis and Deafness in Patients with Recessive Mutations in FOXI1. *J. Am. Soc. Nephrol.* **2018**, *29*, 1041–1048. [CrossRef]
47. Rungroj, N.; Nettuwakul, C.; Sawasdee, N.; Sangnual, S.; Deejai, N.; Misgar, R.A.; Pasena, A.; Khositseth, S.; Kirdpon, S.; Sritippayawan, S.; et al. Distal renal tubular acidosis caused by tryptophan-aspartate repeat domain 72 (WDR72) mutations. *Clin. Genet.* **2018**, *94*, 409–418. [CrossRef] [PubMed]
48. Park, E.; Cho, M.H.; Hyun, H.S.; Shin, J.I.; Lee, J.H.; Park, Y.S.; Choi, H.J.; Kang, H.G.; Cheong, H.I. Genotype-Phenotype Analysis in Pediatric Patients with Distal Renal Tubular Acidosis. *Kidney Blood Press. Res.* **2018**, *43*, 513–521. [CrossRef] [PubMed]
49. Strauss, S.B.; Waltuch, T.; Bivin, W.; Kaskel, F.; Levin, T.L. Primary hyperoxaluria: Spectrum of clinical and imaging findings. *Pediatr. Radiol.* **2017**, *47*, 96–103. [CrossRef] [PubMed]
50. Milliner, D.; Hoppe, B.; Groothoff, J. A randomised Phase II/III study to evaluate the efficacy and safety of orally administered Oxalobacter formigenes to treat primary hyperoxaluria. *Urolithiasis* **2018**, *46*, 313–323. [CrossRef]
51. Cochat, P.; Basmaison, O. Current approaches to the management of primary hyperoxaluria. *Arch. Dis. Child.* **2000**, *82*, 470–473. [CrossRef]
52. Sas, D.J.; Harris, P.C.; Milliner, D.S. Recent advances in the identification and management of inherited hyperoxalurias. *Urolithiasis* **2019**, *47*, 79–89. [CrossRef]
53. Grujic, D.; Salido, E.C.; Shenoy, B.C.; Langman, C.B.; McGrath, M.E.; Patel, R.J.; Rashid, A.; Mandapati, S.; Jung, C.W.; Margolin, A.L. Hyperoxaluria Is Reduced and Nephrocalcinosis Prevented with an Oxalate-Degrading Enzyme in Mice with Hyperoxaluria. *Am. J. Nephrol.* **2009**, *29*, 86–93. [CrossRef]
54. Matthew, L.; Victoria, B.; Meekah, C.; Ming, Y.; Qing-Shan, L.; Haifeng, L. MP03-06 Oxalate decarboxylase enzyme reduces hyperoxaluria in an animal model that mimics primary hyperoxaluria. *J. Urol.* **2019**, *201*, e22.
55. National Kidney Foundation. Medullary Sponge Kidney. Available online: https://www.kidney.org/atoz/content/medullary-sponge-kidney (accessed on 29 December 2019).
56. Fabris, A.; Anglani, F.; Lupo, A.; Gambaro, G. Medullary sponge kidney: State of the art. *Nephrol. Dial. Transplant.* **2012**, *28*, 1111–1119. [CrossRef]
57. Torregrossa, R.; Anglani, F.; Fabris, A.; Gozzini, A.; Tanini, A.; Del Prete, D.; Cristofaro, R.; Artifoni, L.; Abaterusso, C.; Marchionna, N.; et al. Identification of GDNF gene sequence variations in patients with medullary sponge kidney disease. *Clin. J. Am. Soc. Nephrol.* **2010**, *5*, 1205–1210. [CrossRef]
58. Azizi, E.; Eshel, G.; Aladjem, M. Hypercalciuria and nephrolithiasis as a presenting sign in Wilson disease. *Eur. J. Pediatr.* **1989**, *148*, 548–549. [CrossRef] [PubMed]
59. Di Stefano, V.; Lionetti, E.; Rotolo, N.; La Rosa, M.; Leonardi, S. Hypercalciuria and nephrocalcinosis as early feature of Wilson disease onset: Description of a pediatric case and literature review. *Hepat. Mon.* **2012**, *12*, e6233. [CrossRef] [PubMed]
60. Sindhar, S.; Lugo, M.; Levin, M.D.; Danback, J.R.; Brink, B.D.; Yu, E.; Dietzen, D.J.; Clark, A.L.; Purgert, C.A.; Waxler, J.L.; et al. Hypercalcemia in Patients with Williams-Beuren Syndrome. *J. Pediatr.* **2016**, *178*, 254–260. [CrossRef]

61. Katz, S.M.; Krueger, L.J.; Falkner, B. Microscopic Nephrocalcinosis in Cystic Fibrosis. *N. Engl. J. Med.* **1988**, *319*, 263–266. [CrossRef]
62. Elizabeth, J.; Lakshmi Priya, E.; Umadevi, K.M.R.; Ranganathan, K. Amelogenesis imperfecta with renal disease—A report of two cases. *J. Oral Pathol. Med.* **2007**, *36*, 625–628. [CrossRef] [PubMed]

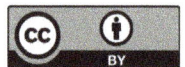

© 2020 by the authors. Licensee MDPI, Basel, Switzerland. This article is an open access article distributed under the terms and conditions of the Creative Commons Attribution (CC BY) license (http://creativecommons.org/licenses/by/4.0/).

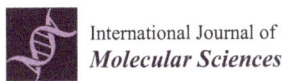

Review

A New Vision of IgA Nephropathy: The Missing Link

Fabio Sallustio [1,2,*], Claudia Curci [2,3,*], Vincenzo Di Leo [3], Anna Gallone [2], Francesco Pesce [3] and Loreto Gesualdo [3]

1. Interdisciplinary Department of Medicine (DIM), University of Bari "Aldo Moro", 70124 Bari, Italy
2. Department of Basic Medical Sciences, Neuroscience and Sense Organs, University of Bari "Aldo Moro", 70124 Bari, Italy; anna.gallone@uniba.it
3. Nephrology, Dialysis and Transplantation Unit, DETO, University "Aldo Moro", 70124 Bari, Italy; vincenzodileo88@yahoo.it (V.D.L.); f.pesce81@gmail.com (F.P.); loreto.gesualdo@uniba.it (L.G.)
* Correspondence: fabio.sallustio@uniba.it (F.S.); claudiacurci@gmail.com (C.C.)

Received: 7 December 2019; Accepted: 24 December 2019; Published: 26 December 2019

Abstract: IgA Nephropathy (IgAN) is a primary glomerulonephritis problem worldwide that develops mainly in the 2nd and 3rd decade of life and reaches end-stage kidney disease after 20 years from the biopsy-proven diagnosis, implying a great socio-economic burden. IgAN may occur in a sporadic or familial form. Studies on familial IgAN have shown that 66% of asymptomatic relatives carry immunological defects such as high IgA serum levels, abnormal spontaneous in vitro production of IgA from peripheral blood mononuclear cells (PBMCs), high serum levels of aberrantly glycosylated IgA1, and an altered PBMC cytokine production profile. Recent findings led us to focus our attention on a new perspective to study the pathogenesis of this disease, and new studies showed the involvement of factors driven by environment, lifestyle or diet that could affect the disease. In this review, we describe the results of studies carried out in IgAN patients derived from genomic and epigenomic studies. Moreover, we discuss the role of the microbiome in the disease. Finally, we suggest a new vision to consider IgA Nephropathy as a disease that is not disconnected from the environment in which we live but influenced, in addition to the genetic background, also by other environmental and behavioral factors that could be useful for developing precision nephrology and personalized therapy.

Keywords: IgA Nephropathy; microbiome; virome; environment

1. Introduction

IgA-Nephropathy (IgA-N) is the most common form of primary glomerulonephritis worldwide. It is characterized by the manifestation of mesangial IgA deposits in the glomeruli leading to frequent episodes of intra-infectious macroscopic hematuria or continuous microscopic hematuria and/or proteinuria. The aberrant synthesis of deglycosylated IgA1, selective mesangial IgA1 deposition with ensuing mesangial cell proliferation and extracellular matrix expansion lead to renal fibrosis, with molecular mechanisms still poorly understood. Approximately 40% of patients older than 20 years develop end-stage renal disease within 20 years after the renal biopsy-proven diagnosis [1,2]. The prevalence of IgA-N ranges widely worldwide, from 16.7% in the USA to 48.7% in Australia of all patients with biopsy-proven primary glomerulonephritis as reported in regional biopsy registries. The frequency of the disease increases from the Western (USA 16.7%) to the Eastern regions of the world (Japan 47.4%) [2,3]. IgAN is the most common glomerulonephritis in Asia, where it accounts for 40% of glomerulonephritis; it is also very common among the native Americans in Manitoba, the Zuni and the Australian aborigines; it is rare in African native populations and in the Indian [2–7]. The family aggregation has been widely described in the world, in sibling pairs, in families and in extensive pedigrees belonging to geographically-isolated populations [8–10]. The difference in percentages in all countries may be only partially attributed to late referral to nephrologists, routine screening of urine in some countries, and disparities in the indication to perform a kidney biopsy in individuals with permanent urinary abnormalities.

Several studies describe immunological abnormalities involving B and T lymphocytes throughout the clinical course of the disease [11]. Naive B cells express surface IgM/IgD and have to go through a process of clonal expansion, isotype switching, affinity maturation, and differentiation before IgA plasma cells develop. During the process of class switching, recombination occurs by looping out and deletions of segments of DNA. In IgA-N patients, B cells not only seem to be increased in number in both bone marrow and tonsils [12–14], but also show reduced susceptibility to Fas-mediated apoptosis with a marked expression of BCL-2 [12]. In addition, B cells produce polymeric IgA1 abnormally glycosylated in response to a variety of antigens that initiate the formation of IgA immune complexes [15,16].

The regulation of IgA production by B cells is regulated in both a T cell-dependent and a T cell-independent manner, through molecular signals involving the TNF-Receptor superfamily, which is expressed on the surface of dendritic cells. In both cases, dendritic cells are thought to play a critical role in this process. A functional defect of these cells has been observed in the nasal mucosa of IgA-N patients, thus inducing dysregulation of the immune response [16].

Mucosal immunity is largely involved in the pathogenesis of the disease, as the exposure of the upper respiratory tract to bacteria or virus is often associated with recurrent episodes of macroscopic hematuria. There is increasing support for the hypothesis of altered cell homing in IgAN patients, in which there is a displacement of mucosal derived plasma cells and a secretion of mucosal-type antibodies in the systemic compartment [17,18]. In particular, $CD4^+$ T cells represent a key component of the mucosal immune defense against pathogens, altered homing from mucosal to systemic sites, and excessive activation of this leukocyte subset has been demonstrated by Batra et al. [19].

Numerous observations point towards an important role for alterations in IgA biology in the pathogenesis of the disease. Deposited IgA is predominantly polymeric IgA (pIgA) of the IgA1 subclass [20] and has been shown to be differently glycosylated [21], since there is a reduced galactosylation of the O-linked glycans in the hinge region of serum IgA1 and in IgA1 located in the mesangial deposits. Levels of plasma IgA1 are elevated in about half of the IgA-N patients [21]. This is the result of a higher production of deglycosylated IgA1 by plasma cells in the bone marrow and by tonsillar lymphocytes [22,23]. IgA1 glycosylation takes place in the Golgi apparatus of the B cells. These IgA1 proteins with altered glycans represent an autologous antigen recognized by ubiquitous, naturally occurring antibodies, mostly of the IgG isotype with anti-glycan or anti-glycopeptide specificities [24]. Thus, the presence of glycan-specific anti-IgA1 antibodies promotes the formation of circulating immune-complexes which are relatively large [25]. Because of their size, they are not efficiently cleared from the circulation, and thus tend to deposit in the renal mesangium. Deposited immune-complexes and/or polymeric IgA1 aggregated for their de-glycosylation stimulate mesangial cell proliferation and production of cytokines (IL-6 or TGFβ) [26]. Continuous deposition of circulating IgA1-IgG immune complexes induces activation of mesangial cells and of the innate immune system with the attraction of macrophages that produce inflammatory mediators leading to renal damage. Interstitial infiltration by T cells at the renal level causes tubular injury and sets in motion irreversible interstitial fibrosis leading to end-stage renal failure. Hence, a dynamic constellation of B and T lymphocytes and their soluble mediators participate at all levels in disease pathogenesis: Initiation, perpetuation, amplification, regulation, disease relapse, and tissue and organ destruction.

2. Genetics Involvement in IgAN

IgA-N may occur in a sporadic or a familial form according to the clinical evidence that one or more subjects belonging to the same family are affected by biopsy-proven IgA-N. The routine urinalysis carried out in first-degree relatives frequently evidences the occurrence of urinary abnormalities. Such abnormalities have been detected in 25% of first-degree relatives of IgA-N patients as compared to 4% of unrelated subjects [27]. Moreover, first-degree relatives have a higher risk of developing the disease, with an odds ratio (OR) of 16.4 (95% CI 5.7–47.8), than second-degree relatives (OR = 2.4; 95% CI 0.7–7.9) [10]. Three loci linked for familial IgA-N have been found by our group [8,9] (7,8), and some genetic variants which may predispose individuals to sporadic IgA-N have been identified [28]. The IGAN 1 locus is located on chromosome 6q22-23, with a LOD score of 5.6 [9]. IGAN 2 and 3 loci are located on chromosome 4q26-31 and 17q12-22, respectively [8]. These chromosomal traits may contain causative and/or susceptibility genes for familial IgAN which may be involved in the development of, or susceptibility to, overt IgA-N.

Advancements in the field of knowledge on the genetics of IgAN have recently been achieved by the application of genome-wide association studies (GWAS) on large cohorts of IgAN cases and controls. GWAS is an approach aimed at providing comprehensive coverage of the entire genome in order to find variants associated with susceptibility to developing the disease. The major limitation of GWAS is that they only identify common variants of susceptibility, and these obviously have only a modest effect. However, a well-conducted GWAS can offer additional bias-free knowledge on the biology of a human disease that could be clinically relevant, allowing for the identification of new unknown pathways and of potential targets of innovative drug therapies. What is needed for an informative GWAS is the collection of very large numbers of sporadic patients affected by IgAN and healthy controls, comparable in age, sex and geographical origin. The recent GWAS have allowed the discovery of common susceptibility variants to IgAN development. To date, several GWAS related to IgAN have been published and, overall, have led to the identification of 15 disability susceptibilities due to illness.

Regarding classical genetics, several hypotheses have been made on the type of inheritance in the course of family IgAN. The autosomal recessive transmission would seem to be the most unlikely. Many families have affected members in different generations of the pedigree; moreover, a high incidence of the disease in children of consanguineous parents has not been found. An X-linked transmission was considered, given that IgAN is more frequent in males; however, this hypothesis can be excluded as the male-male transmission has also been observed. An autosomal dominant transmission with complete penetrance has been excluded because, in the pedigrees there are numerous examples of subjects that should be obligated carriers but that are healthy. Autosomal dominant transmission with incomplete penetrance would seem to be the most plausible hypothesis as it would be a suitable model to explain most pedigrees. This model would explain the presence of cases in many arms of the pedigree and the recurrence of the disease in subsequent generations. Incomplete penetrance may justify the presence of another genetic factor or environmental exposure. The other model that would explain this type of family aggregation is the hypothesis of a multifactorial etiology in which the combined effect of more genes and/or environmental factors is necessary for the development of the disease in each individual [29].

The three major GWAS on IgAN, performed between 2010 and 2012, had shown a strong contribution of the MHC locus in determining the risk of developing the disease; in addition to this locus, the studies had identified 4 additional non-HLA susceptibility loci (chromosome 1q32, containing the CFH cluster; chromosomal 8p23, comprising the DEFA gene cluster, coding α-defensin; chromosome 17p13, including TNFSF13; chromosome 22, including HORMAD2) [8,9,30]. Cumulatively, these 9 loci are responsible for around 5% of the risk of developing IgAN. In addition, the variation in the frequency of risk alleles is able to explain a substantial proportion of the variation observed in the various ethnic groups with regard to the prevalence of the disease, with the risk alleles showing a higher frequency in Asians compared to Europeans.

The 3 loci in the MHC region (with the strongest signal at the HLA DQB1/DQA1/DRB1 locus) suggested pathways involved in antigen processing and presentation [31]; a locus on chromosome 1q32 containing the Complement Factor H (CFH) gene cluster, suggested a metabolic pathway involved in regulating the activation of the complement pathway. However, the locus on chromosome 22 (HORMAD2) is active in the regulation of mucosal immunity, through the regulation of IgA levels. Moreover, the two regions on chromosome 17p13 and 8q23, containing respectively the TNFSF13 genes (Tumor Necrosis Factor ligand superfamily member 13, encoding a protein which plays an important role in the development of B cells) and DEFA (coding a protein, defensin, which has natural antimicrobial properties, having a role in innate immunity) were also involved in the regulation of mucosal immunity [31,32]. TNFSF13 codifies for APRIL, a potent B-cell stimulating cytokine that is stimulated by intestinal bacteria and leads to CD40-independent IgA class switching [33]. APRIL concentrations are high in patients with IgAN [34] and may upregulate intestinal IgA production [32] (Table 1).

Table 1. Evidence of Potential Relationship with Environmental and Alimentary Hit in IgAN.

References	Loci	Chormosomes	Year	Notes on Potential Relationship with Environmental and Alimentary Hit
Sallustio [35]	TRIM27 DUSP3 VTRNA2-1	6p22 17q21.31 5q31.1	2016	TRIM27 and DUSP3 and the hyper-methylation of VTRNA2-1 lead to the overexpression of TGFβ and to a reduced TCR signal strength of the CD4$^+$ T-cells, with a consequent T helper cell imbalance
AI [36]	DEFA	8p23	2016	The DEFA locus may probably regulate intestinal microbial pathogens and inflammation.
Sallustio [37]	GALNT13 COL11A2 TLR9	2q24 6p21 3p21	2015	The TLR9 loss in IgAN may result in impaired elimination of mucosal antigens, prolonged antigen exposure to B cells and an increase in immunologic memory leading to deal with a continuous antigenic challenge that triggers the production of nephritogenic IgA1
Kiryluk [38]	VAV3 HLA-DR HLA-DQ DEFA CARD9 ITGAM-ITGAX	1p13 6p21 8p23 9q34 16p11	2014	MHC class II molecules are critical for antigen presentation and adaptive immunity. MHC class II molecules participate in the regulation of intestinal inflammation and IgA production. VAV3 may modulate the intestinal inflammation, IgA secretion, the glomerular inflammation, the phagocytosis, and the clearance of immune complexes. CARD9 may intervene in the regulation of bacterial infection after intestinal epithelial injury. Integrins codified by ITGAM and ITGAX are expressed in intestinal dendritic cells and bring to T-cell independent IgA class-switch.
Kiryluk [39]	HLA-DR– HLA-DQ	6p21	2012	There are four independent classical HLA alleles associated with IgAN at this locus; two risk alleles (DQA1*0101, DQB1*0301) and two protective alleles (DQA1*0102, DQB1*0201). Some class II alleles have a permissive role in autoimmunity, and thus may be associated with a greater risk of antiglycan response
Yu [32]	DEFA TNFSF13	8p23 17p13	2012	TNFSF13 codify for APRIL, a potent B-cell stimulating cytokine which is stimulated by intestinal bacteria and lead to CD40-independent IgA class switching
Gharavi [31]	HLA-DR– HLA-DQ HLA-DPA1-DPB1-DPB2 TAP1-PSMB9 CFHR3-CFHR1 del HORMAD2	6p21 6p21 6p21 1p32 22q12	2011	HLA-DP are MHC class II molecules, less well studied compared with HLA-DQ and HLA-DR. Some class II alleles have a permissive role in autoimmunity, and thus may be associated with a greater risk of antiglycan response. Elevated expression of TAP2, PSMB8, and PSMB9, may lead to a proinflammatory intestinal state. HORMAD2 regulates mucosal immunity, through the control of IgA levels.
Feehally [40]	HLA-DR– HLA-DQ	6p21	2010	

These data, however, suggested the possible existence of additional loci of susceptibility to developing the disease. For this reason, new GWAS larger than the previous ones were performed [38]. In addition to replicating the 9 loci described in the previous GWAS, including the loci on chromosome 6p21 (HLA-DQ–HLA-DR, TAP1-PSMB8 and HLA-DP), on chromosome 1q32 (CFHR3-CFHR1), on chromosome 8p23 (DEFA), on chromosome 17p13 (TNFSF13) and on chromosome 22q12 (HORMAD2), new signals were identified, 4 of which in three new loci [38]: Integrin alpha M- Integrin alpha X (ITGAM-ITGAX) on the 16p11 chromosome, implicated in the adhesion and migration of leukocytes and in phagocytosis complement-mediated by monocytes and macrophages and associated with the development of erythematous systemic lupus; CARD9, on chromosome 9q34, implicated in the activation of nuclear factor NF-κB in macrophages, which gives an increased risk of ulcerative colitis and Crohn's disease; and VAV3, on chromosome 1p13, implicated in the development of B and T lymphocytes and in the antigen presentation process. PSMB8 and PSMB9 constitute interferon-inducible immunoproteasome mediating intestinal NF-κB activation in inflammatory bowel diseases (IBD) [41,42]. The TAP gene encodes a protein involved in the transport of antigens from the cytoplasm to the endoplasmic reticulum for association with MHC class I molecules. Elevated expression of TAP2, PSMB8, and PSMB9 may lead to a proinflammatory intestinal state [42]. Moreover, two new independent signals (HLA-DQB1 and DEFA, respectively) were identified in previously known regions (Table 1).

Some case-control association studies identified the C1GALT1 as an important gene for the pathogenesis of IgAN and highlighted some C1GALT1 genetic variants associated with the IgAN pathogenesis in the Italian and Chinese populations [43,44]. C1GALT1 codifies for the enzyme core 1,b1,3-galactosyltransferase 1 that adds a galactose to the IgA1 heavy-chain hinge region. In IgAN, IgA1are aberrantly glycosylated, since the hinge-region O-linked glycans of the IgA1 heavy-chain lack galactose. This contributes to the kidney mesangial deposition of IgA1.

In particular, these studies associated the disease to a C1GALT1 SNP (rs1047763) in the gene promoter region. This variant was also correlated with a decreased C1GALT1 expression in homozygous people [43]. Interestingly, the SNP is contained within the gene region binding the microRNA miR-148b that was found regulating the *C1GALT1* expression and the IgA1 O-glycosylation [45–47]. We do not know whether this SNP effectively influences the disease pathogenesis, but probably it can affect the miR-148b binding to C1GALT1.

Overall, the identified loci seem to be implicated in critical mechanisms for the development of IgAN: The maintenance of the intestinal mucosal barrier, the synthesis of IgA at the mucosal level, the modulation of the signal by NF-kB, the defense against intracellular pathogens and complement activation. The innovative finding is that most of these loci are directly associated with the risk of developing inflammatory bowel disease (HLA-DQ, HLA-DR, CARD9, and HORMAD2), or maintenance of intestinal epithelial barrier integrity and response to various pathogenic pathogens (DEFA, TNFSF13, VAV3, ITGAM-ITGAX, and PSMB8) (Table 1). In fact, abnormal glycosylation mainly consists of polymeric IgA1, which is generated by mucosal IgA1-secreting cells. Also, 107 Immunocompetent B cells can migrate to the gut mucosal lamina propria, where they mature into IgA-secreting plasma cells. These plasma cells can release dimeric IgA1, which can form dimeric IgA or polymeric IgA proteins. The risen levels of polymeric IgA1 in the circulation may be the result of 'spillover' from mucosal sites to the vascular space. Instead, the preponderance of the IgA that achieves the circulation from the bone marrow is predominantly in a monomeric form [48,49].

VAV proteins are guanine nucleotide exchange proteins crucial for adaptive immune function and NF-κB triggering in B cells, stimulating IgA production [50]. They are necessary for appropriate differentiation of colonic enterocytes and avoiding natural ulcerations of intestinal mucosa [50]. Moreover, VAV3 may modulate the intestinal inflammation, IgA secretion, the glomerular inflammation, the phagocytosis, and the clearance of immune complexes. DEFA genes codify for α-defensins that are antimicrobial peptides keeping innate immunity against microbial pathogens. α-defensin 1 and 3 are synthesized in neutrophils, whereas α-defensin 5 and 6 (DEFA5 and DEFA6) are synthesized by the intestinal Paneth cells. Whether DEFA IgAN risk alleles constitute a risk haplotype per se or are associated with close variants of DEFA5 or DEFA6 genes is not clear. Anyway, the DEFA locus may probably regulate intestinal microbial pathogens and inflammation. CARD9 codifies for a protein necessary for the assemblage of a BCL10 signaling complex. It triggers NF-κB, which is involved in both innate and adaptive immunity [51]. CARD9 intervenes in intestinal repair, T-helper 17 responses, and regulation of bacterial infection after intestinal epithelial injury in mice [52].

ITGAM and ITGAX codify for integrins αM and αX that, together with the integrin β2 chain, constitute leukocyte-specific complement receptors 3 and 4 (CR3 and CR4, respectively). High quantity of these integrins, expressed in intestinal dendritic cells bringing to T-cell independent IgA class-switch [53,54]. In addition, ITGAM and ITGAX are also present in macrophages and contribute to the phagocytosis process (Table 1).

Indications on the involvement of genes correlated with environmental factors or eating habits have also come from studies on copy number variations (CNV) in IgAN patients. Ai Z. et al. identified CNV of DEFA locus, including DEFA1A3, DEFA3 [36], and Sallustio et al. identified GALNT13, COL11A2, and TLR9 loci that are associated with susceptibility to and progression of IgAN [37] (Table 1). In particular, a TLR9 loss has been found associated with IgAN progression and renal dysfunction. TLR9 is expressed in immune system cells such as B cells, dendritic cells, macrophages, natural killer cells, and other antigen-presenting cells [55]. TLR9 preferentially binds unmethylated CpG dinucleotides (CpG DNA) released by bacteria and viruses and triggers signaling cascades that lead to a pro-inflammatory cytokine response [56,57]. In IgAN, the TLR9 CNV loss may lead to the failure of CpG to induce the proliferation of memory B cells because of the lower expression levels of TLR9, thus exacerbating IgA class switching in naive B cells via BCR. This may result in impaired elimination of mucosal antigens, prolonged antigen exposure to B cells, and an increase in immunologic memory leading to deal with a continuous antigenic challenge that triggers the production of nephritogenic IgA1 [58–61].

Taken together, these data seem to suggest that IgAN is an inflammatory disease with an autoimmune genesis that involves or perhaps even originates in the intestine. GWAS study of the Gharavi group also showed that the frequency of the 15 identified genetic risk factors reflects the different distribution of IgAN frequency in the various areas of the world. It was confirmed that the loci of susceptibility to develop IgAN were, in fact, more frequent in Asian populations, which have the highest incidence of disease, and less frequent in African populations, which have the lowest incidence [38]. This data strongly suggested that the distinctive geographic pattern of IgAN risk alleles could have been modeled by an adaptation to the local environment.

The environmental influence on IgAN is supported also from DNA methylation studies showing that aberrant DNA methylation in IgAN patients influences the expression of some genes involved in the T-cell receptor signaling, the pathway that transfers the signal of the presence of antigens and that activates the T-cells [35]. In particular, the hypo-methylation of TRIM27 and DUSP3 and the hyper-methylation of VTRNA2-1 lead to the overexpression of TGFβ and to a reduced TCR signal strength of the $CD4^+$ T-cells, with a consequent T helper cell imbalance. DNA methylation studies are important because the structural modifications of the DNA can be established through environmental programming. Moreover, the DNA methylation can be dynamic and potentially reversible [62]. For these reasons, further studies about the DNA methylation in IgAN will be needed to better understand environmental influences on this disease.

The last GWAS study of the Gharavi group suggested that the distinctive geographical pattern of IgAN risk alleles could have been modeled by adaptation to the local environment [38]. It was also able to better define potential environmental factors able to explain such an adaptation process. The authors carried out an association analysis of the genetic risk score to develop IgAN with some ecological variables present in the populations enrolled in the study, reflecting the local climate, pathogenic load, and dietary factors. A strong positive association emerged between the score of genetic risk for IgAN and the diversity of local pathogens such as viruses, bacteria, protozoa, helminths. The strongest correlation was the diversity of parasitic worms (helminths), which often infest the intestine. The increased incidence of IgAN in some geographical areas, therefore, could be the accidental consequence of a protective adaptation from intestinal worm mucosal invasion. Helminth infection has been an important source of morbidity and mortality in human history, and still occurs in 25% of the world's population, with the highest global burden of soil-transmitted helminth infections (geo-helminthiasis) in Asia, where it contributes significantly to pediatric mortality. Schistosomiasis, a common helminthic infection that is a long-known cause of secondary IgAN, further supports this hypothesis.

On the other hand, it is known that host-pathogen interactions have exerted a critical influence on the genetic architecture of IBD. According to these data, IgAN susceptibility loci appear to be either directly associated with the risk of IBD or encode proteins involved in maintaining the intestinal mucosal barrier or in regulating the mucosal immune response. Thanks to these latest studies it is possible to link inflammatory diseases of the intestinal mucosa, including IBD, with the risk of IgAN, and to explain why these two diseases occur simultaneously more often than expected. These data are also consistent with the clinical observations that mucosal infections often trigger episodes of acute nephritis during IgAN, with the key role of IgA in defense at the mucosal surface level.

3. Microbiota and IgA Nephropathy: The "Chicken or Egg" Question

The ensemble of bacteria, bacteriophages, fungi, protozoa, and viruses that live in the digestive tract of humans, called microbiota, is in contact with the gut epithelium and plays a role in the development of the mucosal-associated lymphoid tissue (MALT) and, reciprocally, the composition of the commensal microbiota depends on MALT function [63,64]. In humans, the MALT is the primary source of IgA [65], and numerous studies indicate that IgA Nephropathy (IgAN) is closely associated with alterations in the gut microbiota [34,66,67]. To date, it is unclear whether dysbiosis precedes the disease or if the IgAN can lead to gut dysbiosis.

A transgenic mouse model of IgA nephropathy that overexpresses the B cell activation factor of the TNF family (BAFF) fails to develop glomerular IgA deposits when raised in germ-free conditions until gut microbiota are introduced [34].

In a cross-sectional study, Gesualdo et al. [66] identified reduced fecal microbial diversity in patients with progressive IgAN compared to those with non-progressive IgAN and healthy subjects. IgAN patients have been found to have microbial dysbiosis with an increased Firmicutes/Bacteroidetes ratio. Specifically, in the fecal samples of IgAN patients, a high level of Firmicutes has been found. They are characterized by high percentages of some genera/species of Ruminococcaceae, Lachnospiraceae, Eubacteriaceae, and Streptococcaeae. Instead, healthy controls presented a higher level of Clostridium, Enterococcus and Lactobacillus genera.

4. Microbiome Modulation in IgAN: "State of the Art"

In the context of detection of microbiota dysbiosis in IgAN patients, restoring some microbial gaps could lead to new supportive therapeutic strategies, such as the use of antibiotics or dietary implementation with prebiotics and/or probiotics, or through fecal microbiota transplantation (FMT).

In this scenario, the first therapeutic approach was conducted by Monteiro et al. [67]. The authors have demonstrated that antibiotic treatment (ampicillin, vancomycin, neomycin, and metronidazole) of a double transgenic mice model of IgAN reverses the phenotype of the disease; but this antibiotic cocktail may have other collateral effects on the gut and weight. Moreover, it is not feasible to give to patients a broad-spectrum antibiotic mix, and it could generate resistant strains of bacteria.

The use of probiotics, prebiotics or symbiotics may prove to be a viable and low-risk therapeutic strategy in the future. Probiotics have anti-inflammatory, anti-oxidative, and other favorable gut-modulating properties [68]. Especially species from the Lactobacilli and Bifidobacteria genera were shown to support the humoral immune responses against environmental toxins and antigens [69]. The use of probiotics or symbiotics in patients with chronic kidney disease has been shown to have some beneficial effects on the uremic toxins, blood urea nitrogen, oxidative stress, and markers of inflammation also by enhancing barrier function [70–73]. In that regard, the study of Soylu et al. [74] showed that the administration of Saccharomyces boulardii, which is able to decrease intestinal inflammation through modulation of the T-cell [75], reduced systemic IgA response and protected induced IgAN mice from the disease.

Another future weapon against the IgAN could be the FMT. This approach consists of stool transfer from a selected healthy donor to the gastrointestinal tract of a recipient patient suffering from microbial dysbiosis [76]. Currently, FMT is recommended as the most effective therapy for the recurrent Clostridium difficile infection [77]. Although there is no strong evidence that supports the use of the FMT in IgAN, promising studies are focusing on revealing whether this therapeutic option may play a role in the management of this disease. Indeed, an interesting interventional ongoing study (clinical trial NCT03633864) aims to determine the safety and efficacy of FMT in IgAN patients not responding to the standard treatment or not responding to immunosuppressive treatments.

5. The Interplay between the Microbiome and Virome: A New Vision of Human Metagenome

The human gut microbiome is a complex ecosystem that begins with colonization at birth and continues to alter and adapt throughout the life of an individual [78]. The bacterial and archaeal communities of the microbiome provide their host with an array of functions, including immune system development, synthesis of vitamins, and energy generation [79]. The bacterial components are characterized by high temporal stability in a healthy subject but can be transiently affected by events such as travel, sickness, and antibiotic usage [80].

Recently, the scientific community focused attention also on the human virome. The human virome consists of both the viral component of the microbiome, dominated by bacteriophages [80], and a variety of DNA viruses that directly infect eukaryotic cells [81]. Viruses access the human body through mucosal surfaces, where they interact with the host immune defense, commensal bacteria included. Bacteria of microbiota interact with viruses to eliminate or reduce their infectivity, ensuring the homeostasis of the mucosal sites, but viruses had mechanisms to take advantage of the microbiota, and thereby evade the immune system [82]. The concept of the virome as a stable part of the human metagenome has been raised from studies on chronic viral infections. During a chronic viral infection, a dynamic relationship between the host and viral agents occurs, creating a continuous state of immune surveillance. This immune system dynamism is neutral for the host, but it has a critically important role in shaping the "normal" human immune system [83]. The virome is one of the most variable components of the human gut microbiome, changing from childhood to adult life [84] in response to different environments, lifestyles or infections. A number of cross-sectional population studies reported disease-specific alterations of the gut virome in a number of gastrointestinal and systemic disorders, such as inflammatory bowel disease [85,86], AIDS [87], diabetes [88], and malnutrition [89]. However, to date, interpretation of these data is inconsistent, due to the very high variability in the virome composition and the lack of exact taxonomic classification and biological properties of several viral groups [80].

Recent studies have shed light on how resident enteric viruses may affect host physiology beyond causing disease [90]. Despite the partial picture of the taxonomic composition of the mammalian virome, recent investigations showed that the preponderance of viruses residing in the intestine are bacteriophages, which infect bacteria and can be released from them in response to stress signals [91]. As a consequence of the lysis of bacteria by phages, bacterial cell wall components and bacterial and phage DNA can trigger pattern recognition receptors in intestinal or immune cells, influencing intestinal homeostasis and immunity [92,93]. This hypothesis has been investigated in several studies with discordant results. In fact, some in vitro studies showed that phages were internalized by phagocytosis or endocytosis in lysosomes of lymphocytes and degraded without inflammation [94]. A different study performed on mice showed activation of myeloid differentiation primary response 88 (MyD88)-dependent pathway, with consequent involvement of TLRs [95]. Despite controversial results, it is clear that enteric phages have a key role in the modulation of the bacterial microbiome on the intestinal mucosal surface [90].

It is known that IgAN and other glomerulonephritides are clinically associated with viral infections, such as hepatitis B virus [96], respiratory syncytial virus [97] or HIV [98]. Most viral pathogens for mammals produce double-stranded RNA (dsRNA) incidental to viral replication. dsRNAs are recognized by TLR3, which is expressed on the cellular membrane surface of many immune cells [99]. TLR3 binds primarily to dsRNA and induce antiviral and inflammatory responses, mediated by the TNFs system and NFkB [100,101].

Yamashita et al. investigated the cellular podocyte response to dsRNA [102]. Cell cultures of human or murine podocytes were cultured and stimulated with Polyinosinic-polycytidylic acid (Poly(I:C)), a synthetic double-stranded (ds) RNA. RT-PCR, immunoblotting, phenotype characterization and functional assays were then performed to study alterations in podocyte marker expression or cellular functions. They found that human and murine podocytes expressed TLR3 and other proteins of its correlated activation pathway. Stimulation with synthetic dsRNA led to the activation of the TLR3 signaling, and exposed podocytes showed alteration in migration processes and defective expression of proteins podocyte-specific such as nephrin, podocin or CD2AP, and increased transepithelial albumin flux [102]. Although these results need to be validated by in vivo experiments, they support the hypothesis that dsRNA exposure can contribute to glomerular injury associated with immune complex deposition and could be associated with the progression of IgAN.

The group of He L. et al. [103] offered more direct evidence of the involvement of dsRNA in IgAN. In this paper, human leukocytes, isolated from tonsil tissue and whole blood, were cultured with or without poly(I:C) for 1–7 days. They also analyzed lymphomonocyte, urine, kidney and spleen samples from rats administered with or without poly(I:C) in the presence or absence of IgAN. In both in vivo and in vitro experiments, the TLR3-dependent BAFF expression was upregulated after a viral infection, especially in IgAN patients or animals. The TLR3 crosstalk with BAFF plays a vital role in the over-production of IgA and in the Recombinant Class Switch to IgA in IgAN. Thus, the inhibition of TLR3/BAFF axis activation could be an interesting option for preventing IgAN progression [103].

These studies demonstrated that exposure to viral products can directly influence the IgAN progression. However, to date, there are no data available about a direct role of the virome in the modulation of IgAN pathogenesis and/or progression. Specific studies aimed to study the influence of virome in healthy and pathological processes are in very early stages, and efforts must be made to improve our knowledge in this challenging field.

6. Conclusions

The GWAS and the other whole-genome genomic studies, thanks to technological developments in the field of genetics, have allowed researchers to identify multiple susceptibility loci for the IgAN and, consequently, they have shed new light on the pathogenesis of this disease, revealing the close connections with multiple environmental, alimentary and behavioral factors. Nevertheless, these studies have made possible the correlation of the genetic risk to develop IgAN with the geo-epidemiological aspects of the disease. These findings focalize attention on a new perspective to study the IgAN pathogenesis and show the involvement of factors driven by environment, lifestyle, or diet affecting the disease (Table 1). These factors may represent the missing link in IgAN pathogenesis. Many steps forward have been taken in the characterization of IgAN, and new studies through an integrated genomic approach will be needed to deepen the etiopathogenetic mechanisms and to suggest new potential therapeutic targets. Nevertheless, recent data suggest a new vision to consider the IgA Nephropathy as a disease which is not disconnected from the environment in which we live but influenced by, in addition to the genetic background, other environmental and behavioral factors that could be useful for developing precision nephrology and personalized therapy.

Author Contributions: Conceptualization, F.S. and L.G.; investigation, C.C., F.S., F.P.; resources, V.D.L., F.P.; data curation, C.C., V.D.L.; writing—original draft preparation, C.C., F.S., F.P., V.D.L.; writing—review and editing, F.S., A.G., F.P., L.G.; supervision, F.S., F.P., L.G.; funding acquisition, L.G. All authors have read and agreed to the published version of the manuscript.

Funding: This research received no external funding.

Conflicts of Interest: The authors declare no conflict of interest.

Abbreviations

IgAN	IgA Nephropathy
PBMC	Peripheral blood mononuclear cells
OR	Odds ratio
GWAS	Genome-wide association studies
IBD	Inflammatory bowel diseases

References

1. D'Amico, G. The commonest glomerulonephritis in the world: IgA nephropathy. *Q. J. Med.* **1987**, *64*, 709–727. [PubMed]
2. Suzuki, H.; Kiryluk, K.; Novak, J.; Moldoveanu, Z.; Herr, A.B.; Renfrow, M.B.; Wyatt, R.J.; Scolari, F.; Mestecky, J.; Gharavi, A.G.; et al. The Pathophysiology of IgA Nephropathy. *J. Am. Soc. Nephrol.* **2011**, *22*, 1795–1803. [CrossRef] [PubMed]
3. Paolo Schena, F. A retrospective analysis of the natural history of primary IgA nephropathy worldwide. *Am. J. Med.* **1990**, *89*, 209–215. [CrossRef]
4. Julian, B.A.; Waldo, F.B.; Rifai, A.; Mestecky, J. IgA nephropathy, the most common glomerulonephritis worldwide. *Am. J. Med.* **1988**, *84*, 129–132. [CrossRef]
5. Smith, S.M.; Harford, A.M. IgA Nephropathy in Renal Allografts: Increased Frequency in Native American Patients. *Ren. Fail.* **1995**, *17*, 449–456. [CrossRef]
6. Hughson, M.D.; Megill, D.M.; Smith, S.M.; Tung, K.S.; Miller, G.; Hoy, W.E. Mesangiopathic glomerulonephritis in Zuni (New Mexico) Indians. *Arch. Pathol. Lab. Med.* **1989**, *113*, 148–157.
7. O'connell, P.J.; Ibels, L.S.; Thomas, M.A.; Harris, M.; Eckstein, R.P. Familial IgA nephropathy: A Study of renal disease in an australian aboriginal family. *Aust. N. Z. J. Med.* **1987**, *17*, 27–33. [CrossRef]
8. Bisceglia, L.; Cerullo, G.; Forabosco, P.; Torres, D.D.; Scolari, F.; Di Perna, M.; Foramitti, M.; Amoroso, A.; Bertok, S.; Floege, J.; et al. Genetic heterogeneity in Italian families with IgA nephropathy: Suggestive linkage for two novel IgA nephropathy loci. *Am. J. Hum. Genet.* **2006**, *79*, 1130–1134. [CrossRef]
9. Gharavi, A.G.; Yan, Y.; Scolari, F.; Schena, F.P.; Frasca, G.M.; Ghiggeri, G.M.; Cooper, K.; Amoroso, A.; Viola, B.F.; Battini, G.; et al. IgA nephropathy, the most common cause of glomerulonephritis, is linked to 6q22–23. *Nat. Genet.* **2000**, *26*, 354–357. [CrossRef]
10. Schena, F.P.; Cerullo, G.; Rossini, M.; Lanzilotta, S.G.; D'Altri, C.; Manno, C. Increased risk of end-stage renal disease in familial IgA nephropathy. *J. Am. Soc. Nephrol.* **2002**, *13*, 453–460.
11. Emancipator, P. Discussant: S.N. Immunoregulatory factors in the pathogenesis of IgA nephropathy. *Kidney Int.* **1990**, *38*, 1216–1229. [CrossRef] [PubMed]
12. Kodama, S.; Suzuki, M.; Arita, M.; Mogi, G. Increase in tonsillar germinal centre B-1 cell numbers in IgA nephropathy (IgAN) patients and reduced susceptibility to Fas-mediated apoptosis. *Clin. Exp. Immunol.* **2001**, *123*, 301–308. [CrossRef] [PubMed]
13. Harper, S.J.; Allen, A.C.; Pringle, J.H.; Feehally, J. Increased dimeric IgA producing B cells in the bone marrow in IgA nephropathy determined by in situ hybridisation for J chain mRNA. *J. Clin. Pathol.* **1996**, *49*, 38–42. [CrossRef] [PubMed]
14. Harper, S.J.; Allen, A.C.; Béné, M.C.; Pringle, J.H.; Faure, G.; Lauder, I.; Feehally, J. Increased dimeric IgA-producing B cells in tonsils in IgA nephropathy determined by in situ hybridization for J chain mRNA. *Clin. Exp. Immunol.* **2008**, *101*, 442–448. [CrossRef]
15. Suzuki, H.; Moldoveanu, Z.; Hall, S.; Brown, R.; Vu, H.L.; Novak, L.; Julian, B.A.; Tomana, M.; Wyatt, R.J.; Edberg, J.C.; et al. IgA1-secreting cell lines from patients with IgA nephropathy produce aberrantly glycosylated IgA1. *J. Clin. Investig.* **2008**, *118*, 629–639. [CrossRef]
16. Eijgenraam, J.W.; Woltman, A.M.; Kamerling, S.W.A.; Briere, F.; De Fijter, J.W.; Daha, M.R.; Van Kooten, C. Dendritic cells of IgA nephropathy patients have an impaired capacity to induce IgA production in naïve B cells. *Kidney Int.* **2005**, *68*, 1604–1612. [CrossRef]
17. Kennel-de March, A.; Bene, M.C.; Renoult, E.; Kessler, M.; Faure, G.C.; Kolopp-Sarda, M.N. Enhanced expression of L-selectin on peripheral blood lymphocytes from patients with IgA nephropathy. *Clin. Exp. Immunol.* **1999**, *115*, 542–546. [CrossRef]

18. Barratt, J.; Bailey, E.M.; Buck, K.S.; Mailley, J.; Moayyedi, P.; Feehally, J.; Turney, J.H.; Crabtree, J.E.; Allen, A.C. Exaggerated systemic antibody response to mucosal Helicobacter pylori infection in IgA nephropathy. *Am. J. Kidney Dis.* **1999**, *33*, 1049–1057. [CrossRef]
19. Batra, A.; Smith, A.C.; Feehally, J.; Barratt, J. T-cell homing receptor expression in IgA nephropathy. *Nephrol. Dial. Transplant.* **2007**, *22*, 2540–2548. [CrossRef]
20. Allen, A.C.; Bailey, E.M.; Barratt, J.; Buck, K.S.; Feehally, J. Analysis of IgA1 O-glycans in IgA nephropathy by fluorophore-assisted carbohydrate electrophoresis. *J. Am. Soc. Nephrol.* **1999**, *10*, 1763–1771.
21. Allen, A.C.; Bailey, E.M.; Brenchley, P.E.C.; Buck, K.S.; Barratt, J.; Feehally, J. Mesangial IgA1 in IgA nephropathy exhibits aberrant O-glycosylation: Observations in three patients. *Kidney Int.* **2001**, *60*, 969–973. [CrossRef] [PubMed]
22. Horie, A.; Hiki, Y.; Odani, H.; Yasuda, Y.; Takahashi, M.; Kato, M.; Iwase, H.; Kobayashi, Y.; Nakashima, I.; Maeda, K. IgA1 molecules produced by tonsillar lymphocytes are under-O-glycosylated in IgA nephropathy. *Am. J. Kidney Dis.* **2003**, *42*, 486–496. [CrossRef]
23. Van den Wall Bake, A.W.; Daha, M.R.; Valentijn, R.M.; van Es, L.A. The bone marrow as a possible origin of the IgA1 deposited in the mesangium in IgA nephropathy. *Semin. Nephrol.* **1987**, *7*, 329–331. [PubMed]
24. Kokubo, T.; Hashizume, K.; Iwase, H.; Arai, K.; Tanaka, A.; Toma, K.; Hotta, K.; Kobayashi, Y. Humoral immunity against the proline-rich peptide epitope of the IgA1 hinge region in IgA nephropathy. *Nephrol. Dial. Transplant.* **2000**, *15*, 28–33. [CrossRef]
25. Tomana, M.; Novak, J.; Julian, B.A.; Matousovic, K.; Konecny, K.; Mestecky, J. Circulating immune complexes in IgA nephropathy consist of IgA1 with galactose-deficient hinge region and antiglycan antibodies. *J. Clin. Investig.* **1999**, *104*, 73–81. [CrossRef]
26. Gómez-Guerrero, C.; López-Armada, M.J.; González, E.; Egido, J. Soluble IgA and IgG aggregates are catabolized by cultured rat mesangial cells and induce production of TNF-alpha and IL-6, and proliferation. *J. Immunol.* **1994**, *153*, 5247–5255.
27. Schena, F.P. Immunogenetic aspects of primary IgA nephropathy. *Kidney Int.* **1995**, *48*, 1998–2013. [CrossRef]
28. Schena, F.P.; D'Altri, C.; Cerullo, G.; Manno, C.; Gesualdo, L. ACE gene polymorphism and IgA nephropathy: An ethnically homogeneous study and a meta-analysis. *Kidney Int.* **2001**, *60*, 732–740. [CrossRef]
29. Hsu, S.I.-H.; Ramirez, S.B.; Winn, M.P.; Bonventre, J.V.; Owen, W.F. Evidence for genetic factors in the development and progression of IgA nephropathy. *Kidney Int.* **2000**, *57*, 1818–1835. [CrossRef]
30. Paterson, A.D.; Liu, X.Q.; Wang, K.; Magistroni, R.; Song, X.; Kappel, J.; Klassen, J.; Cattran, D.; St George-Hyslop, P.; Pei, Y. Genome-wide linkage scan of a large family with IgA nephropathy localizes a novel susceptibility locus to chromosome 2q36. *J. Am. Soc. Nephrol.* **2007**, *18*, 2408–2415. [CrossRef]
31. Gharavi, A.G.; Kiryluk, K.; Choi, M.; Li, Y.; Hou, P.; Xie, J.; Sanna-Cherchi, S.; Men, C.J.; Julian, B.A.; Wyatt, R.J.; et al. Genome-wide association study identifies susceptibility loci for IgA nephropathy. *Nat. Genet.* **2011**, *43*, 321–327. [CrossRef] [PubMed]
32. Yu, X.Q.; Li, M.; Zhang, H.; Low, H.Q.; Wei, X.; Wang, J.Q.; Sun, L.D.; Sim, K.S.; Li, Y.; Foo, J.N.; et al. A genome-wide association study in Han Chinese identifies multiple susceptibility loci for IgA nephropathy. *Nat. Genet.* **2011**, *44*, 178–182. [CrossRef] [PubMed]
33. Litinskiy, M.B.; Nardelli, B.; Hilbert, D.M.; He, B.; Schaffer, A.; Casali, P.; Cerutti, A. DCs induce CD40-independent immunoglobulin class switching through BLyS and APRIL. *Nat. Immunol.* **2002**, *3*, 822–829. [CrossRef] [PubMed]
34. McCarthy, D.D.; Kujawa, J.; Wilson, C.; Papandile, A.; Poreci, U.; Porfilio, E.A.; Ward, L.; Lawson, M.A.E.; Macpherson, A.J.; McCoy, K.D.; et al. Mice overexpressing BAFF develop a commensal flora–dependent, IgA-associated nephropathy. *J. Clin. Investig.* **2011**, *121*, 3991–4002. [CrossRef]
35. Sallustio, F.; Serino, G.; Cox, S.N.; Gassa, A.D.; Curci, C.; De Palma, G.; Banelli, B.; Zaza, G.; Romani, M.; Schena, F.P. Aberrantly methylated DNA regions lead to low activation of CD4$^+$ T-cells in IgA nephropathy. *Clin. Sci.* **2016**, *130*, 733–746. [CrossRef]
36. Ai, Z.; Li, M.; Liu, W.; Foo, J.N.; Mansouri, O.; Yin, P.; Zhou, Q.; Tang, X.; Dong, X.; Feng, S.; et al. Low alpha-defensin gene copy number increases the risk for IgA nephropathy and renal dysfunction. *Sci. Transl. Med.* **2016**, *8*, 345ra88. [CrossRef]
37. Sallustio, F.; Cox, S.N.; Serino, G.; Curci, C.; Pesce, F.; De Palma, G.; Papagianni, A.; Kirmizis, D.; Falchi, M.; Schena, F.P. Genome-wide scan identifies a copy number variable region at 3p21.1 that influences the TLR9 expression levels in IgA nephropathy patients. *Eur. J. Hum. Genet.* **2015**, *23*, 940–948. [CrossRef]

38. Kiryluk, K.; Li, Y.; Scolari, F.; Sanna-Cherchi, S.; Choi, M.; Verbitsky, M.; Fasel, D.; Lata, S.; Prakash, S.; Shapiro, S.; et al. Discovery of new risk loci for IgA nephropathy implicates genes involved in immunity against intestinal pathogens. *Nat. Genet.* **2014**, *46*, 1187–1196. [CrossRef]
39. Kiryluk, K.; Li, Y.; Sanna-Cherchi, S.; Rohanizadegan, M.; Suzuki, H.; Eitner, F.; Snyder, H.J.; Choi, M.; Hou, P.; Scolari, F.; et al. Geographic differences in genetic susceptibility to IgA nephropathy: GWAS replication study and geospatial risk analysis. *PLoS Genet.* **2012**, *8*, e1002765. [CrossRef]
40. Feehally, J.; Farrall, M.; Boland, A.; Gale, D.P.; Gut, I.; Heath, S.; Kumar, A.; Peden, J.F.; Maxwell, P.H.; Morris, D.L.; et al. HLA has strongest association with IgA nephropathy in genome-wide analysis. *J. Am. Soc. Nephrol.* **2010**, *21*, 1791–1797. [CrossRef]
41. Wu, F.; Dassopoulos, T.; Cope, L.; Maitra, A.; Brant, S.R.; Harris, M.L.; Bayless, T.M.; Parmigiani, G.; Chakravarti, S. Genome-wide gene expression differences in Crohn's disease and ulcerative colitis from endoscopic pinch biopsies: Insights into distinctive pathogenesis. *Inflamm. Bowel. Dis.* **2007**, *13*, 807–821. [CrossRef] [PubMed]
42. Visekruna, A.; Joeris, T.; Seidel, D.; Kroesen, A.; Loddenkemper, C.; Zeitz, M.; Kaufmann, S.H.E.; Schmidt-Ullrich, R.; Steinhoff, U. Proteasome-mediated degradation of IκBα and processing of p105 in Crohn disease and ulcerative colitis. *J. Clin. Investig.* **2006**, *116*, 3195–3203. [CrossRef] [PubMed]
43. Li, G.S.; Zhang, H.; Lv, J.C.; Shen, Y.; Wang, H.Y. Variants of C1GALT1 gene are associated with the genetic susceptibility to IgA nephropathy. *Kidney Int.* **2007**, *71*, 448–453. [CrossRef] [PubMed]
44. Pirulli, D.; Crovella, S.; Ulivi, S.; Zadro, C.; Bertok, S.; Rendine, S.; Scolari, F.; Foramitti, M.; Ravani, P.; Roccatello, D.; et al. Genetic variant of C1GalT1 contributes to the susceptibility to IgA nephropathy. *J. Nephrol.* **2009**, *22*, 152–159.
45. Serino, G.; Sallustio, F.; Cox, S.N.; Pesce, F.; Schena, F.P. Abnormal miR-148b expression promotes aberrant glycosylation of IgA1 in IgA nephropathy. *J. Am. Soc. Nephrol.* **2012**, *23*, 814–824. [CrossRef]
46. Serino, G.; Pesce, F.; Sallustio, F.; De Palma, G.; Cox, S.N.; Curci, C.; Zaza, G.; Lai, K.N.; Leung, J.C.K.; Tang, S.C.W.; et al. In a retrospective international study, circulating miR-148b and let-7b were found to be serum markers for detecting primary IgA nephropathy. *Kidney Int.* **2016**, *89*, 683–692. [CrossRef]
47. Serino, G.; Sallustio, F.; Curci, C.; Cox, S.N.; Pesce, F.; De Palma, G.; Schena, F.P. Role of let-7b in the regulation of N-acetylgalactosaminyltransferase 2 in IgA nephropathy. *Nephrol. Dial. Transplant.* **2015**, *30*, 1132–1139. [CrossRef]
48. Floege, J.; Feehally, J. The mucosa-kidney axis in IgA nephropathy. *Nat. Rev. Nephrol.* **2016**, *12*, 147–156. [CrossRef]
49. Magistroni, R.; D'Agati, V.D.; Appel, G.B.; Kiryluk, K. New developments in the genetics, pathogenesis, and therapy of IgA nephropathy. *Kidney Int.* **2015**, *88*, 974–989. [CrossRef]
50. Vigorito, E.; Gambardella, L.; Colucci, F.; McAdam, S.; Turner, M. Vav proteins regulate peripheral B-cell survival. *Blood* **2005**, *106*, 2391–2398. [CrossRef]
51. Bertin, J.; Guo, Y.; Wang, L.; Srinivasula, S.M.; Jacobson, M.D.; Poyet, J.-L.; Merriam, S.; Du, M.-Q.; Dyer, M.J.S.; Robison, K.E.; et al. CARD9 Is a Novel Caspase Recruitment Domain-containing Protein That Interacts with BCL10/CLAP and Activates NF-κB. *J. Biol. Chem.* **2000**, *275*, 41082–41086. [CrossRef] [PubMed]
52. Sokol, H.; Conway, K.L.; Zhang, M.; Choi, M.; Morin, B.; Cao, Z.; Villablanca, E.J.; Li, C.; Wijmenga, C.; Yun, S.H.; et al. Card9 Mediates Intestinal Epithelial Cell Restitution, T-Helper 17 Responses, and Control of Bacterial Infection in Mice. *Gastroenterology* **2013**, *145*, 591–601.e3. [CrossRef] [PubMed]
53. Uematsu, S.; Fujimoto, K.; Jang, M.H.; Yang, B.-G.; Jung, Y.J.; Nishiyama, M.; Sato, S.; Tsujimura, T.; Yamamoto, M.; Yokota, Y.; et al. Regulation of humoral and cellular gut immunity by lamina propria dendritic cells expressing Toll-like receptor 5. *Nat. Immunol.* **2008**, *9*, 769–776. [CrossRef] [PubMed]
54. Fujimoto, K.; Karuppuchamy, T.; Takemura, N.; Shimohigoshi, M.; Machida, T.; Haseda, Y.; Aoshi, T.; Ishii, K.J.; Akira, S.; Uematsu, S. A New Subset of CD103$^+$ CD8α$^+$ Dendritic Cells in the Small Intestine Expresses TLR3, TLR7, and TLR9 and Induces Th1 Response and CTL Activity. *J. Immunol.* **2011**, *186*, 6287–6295. [CrossRef] [PubMed]
55. Du, X.; Poltorak, A.; Wei, Y.; Beutler, B. Three novel mammalian toll-like receptors: Gene structure, expression, and evolution. *Eur. Cytokine Netw.* **2000**, *11*, 362–371. [PubMed]
56. Notley, C.A.; Jordan, C.K.; McGovern, J.L.; Brown, M.A.; Ehrenstein, M.R. DNA methylation governs the dynamic regulation of inflammation by apoptotic cells during efferocytosis. *Sci. Rep.* **2017**, *7*, 42204. [CrossRef]

57. Martínez-Campos, C.; Burguete-García, A.I.; Madrid-Marina, V. Role of TLR9 in Oncogenic Virus-Produced Cancer. *Viral Immunol.* **2017**, *30*, 98–105. [CrossRef]
58. Bernasconi, N.L.; Onai, N.; Lanzavecchia, A. A role for Toll-like receptors in acquired immunity: Up-regulation of TLR9 by BCR triggering in naive B cells and constitutive expression in memory B cells. *Blood* **2003**, *101*, 4500–4504. [CrossRef]
59. Gesualdo, L.; Lamm, M.E.; Emancipator, S.N. Defective oral tolerance promotes nephritogenesis in experimental IgA nephropathy induced by oral immunization. *J. Immunol.* **1990**, *145*, 3684–3691.
60. Bernasconi, N.L. Maintenance of Serological Memory by Polyclonal Activation of Human Memory B Cells. *Science* **2002**, *298*, 2199–2202. [CrossRef]
61. Blaas, S.H.; Stieber-Gunckel, M.; Falk, W.; Obermeier, F.; Rogler, G. CpG-oligodeoxynucleotides stimulate immunoglobulin A secretion in intestinal mucosal B cells. *Clin. Exp. Immunol.* **2009**, *155*, 534–540. [CrossRef] [PubMed]
62. Nagy, C.; Turecki, G. Sensitive periods in epigenetics: Bringing us closer to complex behavioral phenotypes. *Epigenomics* **2012**, *4*, 445–457. [CrossRef] [PubMed]
63. Nakajima, A.; Vogelzang, A.; Maruya, M.; Miyajima, M.; Murata, M.; Son, A.; Kuwahara, T.; Tsuruyama, T.; Yamada, S.; Matsuura, M.; et al. IgA regulates the composition and metabolic function of gut microbiota by promoting symbiosis between bacteria. *J. Exp. Med.* **2018**, *215*, 2019–2034. [CrossRef] [PubMed]
64. Bunker, J.J.; Erickson, S.A.; Flynn, T.M.; Henry, C.; Koval, J.C.; Meisel, M.; Jabri, B.; Antonopoulos, D.A.; Wilson, P.C.; Bendelac, A. Natural polyreactive IgA antibodies coat the intestinal microbiota. *Science* **2017**, *358*. [CrossRef]
65. Coppo, R. The Gut-Renal Connection in IgA Nephropathy. *Semin. Nephrol.* **2018**, *38*, 504–512. [CrossRef]
66. De Angelis, M.; Montemurno, E.; Piccolo, M.; Vannini, L.; Lauriero, G.; Maranzano, V.; Gozzi, G.; Serrazanetti, D.; Dalfino, G.; Gobbetti, M.; et al. Microbiota and metabolome associated with Immunoglobulin a Nephropathy (IgAN). *PLoS ONE* **2014**. [CrossRef]
67. Chemouny, J.M.; Gleeson, P.J.; Abbad, L.; Lauriero, G.; Boedec, E.; Le Roux, K.; Monot, C.; Bredel, M.; Bex-Coudrat, J.; Sannier, A.; et al. Modulation of the microbiota by oral antibiotics treats immunoglobulin A nephropathy in humanized mice. *Nephrol. Dial. Transpl.* **2018**, *34*, 1135–1144. [CrossRef]
68. Cavalcanti Neto, M.P.; Aquino, J.S.; da Romao Silva, L.F.; de Oliveira Silva, R.; Guimaraes, K.S.L.; de Oliveira, Y.; de Souza, E.L.; Magnani, M.; Vidal, H.; de Brito Alves, J.L. Gut microbiota and probiotics intervention: A potential therapeutic target for management of cardiometabolic disorders and chronic kidney disease? *Pharmacol. Res.* **2018**, *130*, 152–163. [CrossRef]
69. Vitetta, L.; Vitetta, G.; Hall, S. Immunological Tolerance and Function: Associations between Intestinal Bacteria, Probiotics, Prebiotics, and Phages. *Front. Immunol.* **2018**, *9*, 2240. [CrossRef]
70. Rao, R.K.; Samak, G. Protection and Restitution of Gut Barrier by Probiotics: Nutritional and Clinical Implications. *Curr. Nutr. Food Sci.* **2013**, *9*, 99–107.
71. Ranganathan, N.; Friedman, E.A.; Tam, P.; Rao, V.; Ranganathan, P.; Dheer, R. Probiotic dietary supplementation in patients with stage 3 and 4 chronic kidney disease: A 6-month pilot scale trial in Canada. *Curr. Med. Res. Opin.* **2009**, *25*, 1919–1930. [CrossRef] [PubMed]
72. Ranganathan, N.; Ranganathan, P.; Friedman, E.A.; Joseph, A.; Delano, B.; Goldfarb, D.S.; Tam, P.; Rao, A.V.; Anteyi, E.; Musso, C.G. Pilot study of probiotic dietary supplementation for promoting healthy kidney function in patients with chronic kidney disease. *Adv. Ther.* **2010**, *27*, 634–647. [CrossRef] [PubMed]
73. Guida, B.; Germano, R.; Trio, R.; Russo, D.; Memoli, B.; Grumetto, L.; Barbato, F.; Cataldi, M. Effect of short-term synbiotic treatment on plasma p-cresol levels in patients with chronic renal failure: A randomized clinical trial. *Nutr. Metab. Cardiovasc. Dis.* **2014**, *24*, 1043–1049. [CrossRef] [PubMed]
74. Soylu, A.; Berktas, S.; Sarioglu, S.; Erbil, G.; Yilmaz, O.; Demir, B.K.; Tufan, Y.; Yesilirmak, D.; Turkmen, M.; Kavukcu, S. Saccharomyces boulardii prevents oral-poliovirus vaccine-induced IgA nephropathy in mice. *Pediatr. Nephrol.* **2008**, *23*, 1287–1291. [CrossRef] [PubMed]
75. Dalmasso, G.; Cottrez, F.; Imbert, V.; Lagadec, P.; Peyron, J.F.; Rampal, P.; Czerucka, D.; Groux, H.; Foussat, A.; Brun, V. Saccharomyces boulardii inhibits inflammatory bowel disease by trapping T cells in mesenteric lymph nodes. *Gastroenterology* **2006**, *131*, 1812–1825. [CrossRef] [PubMed]
76. Zipursky, J.S.; Sidorsky, T.I.; Freedman, C.A.; Sidorsky, M.N.; Kirkland, K.B. Patient attitudes toward the use of fecal microbiota transplantation in the treatment of recurrent Clostridium difficile infection. *Clin. Infect. Dis.* **2012**, *55*, 1652–1658. [CrossRef]

77. Wortelboer, K.; Nieuwdorp, M.; Herrema, H. Fecal microbiota transplantation beyond Clostridioides difficile infections. *EBioMedicine* **2019**, *44*, 716–729. [CrossRef]
78. Rodríguez, J.M.; Murphy, K.; Stanton, C.; Ross, R.P.; Kober, O.I.; Juge, N.; Avershina, E.; Rudi, K.; Narbad, A.; Jenmalm, M.C.; et al. The composition of the gut microbiota throughout life, with an emphasis on early life. *Microb. Ecol. Health Dis.* **2015**, *26*, 1–17. [CrossRef]
79. Qin, J.; Li, R.; Raes, J.; Arumugam, M.; Burgdorf, S.; Manichanh, C.; Nielsen, T.; Pons, N.; Yamada, T.; Mende, D.R.; et al. Europe PMC Funders Group Europe PMC Funders Author Manuscripts A human gut microbial gene catalog established by metagenomic sequencing. *Nature* **2010**, *464*, 59–65. [CrossRef]
80. Shkoporov, A.N.; Clooney, A.G.; Sutton, T.D.S.; Ryan, F.J.; Daly, K.M.; Nolan, J.A.; McDonnell, S.A.; Khokhlova, E.V.; Draper, L.A.; Forde, A.; et al. The Human Gut Virome Is Highly Diverse, Stable, and Individual Specific. *Cell Host Microbe* **2019**, *26*, 527–541.e5. [CrossRef]
81. Wylie, K.M.; Mihindukulasuriya, K.A.; Zhou, Y.; Sodergren, E.; Storch, G.A.; Weinstock, G.M. Metagenomic analysis of double-stranded DNA viruses in healthy adults. *BMC Med.* **2014**, *12*, 71. [CrossRef] [PubMed]
82. Domínguez-Díaz, C.; García-Orozco, A.; Riera-Leal, A.; Padilla-Arellano, J.R.; Fafutis-Morris, M. Microbiota and Its Role on Viral Evasion: Is It with Us or Against Us? *Front. Cell. Infect. Microbiol.* **2019**, *9*, 1–7. [CrossRef] [PubMed]
83. Virgin, H.W.; Wherry, E.J.; Ahmed, R. Redefining Chronic Viral Infection. *Cell* **2009**, *138*, 30–50. [CrossRef] [PubMed]
84. Moreno-Gallego, J.L.; Chou, S.P.; Di Rienzi, S.C.; Goodrich, J.K.; Spector, T.D.; Bell, J.T.; Youngblut, N.D.; Hewson, I.; Reyes, A.; Ley, R.E. Virome Diversity Correlates with Intestinal Microbiome Diversity in Adult Monozygotic Twins. *Cell Host Microbe* **2019**, *25*, 261–272.e5. [CrossRef]
85. Norman, J.M.; Handley, S.A.; Baldridge, M.T.; Droit, L.; Liu, C.Y.; Keller, B.C.; Kambal, A.; Monaco, C.L.; Zhao, G.; Fleshner, P.; et al. Disease-specific alterations in the enteric virome in inflammatory bowel disease. *Cell* **2015**, *160*, 447–460. [CrossRef]
86. Zuo, T.; Lu, X.J.; Zhang, Y.; Cheung, C.P.; Lam, S.; Zhang, F.; Tang, W.; Ching, J.Y.L.; Zhao, R.; Chan, P.K.S.; et al. Gut mucosal virome alterations in ulcerative colitis. *Gut* **2019**, *68*, 1169–1179. [CrossRef]
87. Monaco, C.L.; Gootenberg, D.B.; Zhao, G.; Handley, S.A.; Musie, S.; Lim, E.S.; Lankowski, A.; Baldridge, M.T.; Wilen, C.B.; Flagg, M.; et al. Altered Virome and Bacterial Microbiome in Human Immuni. *Cell Host Microbe* **2017**, *19*, 311–322. [CrossRef]
88. Ma, Y.; You, X.; Mai, G.; Tokuyasu, T.; Liu, C. A human gut phage catalog correlates the gut phageome with type 2 diabetes. *Microbiome* **2018**, *6*, 1–12. [CrossRef]
89. Reyes, A.; Blanton, L.V.; Cao, S.; Zhao, G.; Manary, M.; Trehan, I.; Smith, M.I.; Wang, D.; Virgin, H.W.; Rohwer, F.; et al. Gut DNA viromes of Malawian twins discordant for severe acute malnutrition. *Proc. Natl. Acad. Sci. USA* **2015**, *112*, 11941–11946. [CrossRef]
90. Metzger, R.N.; Krug, A.B.; Eisenächer, K. Enteric virome sensing—Its role in intestinal homeostasis and immunity. *Viruses* **2018**, *10*, 146. [CrossRef]
91. Duerkop, B.A.; Hooper, L.V. Resident viruses and their interactions with the immune system. *Nat. Immunol.* **2013**, *14*, 654–659. [CrossRef] [PubMed]
92. Duerkop, B.A.; Clements, C.V.; Rollins, D.; Rodrigues, J.L.M.; Hooper, L.V. A composite bacteriophage alters colonization by an intestinal commensal bacterium. *Proc. Natl. Acad. Sci. USA* **2012**, *109*, 17621–17626. [CrossRef] [PubMed]
93. Reyes, A.; Wu, M.; McNulty, N.P.; Rohwer, F.L.; Gordon, J.I. Gnotobiotic mouse model of phage-bacterial host dynamics in the human gut. *Proc. Natl. Acad. Sci. USA* **2013**, *110*, 20236–20241. [CrossRef] [PubMed]
94. Jończyk-Matysiak, E.; Weber-Dąbrowska, B.; Owczarek, B.; Międzybrodzki, R.; Łusiak-Szelchowska, M.; Łodej, N.; Górski, A. Phage-phagocyte interactions and their implications for phage application as therapeutics. *Viruses* **2017**, *9*, 150. [CrossRef] [PubMed]
95. Eriksson, F.; Tsagozis, P.; Lundberg, K.; Parsa, R.; Mangsbo, S.M.; Persson, M.A.A.; Harris, R.A.; Pisa, P. Tumor-Specific Bacteriophages Induce Tumor Destruction through Activation of Tumor-Associated Macrophages. *J. Immunol.* **2009**, *182*, 3105–3111. [CrossRef] [PubMed]
96. Ozdamar, S.O.; Gucer, S.; Tinaztepe, K. Hepatitis-B virus associated nephropathies: A clinicopathological study in 14 children. *Pediatr. Nephrol.* **2003**, *18*, 23–28. [CrossRef] [PubMed]

97. Hu, X.; Feng, J.; Zhou, Q.; Luo, L.; Meng, T.; Zhong, Y.; Tang, W.; Deng, S.; Li, X. Respiratory syncytial virus exacerbates kidney damages in IgA nephropathy mice via the C5a-C5AR1 axis orchestrating Th17 cell responses. *Front. Cell Infect. Microbiol.* **2019**, *9*, 151. [CrossRef]
98. Kupin, W.L. Viral-associated GN hepatitis B and other viral infections. *Clin. J. Am. Soc. Nephrol.* **2017**, *12*, 1529–1533. [CrossRef]
99. Sallustio, F.; Curci, C.; Stasi, A.; De Palma, G.; Divella, C.; Gramignoli, R.; Castellano, G.; Gallone, A.; Gesualdo, L. Role of Toll-Like Receptors in Actuating Stem/Progenitor Cell Repair Mechanisms: Different Functions in Different Cells. *Stem Cells Int.* **2019**, *2019*, 1–12. [CrossRef]
100. Ozato, K.; Tailor, P.; Kubota, T. The interferon regulatory factor family in host defense: Mechanism of action. *J. Biol. Chem.* **2007**, *282*, 20065–20069. [CrossRef]
101. Sarkar, S.N.; Elco, C.P.; Peters, K.L.; Chattopadhyay, S.; Sen, G.C. Two tyrosine residues of toll-like receptor 3 trigger different steps of NF-κB activation. *J. Biol. Chem.* **2007**, *282*, 3423–3427. [CrossRef] [PubMed]
102. Yamashita, M.; Millward, C.A.; Inoshita, H.; Saikia, P.; Chattopadhyay, S.; Sen, G.C.; Emancipator, S.N. Antiviral innate immunity disturbs podocyte cell function. *J. Innate Immun.* **2013**, *5*, 231–241. [CrossRef] [PubMed]
103. He, L.; Peng, X.; Wang, J.; Tang, C.; Zhou, X.; Liu, H.; Liu, F.; Sun, L.; Peng, Y. Synthetic double-stranded RNA Poly(I:C) aggravates IgA nephropathy by triggering IgA class switching recombination through the TLR3-BAFF axis. *Am. J. Nephrol.* **2015**, *42*, 185–197. [CrossRef] [PubMed]

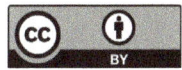

© 2019 by the authors. Licensee MDPI, Basel, Switzerland. This article is an open access article distributed under the terms and conditions of the Creative Commons Attribution (CC BY) license (http://creativecommons.org/licenses/by/4.0/).

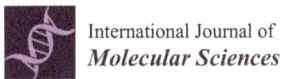

Review

Pseudoxanthoma Elasticum, Kidney Stones and Pyrophosphate: From a Rare Disease to Urolithiasis and Vascular Calcifications

Emmanuel Letavernier [1,*], Elise Bouderlique [1], Jeremy Zaworski [1], Ludovic Martin [2] and Michel Daudon [1]

1. UMR S 1155 and Physiology Unit, AP-HP, Hôpital Tenon, Sorbonne Université and INSERM, F-75020 Paris, France; eliseboud@aol.com (E.B.); jyzaworski@gmail.com (J.Z.); michel.daudon@aphp.fr (M.D.)
2. PXE Consultation Center, MAGEC Reference Center for Rare Skin Diseases, Angers University Hospital, MITOVASC Institute, UMR CNRS 6015 INSERM U1083 Angers University, 49000 Angers, France; lumartin@chu-angers.fr
* Correspondence: emmanuel.letavernier@aphp.fr

Received: 19 November 2019; Accepted: 11 December 2019; Published: 17 December 2019

Abstract: Pseudoxanthoma elasticum is a rare disease mainly due to *ABCC6* gene mutations and characterized by ectopic biomineralization and fragmentation of elastic fibers resulting in skin, cardiovascular and retinal calcifications. It has been recently described that pyrophosphate (a calcification inhibitor) deficiency could be the main cause of ectopic calcifications in this disease and in other genetic disorders associated to mutations of *ENPP1* or *CD73*. Patients affected by Pseudoxanthoma Elasticum seem also prone to develop kidney stones originating from papillary calcifications named Randall's plaque, and to a lesser extent may be affected by nephrocalcinosis. In this narrative review, we summarize some recent discoveries relative to the pathophysiology of this mendelian disease responsible for both cardiovascular and renal papillary calcifications, and we discuss the potential implications of pyrophosphate deficiency as a promoter of vascular calcifications in kidney stone formers and in patients affected by chronic kidney disease.

Keywords: pseudoxanthoma elasticum; pyrophosphate; kidney; Randall's plaque

1. Introduction: Pseudoxanthoma Elasticum and Related Diseases

1.1. Clinical Manifestations

Pseudoxanthoma elasticum (PXE; OMIM #264800, prevalence 1/25,000 to 1/50,000) is an autosomal recessive disease resulting mainly from mutations in *ABCC6* gene [1,2]. PXE is characterized by the fragmentation of elastin fibers, elastorrhexis, and calcifications of soft tissues involving mainly skin, arteries and retina [3,4]. The 2/3 female to 1/3 male ratio in patients diagnosed with PXE remains unexplained to date.

The disease may present during infancy but is classically discovered in teenagers or young adults, because of cutaneous manifestations [3–6].

Xanthoma-like papules may be sparse or form coalescent plaques and folds of esthetic concern. They give the name to the disease and predominate in flexion zones and neck. Skin biopsy and histopathological examination reveal calcifications with destruction of the elastic fibers [7]. It remains uncertain whether elastorrhexis precedes calcifications or whether calcified elastin fibers are broken in a second step.

PXE also affects retina, inducing fragmentation and rupture of calcified elastin fibers of the Bruch's membrane. The examination of the fundus of the eye reveals a typical "peau d'orange" aspect in

PXE patients, with angioid streaks and choroidal neovascularization leading to hemorrhages [8,9]. When affecting the macula, these lesions lead to the loss of central vision.

Cardiovascular calcifications are a hallmark of PXE but clinical manifestations are relatively delayed, predominating after the fourth decade of life, and their severity is extremely variable among PXE patients [5]. Peripheral arterial disease is frequent and there is a significantly increased risk of stroke [10,11]. Coronary calcifications are also frequent but the risk of cardiac infarction seems only mildly increased (if any) in comparison to the general population [5,12]. The earliest arterial calcifications observed in PXE affect elastic fibers of the medial layer, and predominate in medium and small-sized musculo-elastic arteries. Cardiovascular remodeling in large and medium sized musculo-elastic arteries is characterized by an increased intima-media thickening [13,14]. The arterial lesions affecting PXE peripheral arteries differ from those due to aging, hypertension or classic atherosclerosis and share similarities with calcifications and remodeling observed in chronic kidney disease [5,15].

To date, there is no specific curative or preventive therapy for PXE patients. Bisphosphonates such as Etidronate seem promising to prevent cardiovascular calcifications and anti-Vascular Endothelial Growth Factor (VEGF) intraocular injections limit neoangiogenesis [9,16,17].

Two other autosomal recessive mendelian diseases share phenotypic similarities with PXE: the generalized arterial calcifications of infancy (GACI), caused by mutations of the ectonucleotide pyrophosphatase phosphodiesterase NPP1 encoded by the *ENPP1* gene (OMIM 208000) and Arterial calcification due to deficiency of CD73 (ACDC, OMIM 211800), due to mutation of the *NT5E* gene encoding CD73, an ecto 5′-nucleotidase adenosine (ADO)-generating enzyme [18–21] GACI is an extremely severe but fortunately rare disorder characterized by extensive arterial calcification and stenosis affecting young children leading to heart failure. In some cases, the disease is less severe and patients with *ENPP1* mutations may present with the PXE phenotype. ACDC has been discovered more recently in a few families and is also characterized by cardiovascular calcifications and stenosis [19,20].

In addition to phenotypic resemblances, these three diseases share a common pathophysiological link: pyrophosphate (PPi) deficiency.

1.2. Pathophysiology of PXE, GACI and ACDC: Pyrophosphate Deficiency

During decades, the mechanism responsible for ectopic calcifications in PXE patients remained a mystery. *ABCC6* mutations are responsible for most of the PXE syndromes diagnosed. *ABCC6* encodes an adenosine triphosphate (ATP)-binding cassette transporter mainly expressed in the liver and to a lesser extent in kidney proximal tubular cells [1,22,23]. This specific expression raised the hypothesis that PXE would be a metabolic disease responsible for distant manifestations, i.e., connective tissue calcifications [24]. Due to its structure, close to other ABC-type transporters, ABCC6 could promote the efflux of calcification inhibitors from hepatocytes and tubular cells toward the systemic circulation [24].

A role for vitamin K has been suggested by several observations [25]. First, antivitamin K therapy is associated with vascular calcifications and sometimes calciphylaxis in hemodialyzed patients [26]. Second, *GGCX* mutations cause a PXE-like calcification phenotype and are associated with deficiency in vitamin K clotting factors [25]. The *GGCX* gene encodes a gamma-glutamyl carboxylase which catalyzes the conversion of glutamate residues to gamma-carboxyglutamate residues (gamma-carboxylation). This posttranslational modification process uses vitamin K as an essential cofactor. Gamma-carboxylation is necessary to activate multiple vitamin K-dependent proteins including coagulation factors (Factors II, VII, IX and X) and proteins such as Matrix Gla Protein (MGP). Third, PXE patients have lower serum levels of vitamin K in comparison with a control population [25]. Finally, MGP is a vitamin K-dependent mineralization inhibitor. *MGP* homozygous mutations are responsible for Keutel syndrome, characterized by cartilage calcification and pulmonary artery stenoses [27]. Nevertheless, administration of vitamin K was not efficient to reduce clinical manifestations in patients or to improve significantly the ectopic calcification which also occur in *Abcc6*$^{-/-}$ mice [28,29].

A major breakthrough in the field of calcifying diseases has been the identification that the hepatic (and probably tubular) ABCC6 transporter promotes the release of extracellular adenosine triphosphate (ATP), which serves as a substrate for NPP1 in the vasculature to generate adenosine monophosphate (AMP) and PPi, a potent anticalcifying molecule [30,31]. This process is the main source of circulating PPi, that counteracts the formation of calcium phosphate ectopic calcifications. PPi inhibits the crystallization and the growth of calcium phosphate crystalline phases such as hydroxyapatite [32]. Patients with PXE and GACI as well as $Abcc6^{-/-}$ and $Enpp1$ mutant (tiptoe walking: ttw/ttw) mice have a reduced plasma PPi level, explaining, at least in part, their mineralization disorder [22]. Of note, PPi treatment is sufficient to prevent ectopic mineralization in both $Abcc6^{-/-}$ and $Enpp1^{ttw/ttw}$ murine models [33–35].

Moreover, ABCC6 and NPP1 combined activity generates AMP in addition to PPi. AMP is rapidly converted into adenosine by CD73, which exerts a tonic inhibition on tissue non-specific alkaline enzyme (TNAP). In ACDC, mutations in $NT5E/CD73$ lead to insufficient adenosine levels, increasing TNAP activity: TNAP degrades PPi to generate inorganic phosphate and eventually promotes hydroxyapatite precipitation in ectopic tissues [22,33,35].

Thus, ABCC6, NPP1 and CD73 increase PPi systemic synthesis and decrease endogenous PPi degradation through TNAP inhibition (Figure 1).

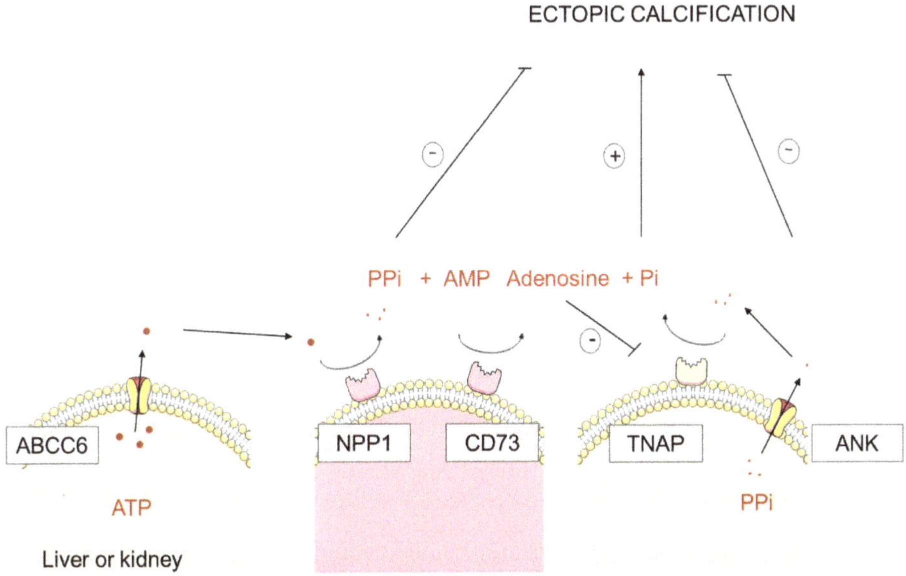

Figure 1. Systemic Pyrophosphate (PPi) synthesis. ABCC6 (expressed in hepatocytes and proximal tubular cells) and NPP1 (in arteries and capillaries) combined activity generates AMP in addition to PPi. AMP is rapidly converted into adenosine by CD73, which exerts a tonic inhibition on tissue non-specific alkaline enzyme (TNAP). TNAP degrades PPi to generate inorganic phosphate and promotes hydroxyapatite precipitation in ectopic tissues. ANK allows PPi externalization from cells, its role in ectopic calcifications is unclear.

2. Pseudoxanthoma Elasticum and Kidney Calcifications

2.1. Nephrocalcinosis and Kidney Stones: Preliminary Reports

A few preliminary and sparse reports have suggested that PXE patients may be affected by kidney stones [36]. In addition to kidney stones, the presence of typical nephrocalcinosis has been reported in a few patients affected by PXE [37–39]. When exposed to a procalcifying diet (high phosphate, vitamin D and low magnesium), $Abcc6^{-/-}$ and $Enpp1^{-/-}$ mice develop rapidly a nephrocalcinosis consisting in multiple calcium phosphate tubular plugs [40].

2.2. High Prevalence of Kidney Stones in PXE Patients

In a recent PXE cohort study that was not specifically designed to record kidney stone prevalence, observations suggested that nephrolithiasis was an unrecognized but a prevalent feature of PXE, affecting at least 10% of patients [11]. To better characterize the prevalence of kidney stones among patients with PXE, we conducted a retrospective study in 170 patients participating in the Angers PXE cohort [41]. Among the 164 patients who received the survey, 113 fulfilled the questionaire (33 men and 80 women). Among these patients, 45 (39.8%) declared they had a past medical history of kidney stones (asymptomatic stones in four patients or renal colic in 41 patients). Although this type of study may be biased, as patients affected by kidney stones may be more prone to fulfill the survey, the prevalence of kidney stones and renal colic in PXE patients appears to be extremely high. As a matter of comparison, the lifetime expected incidence of kidney stones is nearing 10% in the general population. Usually, urolithiasis is more frequent in males than females but in PXE patients approximately two thirds of the patients are women. This is consistent with the higher prevalence of PXE in women.

The analysis of six computed tomography (CT)-scans from PXE patients revealed the presence of papillary calcifications, Randall's plaques, the first step of kidney stone formation in five of them [41]. This is remarkable as only the presence of massive plaques can be determined by imaging. These calcifications affected rather the tip of the renal papilla than the renal medulla. One patient had both papillary calcifications and medullary calcifications, i.e., nephrocalcinosis. CT scans had been performed in patients with a past medical history of kidney stones, but one may hypothesize that patients with PXE and without a past medical history of urolithiasis may also be affected by asymptomatic papillary calcifications. We examined a limited number of CT-scans so that we cannot estimate the prevalence of papillary calcifications/Randall's plaque and nephrocalcinosis in PXE patients. A few stones from PXE patients have been analyzed and presented Randall's plaque fragments made of carbonated apatite, suggesting that stone formation in these individuals was initiated by these plaques. No specific study dedicated to the biological risk factors of kidney stone formation in PXE has been performed to date. In the same way, chronic kidney disease (CKD) is not a classic feature of PXE and we still ignore whether some PXE patients affected by kidney stones and papillary calcifications may be at risk to develop CKD.

2.3. $Abcc6^{-/-}$ Mice: A Murine Model of Randall's Plaque

$Abcc6^{-/-}$ mice recapitulate many of the phenotypical characteristics of the human PXE disease [42]. Mice are affected by ectopic calcifications involving aorta, heart, retina and vibrissae and their PPi serum level is lower than in control mice. As renal cortical and medullary calcifications had been described in these animals, especially after an "acceleration diet", we hypothesized that papillary calcification could develop in this model [40]. Aging $Abcc6^{-/-}$ mice actually developed kidney calcifications electively at the tip of the papilla, mainly in the interstitial tissue, round shaped and surrounding the loops of Henle and the vasa recta: they differed from the tubular plugs observed after an acceleration diet. These calcifications were made of carbonated apatite spheres as evidenced by scanning electron microscopy and Fourier transform infrared microspectroscopy [41]. At the nanometer scale, by using transmission electron microscopy coupled to electron energy loss spectroscopy, we evidenced that incipient calcifications were made of concentric layers containing calcium and phosphate alternating with organic compounds, as described in incipient human calcifications forming the Randall's plaque. Remarkably, the renal calcification observed in aging $Abcc6^{-/-}$ mice met the four essential criteria of Randall's plaque: (i) interstitial deposits surrounding tubules and vasa recta, (ii) electively located at the tip of the renal papilla, (iii) made of carbonated apatite, and (iv) forming nanometer-scale elementary structures made of minerals and organic compounds.

$Abcc6^{-/-}$ mice had also a lower urinary excretion of PPi than control mice, and as previously described lower serum levels of PPi [41]. $Abcc6^{-/-}$ mice expressing a functional human ABCC6 protein in the liver had an increase in serum PPi circulating levels and were protected against kidney calcifications at 18 months of age [33]. It seems therefore very likely that the systemic PPi deficiency in these mice was at the origin of calcium phosphate supersaturation at the tip of the papilla, leading to papillary calcification.

3. The Mystery of Randall's Plaque Formation: A Role for Calcification Inhibitors and Pyrophosphate?

3.1. Randall's Plaque: the Origin of Renal Calculi

Randall's plaque is the first step of calcium oxalate stone formation in many cases. Alexander Randall proposed its original theory in 1936 when he claimed the identification of the origin of renal calculi [43]. He performed extensive forensic studies and observed, at the tip of the renal papilla, whitish deposits made of calcium phosphate and carbonate, originating from the renal interstitium. In some cases, these lesions disrupted the urothelium cellular barrier and brown calcium oxalate stones were attached to these "Randall's" plaques, forming a heterogeneous nucleation process. He identified that the calcium oxalate stones had an umbilication due the shape of the papilla and that calcium phosphate remnants, fragments of Randall's plaque, were present in this umbilication once the stone was passed, identifying the origin of the stone. Other authors performed similar studies during this period [44]. It has been postulated early that the high concentration in calcium in renal papilla could be at the origin of the plaque. The interest in Randall's plaque has grown during the last decades, as the development of endourology evidenced the presence of stones attached to Randall's plaque in situ. Randall's plaque was found in stone formers in 57%–99% of patients when reno-ureterocopy was performed. The prevalence seems lower in France than in North American studies [45–49]. Although Randall's plaques seem to be very frequent, common papillary calcifications are usually too small to be evidenced by CT-scan (unlike PXE patients).

3.2. Determinants of Randall's Plaque Formation

The main risk factors responsible for calcium oxalate supersaturation and crystals or stone formation are relatively well identified: low diuresis, hypercalciuria, hyperoxaluria and/or hypocitraturia [47,50]. However, the origin of the Randall's plaque itself is less understood. The prevalence of calcium oxalate stones is increasing worldwide [47,51]. As there is no longitudinal study taking into account stone morphology or papillary plaque coverage, the role of Randall's plaque in this epidemic is difficult to assess. However, we identified that the proportion of stones with a papillary umbilication and typical plaque remnants was three times more frequent in recent years than three decades ago, especially in young adults [52]. In 2003, Evan et al. analyzed papilla biopsies and identified that incipient Randall's plaque at the tip of the renal papillae were made of subepithelial apatite deposits surrounding the loop of Henle [53]. These observations suggested that apatite droplets formed in around the loop of Henle in contact with basement membrane could spread in the interstitium and form plaques. It has been suggested that calcium phosphate supersaturation in the thin limb of the loop of Henle could promote calcium phosphate particle precipitation and that some of these particles attached to epithelial cells could migrate by endocytosis to the interstitial tissue and form plaques [54,55]. We performed analyses of incipient Randall's plaque in dozens of healthy papillae and identified that early calcifications could also appear around vasa recta at the tip of renal papilla, as previously highlighted by Stoller et al. [56,57]. This suggests that calcium phosphate supersaturation should be extremely high in this environment. Kuo et al. have identified that hypercalciuria, low diuresis and low urine pH correlated with the surface of Randall's plaque in kidney stone formers [58]. More than seven decades ago, Vermooten had performed forensic studies in South Africa and identified Randall's plaque in 17% of whites and only in 4% of the local native Bantus, known to have low calciuria and to be rarely affected by calcium-related stones [44,59]. Hypercalciuria could therefore be involved first in Randall's plaque formation and several years or decades later in calcium oxalate stone formation, once plaque has developed and eroded urothelium locally.

3.3. Randall's Plaque and Calcification Inhibitors

Calcium concentration is predicted to be extremely high at the tip of the renal papilla, especially around vasa recta [60,61]. Considering (i) that phosphate concentration is certainly significant, although reabsorbed partly in the proximal tubule, and (ii) that papillary pH should stand within physiological range (7.4), calcium phosphate supersaturation should be extremely high at the tip of the papilla. This suggests that calcification inhibitors play a key role to prevent Randall's plaque formation. A very large number of low-weight and macromolecular calcification inhibitors have been studied in the field of urolithiasis [62]. Currently, there is no monogenic mendelian disease responsible for calcification inhibitor deficiency and kidney stone formation, maybe with the exception of distal renal tubular acidosis, which is responsible for hypocitraturia and nephrocalcinosis [63]. Interestingly, ABCC6 mutation in PXE patients and $Abcc6$ knock-out murine models are sufficient to induce papillary calcification [41]. This monogenic defect responsible for PPi deficiency is clearly not compensated by other calcification inhibitors. This observation is remarkable as the development of kidney tissue calcifications is extremely difficult to achieve in rodent models. We previously tried to induce Randall's plaque in Sprague Dawley rats exposed to vitamin D and calcium supplementation for 6 months. These animals developed tubular plugs and stones but none of them developed papillary interstitial calcifications [64]. Similar observations have been performed in the genetic hypercalciuric stone forming rat extensively studied by Bushinsky et al. [65]. These data confirm that calcification inhibitors, especially PPi, play a major role to prevent Randall's plaque formation.

Further studies are required to assess whether kidney stone formers affected by Randall's plaque have lower urine (or serum) PPi levels than kidney stone formers without Randall's plaque or than general population. Of note, seminal studies had previously highlighted that kidney stone formers may have lower urinary PPi excretion than matched subjects [66]. However, this field of research has probably been limited during the last decades by the lack of reliable methods to measure PPi, due to pre-analytic pitfalls and to the very low concentration of PPi in biological fluids.

3.4. The $Abcc6^{-/-}$ Murine Model: A Tool to Identify Randall's Plaque Determinants and New Therapeutics

$Abcc6^{-/-}$ mice expressing a functional human ABCC6 protein in the liver or supplemented with PPi were protected against kidney calcification [33,34]. It has been shown that oral PPi is partly absorbed in human subjects and increases serum PPi circulating levels. Taken together, these data suggest that PPi or drugs increasing PPi synthesis could potentially be used as a treatment against kidney calcifications and Randall's plaque.

$Abcc6^{-/-}$ mice can also be used to test whether drugs or dietary factors could influence Randall's plaque formation. We hypothesized that the increased proportion of stones grown on Randall's plaque during the past decades could, at least partly, be explained by the widespread use of vitamin D supplementation in the general population [52]. Although the question is extremely controversial, some studies highlighted a relationship between vitamin D intakes, especially in addition with calcium supplementation, and stone formation [67]. $Abcc6^{-/-}$ and wild-type mice were exposed to vitamin D supplementation, with or without a calcium-rich diet, to promote the formation of Randall's plaque. The combined administration of vitamin D and calcium accelerated significantly Randall's plaque formation in $Abcc6^{-/-}$ mice, although the animal did not develop hypercalcemia or even a significant increase in urine calcium excretion [68]. This model raises some concerns regarding the potential role of long-term vitamin D supplementation and calcium intakes in predisposed individuals.

4. Pyrophosphate Deficiency, the Common Link between Vascular Calcifications, Kidney Stones and Chronic Kidney Disease?

Epidemiological studies have highlighted an association between nephrolithiasis and systemic conditions including cardiovascular diseases but the underlying mechanisms remain unidentified [69]. Vascular calcifications are highly associated with cardiovascular mortality. Kidney stone formers, even young patients, have an increased carotid intima-media wall thickness and an increased arterial stiffness in comparison with matched populations [70,71]. Kidney stone formers have a higher degree of aortic calcification than age- and sex-matched non-stone formers and more severe coronary artery calcification, suggesting that vascular calcifications and kidney stones may have a common underlying mechanism [72].

The potential implication of PPi in vascular calcification is not a novel hypothesis, as Schibler et al. have reported in 1968 that PPi and polyphosphate can inhibit the induction of aortic calcifications by vitamin D, but the recent evidence that PXE patients are affected by both cardiovascular calcifications and kidney stones and Randall's plaque suggests that PPi deficiency could be involved in the development of vascular calcifications in kidney stone formers [41,73]. Here again, further studies based upon a reliable assay of serum PPi levels would be necessary to assess whether PPi deficiency is the missing link between kidney stone/Randall's plaque and vascular calcifications.

Moreover, a relative deficiency in PPi could be involved in the vascular calcifications observed in patients affected by CKD, responsible for an increased cardiovascular morbidity and mortality [74]. TNAP activity is increased in uremic rats, reducing PPi/inorganic phosphate ratio and ABCC6 expression is reduced in uremic mice and rats [75,76]. Exogenous PPi could in theory be of help to protect against vascular calcifications in CKD.

5. Conclusions

An increased prevalence of kidney stones has been reported recently in patients affected by PXE, a disease characterized by low circulating PPi levels and vascular calcifications. These patients are affected by massive Randall's plaques and in some cases by nephrocalcinosis. In clinical practice, patients affected by PXE should be aware that they are at high risk to form kidney stones, and preventive measures should be considered, as for any kidney stone former (increased diuresis, decreased urine calcium excretion, etc.). These observations from a rare monogenic disease evidence that PPi probably prevents the development of Randall's plaque and, in the long term, the formation of kidney stones, a disease with a lifetime incidence nearing 10% of the population. Further studies are required to assess whether PPi deficiency is involved in Randall's plaque and kidney stone formation in the general population, but also whether administration of PPi could be protective in that setting. $Abcc6^{-/-}$ mice can also be used as a model of Randall's plaque to test new drugs or identify potential determinants of plaque formation or worsening. In addition, PPi could be a missing link between kidney stones and the high prevalence of cardiovascular calcifications observed in kidney stone formers, a deficiency in PPi and potentially in other calcification inhibitors could promote both papillary and vascular mineralization.

Funding: This research received no external funding.

Acknowledgments: The authors thank Georges Leftheriotis (Nice, France) and Olivier Le Saux (Hawai'i, USA), all the colleagues that participated in the studies dedicated to the role of Abcc6 in kidney stone formation, the COST action CA16115 EuroSoftCalcNet and Patients associations.

Conflicts of Interest: The authors declare no conflict of interest. The funders had no role in the design of the study; in the collection, analyses, or interpretation of data; in the writing of the manuscript, or in the decision to publish the results.

Abbreviations

PXE	Pseudoxanthoma elasticum
VEGF	Vascular Endothelial Growth Factor
GACI	Generalized arterial calcification of infancy
(E)NPP1	ectonucleotide pyrophosphatase phosphodiesterase
ACDC	Arterial calcification due to deficiency of CD73
PPi	Pyrophosphate
CT	Computed Tomography
CKD	Chronic kidney disease
TNAP	Tissue nonspecific alkaline phosphatase

References

1. Le Saux, O.; Urban, Z.; Tschuch, C.; Csiszar, K.; Bacchelli, B.; Quaglino, D.; Pasquali-Ronchetti, I.; Pope, F.M.; Richards, A.; Terry, S.; et al. Mutations in a gene encoding an ABC transporter cause pseudoxanthoma elasticum. *Nat. Genet.* **2000**, *25*, 223–227. [CrossRef] [PubMed]
2. Le Saux, O.; Beck, K.; Sachsinger, C.; Silvestri, C.; Treiber, C.; Göring, H.H.; Johnson, E.W.; De Paepe, A.; Pope, F.M.; Pasquali-Ronchetti, I.; et al. A spectrum of ABCC6 mutations is responsible for pseudoxanthoma elasticum. *Am. J. Hum. Genet.* **2001**, *69*, 749–764. [CrossRef]
3. Neidner, K.H. History. *Clin. Dermatol.* **1988**, *6*, 1–4. [CrossRef]
4. Uitto, J.; Li, Q.; Jiang, Q. Pseudoxanthoma Elasticum: Molecular Genetics and Putative Pathomechanisms. *J. Investig. Dermatol.* **2010**, *130*, 661–670. [CrossRef] [PubMed]
5. Leftheriotis, G.; Omarjee, L.; Le Saux, O.; Henrion, D.; Abraham, P.; Prunier, F.; Willoteaux, S.; Martin, L. The vascular phenotype in Pseudoxanthoma elasticum and related disorders: Contribution of a genetic disease to the understanding of vascular calcification. *Front. Genet.* **2013**, *4*, 4. [CrossRef] [PubMed]
6. Naouri, M.; Boisseau, C.; Bonicel, P.; Daudon, P.; Bonneau, D.; Chassaing, N.; Martin, L. Manifestations of pseudoxanthoma elasticum in childhood. *Br. J. Dermatol.* **2009**, *161*, 635–639. [CrossRef]
7. Hosen, M.J.; Lamoen, A.; De Paepe, A.; Vanakker, O.M. Histopathology of Pseudoxanthoma Elasticum and Related Disorders: Histological Hallmarks and Diagnostic Clues. *Scientifica* **2012**, *2012*, 598262. [CrossRef]
8. Audo, I.; Vanakker, O.M.; Smith, A.; Leroy, B.P.; Robson, A.G.; Jenkins, S.A.; Coucke, P.J.; Bird, A.C.; Paepe, A.D.; Holder, G.E.; et al. Pseudoxanthoma Elasticum with Generalized Retinal Dysfunction, a Common Finding? *Investig. Ophthalmol. Vis. Sci.* **2007**, *48*, 4250–4256. [CrossRef]
9. Ebran, J.-M.; Milea, D.; Trelohan, A.; Bonicel, P.; Hamel, J.-F.; Leftheriotis, G.; Martin, L. New insights into the visual prognosis of pseudoxanthoma elasticum. *Br. J. Ophthalmol.* **2014**, *98*, 142–143. [CrossRef]
10. De Vilder, E.Y.G.; Cardoen, S.; Hosen, M.J.; Le Saux, O.; De Zaeytijd, J.; Leroy, B.P.; De Reuck, J.; Coucke, P.J.; De Paepe, A.; Hemelsoet, D.; et al. Pathogenic variants in the ABCC6 gene are associated with an increased risk for ischemic stroke. *Brain Pathol. Zurich Switz.* **2018**, *28*, 822–831. [CrossRef]
11. Legrand, A.; Cornez, L.; Samkari, W.; Mazzella, J.-M.; Venisse, A.; Boccio, V.; Auribault, K.; Keren, B.; Benistan, K.; Germain, D.P.; et al. Mutation spectrum in the ABCC6 gene and genotype-phenotype correlations in a French cohort with pseudoxanthoma elasticum. *Genet. Med. Off. J. Am. Coll. Med. Genet.* **2017**, *19*, 909–917. [CrossRef] [PubMed]
12. Prunier, F.; Terrien, G.; Le Corre, Y.; Apana, A.L.Y.; Bière, L.; Kauffenstein, G.; Furber, A.; Bergen, A.A.B.; Gorgels, T.G.M.F.; Le Saux, O.; et al. Pseudoxanthoma elasticum: Cardiac findings in patients and Abcc6-deficient mouse model. *PLoS ONE* **2013**, *8*, e68700. [CrossRef] [PubMed]
13. Germain, D.P.; Boutouyrie, P.; Laloux, B.; Laurent, S. Arterial Remodeling and Stiffness in Patients With Pseudoxanthoma Elasticum. *Arterioscler. Thromb. Vasc. Biol.* **2003**, *23*, 836–841. [CrossRef] [PubMed]
14. Germain, D.P. Pseudoxanthoma elasticum. *Orphanet J. Rare Dis.* **2017**, *12*, 85. [CrossRef] [PubMed]
15. Leftheriotis, G.; Kauffenstein, G.; Hamel, J.F.; Abraham, P.; Le Saux, O.; Willoteaux, S.; Henrion, D.; Martin, L. The contribution of arterial calcification to peripheral arterial disease in pseudoxanthoma elasticum. *PLoS ONE* **2014**, *9*, e96003. [CrossRef] [PubMed]
16. Kranenburg, G.; de Jong, P.A.; Bartstra, J.W.; Lagerweij, S.J.; Lam, M.G.; Ossewaarde-van Norel, J.; Risseeuw, S.; van Leeuwen, R.; Imhof, S.M.; Verhaar, H.J.; et al. Etidronate for Prevention of Ectopic Mineralization in Patients With Pseudoxanthoma Elasticum. *J. Am. Coll. Cardiol.* **2018**, *71*, 1117–1126. [CrossRef] [PubMed]

17. Bauer, C.; le Saux, O.; Pomozi, V.; Aherrahrou, R.; Kriesen, R.; Stölting, S.; Liebers, A.; Kessler, T.; Schunkert, H.; Erdmann, J.; et al. Etidronate prevents dystrophic cardiac calcification by inhibiting macrophage aggregation. *Sci. Rep.* **2018**, *8*, 5812. [CrossRef]
18. Ruf, N.; Uhlenberg, B.; Terkeltaub, R.; Nürnberg, P.; Rutsch, F. The mutational spectrum of ENPP1 as arising after the analysis of 23 unrelated patients with generalized arterial calcification of infancy (GACI). *Hum. Mutat.* **2005**, *25*, 98. [CrossRef]
19. Nitschke, Y.; Baujat, G.; Botschen, U.; Wittkampf, T.; du Moulin, M.; Stella, J.; Le Merrer, M.; Guest, G.; Lambot, K.; Tazarourte-Pinturier, M.-F.; et al. Generalized arterial calcification of infancy and pseudoxanthoma elasticum can be caused by mutations in either ENPP1 or ABCC6. *Am. J. Hum. Genet.* **2012**, *90*, 25–39. [CrossRef]
20. St Hilaire, C.; Ziegler, S.G.; Markello, T.C.; Brusco, A.; Groden, C.; Gill, F.; Carlson-Donohoe, H.; Lederman, R.J.; Chen, M.Y.; Yang, D.; et al. NT5E mutations and arterial calcifications. *N. Engl. J. Med.* **2011**, *364*, 432–442. [CrossRef]
21. Nitschke, Y.; Rutsch, F. Inherited Arterial Calcification Syndromes: Etiologies and Treatment Concepts. *Curr. Osteoporos. Rep.* **2017**, *15*, 255–270. [CrossRef] [PubMed]
22. Favre, G.; Laurain, A.; Aranyi, T.; Szeri, F.; Fulop, K.; Le Saux, O.; Duranton, C.; Kauffenstein, G.; Martin, L.; Leftheriotis, G. The ABCC6 Transporter: A New Player in Biomineralization. *Int. J. Mol. Sci.* **2017**, *18*, 1941. [CrossRef] [PubMed]
23. Pomozi, V.; Le Saux, O.; Brampton, C.; Apana, A.; Iliás, A.; Szeri, F.; Martin, L.; Monostory, K.; Paku, S.; Sarkadi, B.; et al. ABCC6 is a basolateral plasma membrane protein. *Circ. Res.* **2013**, *112*, e148–e151. [CrossRef] [PubMed]
24. Le Saux, O.; Bunda, S.; VanWart, C.M.; Douet, V.; Got, L.; Martin, L.; Hinek, A. Serum factors from pseudoxanthoma elasticum patients alter elastic fiber formation in vitro. *J. Investig. Dermatol.* **2006**, *126*, 1497–1505. [CrossRef] [PubMed]
25. Vanakker, O.M.; Martin, L.; Schurgers, L.J.; Quaglino, D.; Costrop, L.; Vermeer, C.; Pasquali-Ronchetti, I.; Coucke, P.J.; De Paepe, A. Low serum vitamin K in PXE results in defective carboxylation of mineralization inhibitors similar to the GGCX mutations in the PXE-like syndrome. *Lab. Investig. J. Tech. Methods Pathol.* **2010**, *90*, 895–905. [CrossRef] [PubMed]
26. Nigwekar, S.U.; Bloch, D.B.; Nazarian, R.M.; Vermeer, C.; Booth, S.L.; Xu, D.; Thadhani, R.I.; Malhotra, R. Vitamin K-Dependent Carboxylation of Matrix Gla Protein Influences the Risk of Calciphylaxis. *J. Am. Soc. Nephrol. JASN* **2017**, *28*, 1717–1722. [CrossRef] [PubMed]
27. Munroe, P.B.; Olgunturk, R.O.; Fryns, J.P.; Van Maldergem, L.; Ziereisen, F.; Yuksel, B.; Gardiner, R.M.; Chung, E. Mutations in the gene encoding the human matrix Gla protein cause Keutel syndrome. *Nat. Genet.* **1999**, *21*, 142–144. [CrossRef]
28. Brampton, C.; Yamaguchi, Y.; Vanakker, O.; Van Laer, L.; Chen, L.-H.; Thakore, M.; De Paepe, A.; Pomozi, V.; Szabó, P.T.; Martin, L.; et al. Vitamin K does not prevent soft tissue mineralization in a mouse model of pseudoxanthoma elasticum. *Cell Cycle Georget. Tex* **2011**, *10*, 1810–1820. [CrossRef]
29. Gorgels, T.G.M.F.; Waarsing, J.H.; Herfs, M.; Versteeg, D.; Schoensiegel, F.; Sato, T.; Schlingemann, R.O.; Ivandic, B.T.; Vermeer, C.; Schurgers, L.J.; et al. Vitamin K supplementation increases vitamin K tissue levels but fails to counteract ectopic calcification in a mouse model for pseudoxanthoma elasticum. *J. Mol. Med.* **2011**, *89*, 1125–1135. [CrossRef]
30. Jansen, R.S.; Küçükosmanoglu, A.; de Haas, M.; Sapthu, S.; Otero, J.A.; Hegman, I.E.M.; Bergen, A.A.B.; Gorgels, T.G.M.F.; Borst, P.; van de Wetering, K. ABCC6 prevents ectopic mineralization seen in pseudoxanthoma elasticum by inducing cellular nucleotide release. *Proc. Natl. Acad. Sci. USA* **2013**, *110*, 20206–20211. [CrossRef]
31. Jansen, R.S.; Duijst, S.; Mahakena, S.; Sommer, D.; Szeri, F.; Váradi, A.; Plomp, A.; Bergen, A.A.; Oude Elferink, R.P.J.; Borst, P.; et al. ABCC6-mediated ATP secretion by the liver is the main source of the mineralization inhibitor inorganic pyrophosphate in the systemic circulation-brief report. *Arterioscler. Thromb. Vasc. Biol.* **2014**, *34*, 1985–1989. [CrossRef] [PubMed]
32. Fleisch, H.; Bisaz, S. Mechanism of calcification: Inhibitory role of pyrophosphate. *Nature* **1962**, *195*, 911. [CrossRef] [PubMed]

33. Pomozi, V.; Brampton, C.; van de Wetering, K.; Zoll, J.; Calio, B.; Pham, K.; Owens, J.B.; Marh, J.; Moisyadi, S.; Váradi, A.; et al. Pyrophosphate Supplementation Prevents Chronic and Acute Calcification in ABCC6-Deficient Mice. *Am. J. Pathol.* **2017**, *187*, 1258–1272. [CrossRef] [PubMed]
34. Pomozi, V.; Julian, C.B.; Zoll, J.; Pham, K.; Kuo, S.; Tőkési, N.; Martin, L.; Váradi, A.; Le Saux, O. Dietary Pyrophosphate Modulates Calcification in a Mouse Model of Pseudoxanthoma Elasticum: Implication for Treatment of Patients. *J. Investig. Dermatol.* **2019**, *139*, 1082–1088. [CrossRef] [PubMed]
35. Dedinszki, D.; Szeri, F.; Kozák, E.; Pomozi, V.; Tőkési, N.; Mezei, T.R.; Merczel, K.; Letavernier, E.; Tang, E.; Le Saux, O.; et al. Oral administration of pyrophosphate inhibits connective tissue calcification. *EMBO Mol. Med.* **2017**, *9*, 1463–1470. [CrossRef] [PubMed]
36. Fabre, B.; Bayle, P.; Bazex, J.; Durand, D.; Lamant, L.; Chassaing, N. Pseudoxanthoma elasticum and nephrolithiasis. *J. Eur. Acad. Dermatol. Venereol.* **2005**, *19*, 212–215. [CrossRef] [PubMed]
37. Chraïbi, R.; Ismaili, N.; Belgnaoui, F.; Akallal, N.; Bouhllab, J.; Senouci, K.; Hassam, B. Pseudoxanthoma elasticum and nephrocalcinosis. *Ann. Dermatol. Venereol.* **2007**, *134*, 764–766. [CrossRef]
38. Gayen, T.; Das, A.; Roy, S.; Biswas, S.; Shome, K.; Chowdhury, S.N. Pseudoxanthoma elasticum and nephrocalcinosis: Incidental finding or an infrequent manifestation? *Indian Dermatol. Online J.* **2014**, *5*, 176–178.
39. Seeger, H.; Mohebbi, N. Pseudoxanthoma elasticum and nephrocalcinosis. *Kidney Int.* **2016**, *89*, 1407. [CrossRef]
40. Li, Q.; Chou, D.W.; Price, T.P.; Sundberg, J.P.; Uitto, J. Genetic modulation of nephrocalcinosis in mouse models of ectopic mineralization: The Abcc6(tm1Jfk) and Enpp1(asj) mutant mice. *Lab. Investig. J. Tech. Methods Pathol.* **2014**, *94*, 623–632. [CrossRef]
41. Letavernier, E.; Kauffenstein, G.; Huguet, L.; Navasiolava, N.; Bouderlique, E.; Tang, E.; Delaitre, L.; Bazin, D.; de Frutos, M.; Gay, C.; et al. ABCC6 Deficiency Promotes Development of Randall Plaque. *J. Am. Soc. Nephrol.* **2018**, *29*, 2337–2347. [CrossRef] [PubMed]
42. Gorgels, T.G.M.F.; Hu, X.; Scheffer, G.L.; van der Wal, A.C.; Toonstra, J.; de Jong, P.T.V.M.; van Kuppevelt, T.H.; Levelt, C.N.; de Wolf, A.; Loves, W.J.P.; et al. Disruption of Abcc6 in the mouse: Novel insight in the pathogenesis of pseudoxanthoma elasticum. *Hum. Mol. Genet.* **2005**, *14*, 1763–1773. [CrossRef] [PubMed]
43. Randall, A. THE ORIGIN AND GROWTH OF RENAL CALCULI. *Ann. Surg.* **1937**, *105*, 1009–1027. [CrossRef] [PubMed]
44. Vermooten, V. The incidence and significance of the deposition of calcium plaques in the renal papilla as observed in the Caucasian and Bantu population in South Africa. *J. Urol.* **1941**, 193–196. [CrossRef]
45. Low, R.K.; Stoller, M.L. Endoscopic mapping of renal papillae for Randall's plaques in patients with urinary stone disease. *J. Urol.* **1997**, *158*, 2062–2064. [CrossRef]
46. Matlaga, B.R.; Williams, J.C.; Kim, S.C.; Kuo, R.L.; Evan, A.P.; Bledsoe, S.B.; Coe, F.L.; Worcester, E.M.; Munch, L.C.; Lingeman, J.E. Endoscopic evidence of calculus attachment to Randall's plaque. *J. Urol.* **2006**, *175*, 1720–1724. [CrossRef]
47. Khan, S.R.; Pearle, M.S.; Robertson, W.G.; Gambaro, G.; Canales, B.K.; Doizi, S.; Traxer, O.; Tiselius, H.-G. Kidney stones. *Nat. Rev. Dis. Primer* **2016**, *2*, 16008. [CrossRef]
48. Daudon, M.; Bazin, D.; Letavernier, E. Randall's plaque as the origin of calcium oxalate kidney stones. *Urolithiasis* **2015**, *43*, 5–11. [CrossRef]
49. Letavernier, E.; Bazin, D.; Daudon, M. Randall's plaque and kidney stones: Recent advances and future challenges. *Comptes Rendus Chim.* **2016**, *19*, 1456–1460. [CrossRef]
50. Daudon, M.; Letavernier, E.; Frochot, V.; Haymann, J.-P.; Bazin, D.; Jungers, P. Respective influence of calcium and oxalate urine concentration on the formation of calcium oxalate monohydrate or dihydrate crystals. *Comptes Rendus Chim.* **2016**, *19*, 1504–1513. [CrossRef]
51. Ziemba, J.B.; Matlaga, B.R. Epidemiology and economics of nephrolithiasis. *Investig. Clin. Urol.* **2017**, *58*, 299–306. [CrossRef] [PubMed]
52. Letavernier, E.; Vandermeersch, S.; Traxer, O.; Tligui, M.; Baud, L.; Ronco, P.; Haymann, J.-P.; Daudon, M. Demographics and characterization of 10,282 Randall plaque-related kidney stones: A new epidemic? *Medicine (Baltimore)* **2015**, *94*, e566. [CrossRef]

53. Evan, A.P.; Lingeman, J.E.; Coe, F.L.; Parks, J.H.; Bledsoe, S.B.; Shao, Y.; Sommer, A.J.; Paterson, R.F.; Kuo, R.L.; Grynpas, M. Randall's plaque of patients with nephrolithiasis begins in basement membranes of thin loops of Henle. *J. Clin. Investig.* **2003**, *111*, 607–616. [CrossRef]
54. Asplin, J.R.; Mandel, N.S.; Coe, F.L. Evidence of calcium phosphate supersaturation in the loop of Henle. *Am. J. Physiol.* **1996**, *270*, F604–F613. [CrossRef]
55. Lieske, J.C.; Norris, R.; Swift, H.; Toback, F.G. Adhesion, internalization and metabolism of calcium oxalate monohydrate crystals by renal epithelial cells. *Kidney Int.* **1997**, *52*, 1291–1301. [CrossRef]
56. Verrier, C.; Bazin, D.; Huguet, L.; Stéphan, O.; Gloter, A.; Verpont, M.-C.; Frochot, V.; Haymann, J.-P.; Brocheriou, I.; Traxer, O.; et al. Topography, Composition and Structure of Incipient Randall Plaque at the Nanoscale Level. *J. Urol.* **2016**, *196*, 1566–1574. [CrossRef]
57. Stoller, M.L.; Low, R.K.; Shami, G.S.; McCormick, V.D.; Kerschmann, R.L. High resolution radiography of cadaveric kidneys: Unraveling the mystery of Randall's plaque formation. *J. Urol.* **1996**, *156*, 1263–1266. [CrossRef]
58. Kuo, R.L.; Lingeman, J.E.; Evan, A.P.; Paterson, R.F.; Parks, J.H.; Bledsoe, S.B.; Munch, L.C.; Coe, F.L. Urine calcium and volume predict coverage of renal papilla by Randall's plaque. *Kidney Int.* **2003**, *64*, 2150–2154. [CrossRef]
59. Vermooten, V. The Origin and Development in the Renal Papilla of Randall's Calcium Plaques. *J. Urol.* **1942**, *48*, 27–37. [CrossRef]
60. Tournus, M.; Seguin, N.; Perthame, B.; Thomas, S.R.; Edwards, A. A model of calcium transport along the rat nephron. *Am. J. Physiol. Renal Physiol.* **2013**, *305*, F979–F994. [CrossRef]
61. Granjon, D.; Bonny, O.; Edwards, A. A model of calcium homeostasis in the rat. *Am. J. Physiol. Renal Physiol.* **2016**, *311*, F1047–F1062. [CrossRef]
62. Jungers, D. *Lithiase Urinaire*, 2nd ed.; Lavoisier: Paris, France, 2012; pp. 145–150, ISBN 978-2-257-22597-9.
63. Batlle, D.; Haque, S.K. Genetic causes and mechanisms of distal renal tubular acidosis. *Nephrol. Dial. Transplant.* **2012**, *27*, 3691–3704. [CrossRef]
64. Letavernier, E.; Verrier, C.; Goussard, F.; Perez, J.; Huguet, L.; Haymann, J.-P.; Baud, L.; Bazin, D.; Daudon, M. Calcium and vitamin D have a synergistic role in a rat model of kidney stone disease. *Kidney Int.* **2016**, *90*, 809–817. [CrossRef]
65. Bushinsky, D.A.; Grynpas, M.D.; Nilsson, E.L.; Nakagawa, Y.; Coe, F.L. Stone formation in genetic hypercalciuric rats. *Kidney Int.* **1995**, *48*, 1705–1713. [CrossRef]
66. Russell, R.G.; Hodgkinson, A. The urinary excretion of inorganic pyrophosphate by normal subjects and patients with renal calculus. *Clin. Sci.* **1966**, *31*, 51–62.
67. Letavernier, E.; Daudon, M. Vitamin D, Hypercalciuria and Kidney Stones. *Nutrients* **2018**, *10*, 366. [CrossRef]
68. Bouderlique, E.; Tang, E.; Perez, J.; Coudert, A.; Bazin, D.; Verpont, M.-C.; Duranton, C.; Rubera, I.; Haymann, J.-P.; Leftheriotis, G.; et al. Vitamin D and Calcium Supplementation Accelerates Randall's Plaque Formation in a Murine Model. *Am. J. Pathol.* **2019**, *189*, 2171–2180. [CrossRef]
69. Cheungpasitporn, W.; Thongprayoon, C.; Mao, M.A.; O'Corragain, O.A.; Edmonds, P.J.; Erickson, S.B. The Risk of Coronary Heart Disease in Patients with Kidney Stones: A Systematic Review and Meta-analysis. *N. Am. J. Med. Sci.* **2014**, *6*, 580–585. [CrossRef]
70. Reiner, A.P.; Kahn, A.; Eisner, B.H.; Pletcher, M.J.; Sadetsky, N.; Williams, O.D.; Polak, J.F.; Jacobs, D.R.; Stoller, M.L. Kidney stones and subclinical atherosclerosis in young adults: Coronary Artery Risk Development in Young Adults (CARDIA) study. *J. Urol.* **2011**, *185*. [CrossRef]
71. Fabris, A.; Ferraro, P.M.; Comellato, G.; Caletti, C.; Fantin, F.; Zaza, G.; Zamboni, M.; Lupo, A.; Gambaro, G. The relationship between calcium kidney stones, arterial stiffness and bone density: Unraveling the stone-bone-vessel liaison. *J. Nephrol.* **2015**, *28*, 549–555. [CrossRef]
72. Shavit, L.; Girfoglio, D.; Vijay, V.; Goldsmith, D.; Ferraro, P.M.; Moochhala, S.H.; Unwin, R. Vascular Calcification and Bone Mineral Density in Recurrent Kidney Stone Formers. *Clin. J. Am. Soc. Nephrol.* **2015**, *10*, 278–285. [CrossRef]
73. Schibler, D.; Russell, R.G.; Fleisch, H. Inhibition by pyrophosphate and polyphosphate of aortic calcification induced by vitamin D3 in rats. *Clin. Sci.* **1968**, *35*, 363–372.
74. Villa-Bellosta, R.; O'Neill, W.C. Pyrophosphate deficiency in vascular calcification. *Kidney Int.* **2018**, *93*, 1293–1297. [CrossRef]

75. Lomashvili, K.A.; Garg, P.; Narisawa, S.; Millan, J.L.; O'Neill, W.C. Upregulation of alkaline phosphatase and pyrophosphate hydrolysis: Potential mechanism for uremic vascular calcification. *Kidney Int.* **2008**, *73*, 1024–1030. [CrossRef]
76. Lau, W.L.; Liu, S.; Vaziri, N.D. Chronic kidney disease results in deficiency of ABCC6, the novel inhibitor of vascular calcification. *Am. J. Nephrol.* **2014**, *40*, 51–55. [CrossRef]

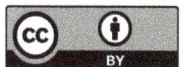

© 2019 by the authors. Licensee MDPI, Basel, Switzerland. This article is an open access article distributed under the terms and conditions of the Creative Commons Attribution (CC BY) license (http://creativecommons.org/licenses/by/4.0/).

MDPI
St. Alban-Anlage 66
4052 Basel
Switzerland
Tel. +41 61 683 77 34
Fax +41 61 302 89 18
www.mdpi.com

International Journal of Molecular Sciences Editorial Office
E-mail: ijms@mdpi.com
www.mdpi.com/journal/ijms

www.ingramcontent.com/pod-product-compliance
Lightning Source LLC
LaVergne TN
LVHW070633100526
838202LV00012B/793